COCHLEAR IMPLANT RESEARCH UPDATES

Edited by **Cila Umat** and **Rinze Anthony Tange**

Cochlear Implant Research Updates
Edited by Cila Umat and Rinze Anthony Tange

Published by InTech
Janeza Trdine 9, 51000 Rijeka, Croatia

Publishing Process Manager Ana Skalamera

Technical Editor Teodora Smiljanic

Cover Designer InTech Design Team

Additional hard copies can be obtained from orders@intechopen.com

Cochlear Implant Research Updates, Edited by Cila Umat and Rinze Anthony Tange
p. cm.
ISBN 978-953-51-0582-4

For EU product safety concerns:
IN TECH d.o.o., Prolaz Marije Krucifikse Kozulić 3, 51000 Rijeka, Croatia,
info@intechopen.com or visit our website at intechopen.com.

Meet the editors

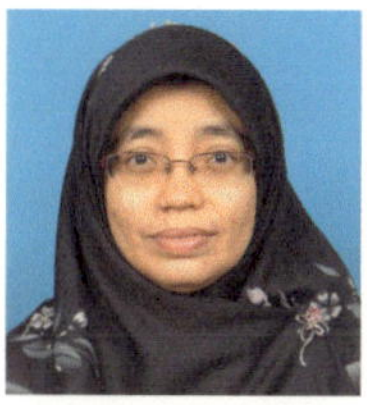

Dr Cila Umat is an Associate Professor and Head of the Audiology Program at the School of Rehabilitation Sciences, Faculty of Health Sciences, Universiti Kebangsaan Malaysia (UKM) Kuala Lumpur, Malaysia. She obtained her first degree in Physics from UKM in 1993, Postgraduate Diploma of Audiology and Masters of Audiology from Macquarie University, Sydney, Australia in 1995 and 1996, respectively. She went on to do her doctorate study at the University of Melbourne in the area of cochlear implant psychophysics in 2002 and obtained her PhD in 2005. She is the first audiologist in Malaysia to obtain her PhD degree in audiology. Associate Professor Dr Cila Umat has worked as a lecturer and audiologist in UKM since 1996 after finishing her Master degree. She has also been appointed as the Head of the Audiology & Speech Sciences Department, the UKM Audiology Program Coordinator and she currently holds position as the Head of the Audiology Program at UKM. Her research interest is in the area of cochlear implantation especially on auditory perception through the cochlear implant device. Associate Professor Dr. Cila Umat has been in the UKM Cochlear Implant Team since 1997. The UKM Cochlear Implant Program which started in 1995 is the first and the largest Cochlear Implant program in Malaysia.

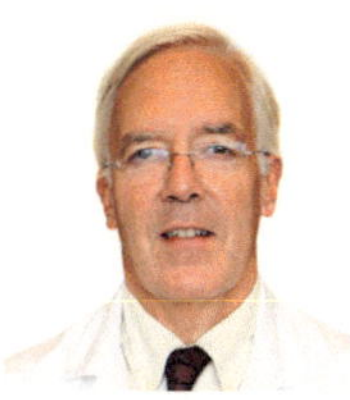

Dr Rinze Anthony Tange was born on 8 January 1950 in Utrecht, the Netherlands. He studied medicine at the Utrecht University where he graduated in 1976 and became specialist in otolaryngology at the Erasmus University in Rotterdam. In 1981 Dr Tange moved from Rotterdam to the ENT department of the University of Amsterdam. In 1983 he published his thesis "Degenerative ototoxic changes in the cochlea as seen in microdissections and surface preparations". The thesis was awarded with two prizes. On 4 September 1996 Dr Tange was appointed associate professor (UHD) at Universiteit van Amsterdam. In 2001 he founded the cochlear implant team of Amsterdam. He introduced an innovative non-invasive surgical approach to implant the cochlea implants. Almost 300 implantations have been performed up until now. Dr Tange has published over 170 papers of which more than 80 are cited. He has been the founder of the Dutch Journal of Otolaryngology and co-founder member of European Academy of Otology and Neurotology (EAONO). In 2003 he organized the 24th Politzer Society Meeting in Amsterdam. Dr Tange is a co-founder member of the LION project a Global Visio conference Network for Otolaryngology. In 2009 he was invited to join the ENT department of Utrecht University.

Contents

Preface

For many years or decades, cochlear implants have been an exciting research area covering multiple disciplines which include otology, engineering, audiology, speech language pathology, education and psychology, among others. Through these research studies, we have started to learn or have better understanding on various aspects of cochlear implant surgery and what follows after the surgery, the implant technology and other related aspects of cochlear implantation. Some are much better than the others but nevertheless, many are yet to be learnt. This book is intended to fill up some gaps in cochlear implant research studies. The compilation of the studies cover a fairly wide range of topics including surgical issues, some basic auditory research, studies to improve the speech or sound processing strategies used in cochlear implants, some ethical issues in language development and cochlear implantation in cases with auditory neuropathy spectrum disorder. The book is meant for postgraduate students, researchers and clinicians in the field to get some updates in their respective areas.

To all the contributing authors, your efforts and patience are very much appreciated. We consider that one of the uniqueness of this publication is that the contributing authors are people who are experts and renowned in their fields. We have learned a lot throughout this whole process of involvement as book editors, just by reading and commenting on these superb-written chapters.

We changed the earlier book title to *'Cochlear Implant Research Updates'* to better define or reflect its content. In facilitating the expected diverse readers of this book, we have divided it into three sections: *Surgical Techniques, Speech Processing Strategies,* and *Other Research Updates.* We hope the readers will find the chapters in the book as much interesting and informative as we personally have. They are stimulating new findings and hold for the future of improving the technology, and better understanding of how the users hear through the cochlear implant device. One of the studies also discusses on the contra aspect of what we generally believe on the usefulness of the cochlear implant technology in facilitating speech and language development of young children with severe and profound hearing impairment. Reading the chapter is refreshing as we, in the excitement to observe how the cochlear implant technology changes the lives of many people who use this hearing device, tend to forget that there are people with different views on cochlear implantation especially for young children. Including this chapter in this book hopefully will allow readers to critically analyze the arguments or concerns put forward by this group of people.

We would like to thank Ms Ana Skalamera as the book manager of this project and her dedicated publication team at InTech for this opportunity, their help and patience in finishing this project. Dr Cila Umat would like to thank her colleague Prof Dr. Siti Zamratol-Mai Sarah Mukari who has been a mentor and a friend and has consistently encouraged her to put up to this academic research exercise and challenges. Last but not least, her very special gratitude goes to her father Hj. Umat bin Hj. Baba, her loving mother Hjh. Maznah bt Hj. Abdullah and her siblings Along Anum Umat & family, Angah Bahia Umat & family, Achik Dauza Umat & family, Ezamudin Umat, Far'ain Umat and Gazlia Umat for their ever-lasting, undivided loves, support and encouragement.

We hope that everyone who reads this book will benefit from the collection of studies presented here. *Happy reading!*

Cila Umat, PhD
School of Rehabilitation Sciences
Faculty of Health Sciences
Universiti Kebangsaan Malaysia
Kuala Lumpur
Malasyia

Rinze Anthony Tange MD PhD
Associate Professor Otology (UHD)
Dept. of Otorhinolaryngology
University Medical Center
Utrecht
Netherlands

Section 1

Surgical Techniques

1

Cochlear Implant Surgery

Hakan Soken, Sarah E. Mowry and Marlan R. Hansen
Department of Otolaryngology, University of Iowa Hospitals and Clinics, Iowa City, Iowa USA

1. Introduction

Over the past quarter of a century, cochlear implants (CIs) have become recognized as highly successful auditory rehabilitation devices for individuals with severe to profound hearing impairment. There is ample evidence of the success of electrical stimulation of the inner ear as a treatment for profound deafness.

However, the majority of persons with hearing loss are not profoundly deaf and they have some remaining usable hearing. Encouraged by promising results in traditional cochlear implant patients and by improvements in the electrode design and the signal processing, investigators have expanded the indications for implantation. Now in addition to completely deaf patients, selected subjects with residual hearing are eligible for cochlear implantation with modified electrodes. The approach involves preserving existing residual acoustic hearing (low-frequency) in an ear to be implanted. Electrical stimulation is provided via a modified CI for the missing high frequencies to improve speech understanding via combined acoustic and electric (A + E) hearing. The prerequisite for this form of combined stimulation (ipsilateral A + E) is a sufficient degree of residual low frequency hearing in the implanted ear. Most patients with the modified electrodes are able to achieve improved sound perception and word understanding while preserving their residual acoustic hearing (Ching et al., 1998; Hogan & Turner, 1998). The listening condition using only A+E hearing and no hearing aid in the contralateral ear is referred to as "hybrid mode". However, these implant recipients benefit from using a hearing aid in their contralateral ear, a listening condition referred to as "combined mode". This listening situation has the potential to improve speech recognition in both quiet and noise (Gstoettner et al., 2006; Turner & Cummings, 1999).

Since Gantz and von Ilberg first discussed the possibility of using A+ E stimulation simultaneously in patients with significant residual hearing, the concept of combined electric and acoustic stimulation has provided a focus of interest and research (von Ilberg et al., 1999; Gantz & Turner, 2003). The Iowa Hybrid project stemmed from work by Shepherd and colleagues that showed that preservation of the apical regions of the feline cochlea could be spared anatomically and functionally following limited electrode insertion (Ni et al., 1992; Xu et al., 1997). Developments in technology and "soft" surgery techniques, combined with a better understanding of the structure and function of the inner ear allowed the first patient to be implanted with a modified electrode in 1999 (Gantz & Turner, 2003). Work by groups in Iowa and Frankfurt have targeted hearing-impaired patients who are not traditionally considered CI candidates (Gantz & Turner, 2003; Cohen et al., 2002). These patients are characterized by severe and profound thresholds at frequencies ≥1000 Hz, with near-normal or mild hearing losses in the low frequencies. These patients commonly present with monosyllabic word recognition scores <50%. In these cases the aim is to preserve functional low frequency hearing while providing additional high frequency information via the CI.

Successful implantation of this group of hearing impaired patients requires meticulous microsurgical techniques. This chapter will explore the indications for use of A+E stimulation, patient outcomes, microsurgical techniques, electrode design and possibilities for future interventions.

2. Indications for combined acoustic and electric stimulation

Cochlear implantation is traditionally offered to individuals who receive limited hearing benefit from well-fit hearing aids (HAs). The definition of "limited benefit" for patients has changed appreciably in the past 15 years. The audiologic selection criteria have been expanded for both adults and pediatric patients. For adults, selection criteria have changed from a profound hearing loss and limited open-set speech recognition in the early 1990s to a 70 dB hearing loss and up to 50% open-set sentence speech perception. Although the broadening of the selection criteria to a 70 dB pure-tone-average hearing loss occurred in 1995 for the adult population, the criteria for children remain a pure-tone-average of less than or equal to 90 dB hearing level. As cochlear implant technology progressed and documented outcomes exceeded early expectations, the audiologic boundaries of candidacy broadened to include patients with more residual hearing (Kiefer et al., 1998; Klenzner et al., 1999).

Severe to profound hearing impaired individuals typically derive substantial benefit from a CI for speech understanding and quality of life. Conventional CI users may use a HA in the contralateral ear (bimodal condition) if sufficient residual hearing is present. This listening condition has the potential to improve speech recognition, particularly in noise. Results in these patients show that bimodal listening is of significant benefit, and a strong synergistic effect of using both devices is particularly noticeable during speech testing in noise (Gantz & Turner, 2003; Turner et al., 2004; Gstoettner et al., 2008). Ipsilateral combination of A+E hearing (hybrid listening mode) provides similar benefits for speech recognition in noise and subjective improvements in sound quality (Gstoettner et al., 2006).

Several recent studies demonstrated that acoustic amplification for hearing loss above 60 dB HL for frequencies greater than 2500 Hz usually provides no enhancements of speech recognition (Hogan & Turner, 1998; Turner & Cummings, 1999). Thus, candidates for A+E stimulation must have pure tone detection <60dB HL between 125-500 Hz and <80dB HL above 2000 Hz. They may have substantial word understanding scores (consonant nucleus consonant (CNC)) in the best aided situation between 10-60% correct in the worse hearing ear and up to 80% correct in the better hearing ear (Fig. 1). Other selection criteria include: no evidence of progressive hearing loss; no evidence of autoimmune inner ear disease; and no history of meningitis, otosclerosis or cochlear ossification. The maximum air-bone gap allowed is 15 dB. There should also be no contraindications to use amplification devices in the implanted ear such as chronic otitis externa or a chronically draining ear.

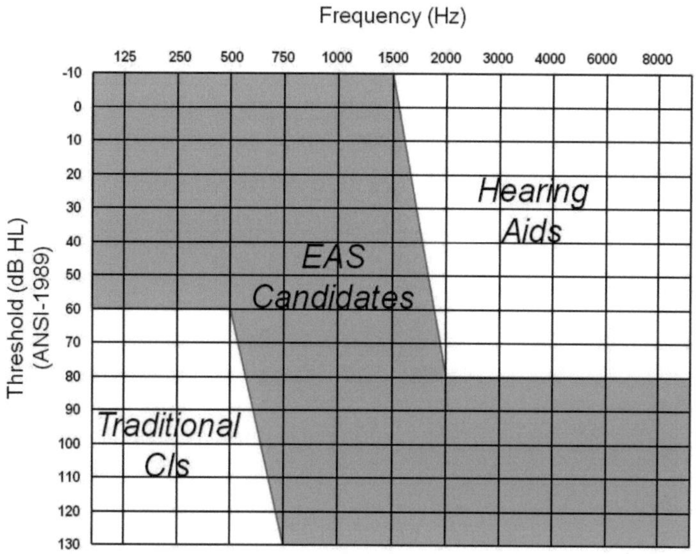

Fig. 1. Expanded audiometric selection criteria for combined electric and acoustic stimulation candidacy. HL=Hearing Level, Hz=Hertz.

3. Outcomes

In 2003, Gantz and Turner reported on 9 adults with severe high-frequency impairment received implants with either 6-mm or 10-mm length hybrid electrodes. Monosyllabic word understanding and consonant identification in a recorded sound-only condition were used to assess changes in speech perception. Acoustic hearing was preserved in all subjects and preoperative monosyllabic word and sentence scores were unchanged in all subjects following implantation. The scores were more than doubled using the 10-mm implant when compared with preoperative scores achieved with hearing aids only. In the subsequent FDA trial of the Hybrid S12 10mm electrode, 87 subjects were enrolled in a larger multi-central clinical trial. Immediate hearing preservation accomplished in 85/87 (98%) subjects. Over time (3 months to 5 years), some hearing was maintained in 91% of the group (Gantz et al., 2009).

Other modified electrodes (Cochlear Hybrid L24 and Med-El Flex^{EAS}) are also designed to preserve hearing. Lenarz et al. (2009) recently published the preliminary data for the European trial of the L24. Of the 32 patients implanted; 24 patients were hybrid candidates and 8 patients were standard electrode candidates. Hearing was preserved within 30 dB of preoperative thresholds in 96% of patients and 68% were within 15 dB. These results were stable over time. Of the 16 patients with 12 months of experience, 94% retained hearing within 30 dB of preoperative thresholds. Those in the European trial showed significant improvement on word scores between the 6- and 12-month post-activation marks.

As discussed previously, patients with preserved LF hearing have significant improvements in their discrimination scores following cochlear implantation. Those implanted with shorter electrode arrays, such as the Hybrid S/L or Med-El M/FLEX^{EAS} electrodes, are achieving significant improvements in discrimination tasks as well. Patients implanted with the Hybrid S electrode continue to demonstrate improvement in CNC scores beyond 1-2 years after activation in the combined mode (Reiss et al., 2007). At the time of publication of the Hybrid 10 clinical trial, 68 of 87 patients in the multi-center trial had follow-up lengths of greater than 9 months. Improvements in speech reception threshold (SRT) or CNC word score occurred in 74% of patients. Nearly half of patients (48%) had improvement in both SRT and CNC scores. Improvement on CNC testing ranged from 10% to 70% better than preoperative scores for 45 of 61 patients with long term follow-up (Gantz et al., 2009).

For those implanted with the Hybrid L24, word recognition scores improved by 21% on average; one patient demonstrated improvement from 5% to 95% on the Freiburg Monosyllabic word test (Lenarz et al., 2009).

Some patients score above 90% on the CNC monosyllabic word test in the combined mode with all electrodes. Patients implanted with the FLEX^{EAS} electrode also scored well. Preoperative open set sentence recognition was 24% and after 12 months of use scores averaged 71% ($p<0.05$). Monosyllable recognition also improved; preoperative scores averaged 16% on the FMS test and postoperative scores averaged 44% ($p<0.05$). One patient in this cohort achieved scores over 90% discrimination post-operatively (Gstoettner et al., 2008).

Although cochlear implants significantly improve speech understanding in quiet, traditional CI users have difficulty in noisy environments. Distinguishing the correct words in a background of competing talkers is an even more difficult task. Normal hearing listeners are able to understand 50% of the presented words when the background noise is 30 dB louder; thus normal hearing listeners have a signal to noise ratio (SNR) of -30 dB (lower numbers are better). For competing talkers, the average SNR in normal hearing listeners is -15 dB (Turner et al., 2004). The average long electrode user requires a SNR of +3 dB for unmodulated background noise and +8 for multitalker babble (MTB), meaning that the talker has to be 3 dB louder than competing noise or 8 dB louder than MTB (Nelson et al., 2003; Gantz et al., 2006).

Hybrid S recipients perform much better than traditional CI patients but not as well as normal hearing listeners in background noise. SNRs varied from -12 to +17 dB in a subgroup of 27 Hybrid S patients with 12 months or greater experience. The average SNR for the Hybrid S group was -9 dB (Gantz et al., 2009). Elevated SNRs occurred in those patients who experienced >30 dB changes to their LF hearing. The results for Hybrid S patients in MTB are similar to hearing impaired patients with SRTs between 81-100 dB (severe/profound).

Patients receiving the Hybrid L electrode also improved their SNR when tested in the combined mode. The average SNR preoperatively was +12.1 dB and postoperatively the SNR dropped to +2.1 dB (Lenarz et al., 2009).

Those with the FLEX^{EAS} electrode also improved speech understanding in noise. Preoperative open set sentence scores in SNR of +10 were 14% and after 1 year in the EAS mode scores averaged 60% ($p<0.05$) (Gstoettner et al., 2008).

Music appreciation has been a part of the research protocol for the Hybrid S/L trials. Subjects with preserved LF hearing have a distinct advantage in a number of music processing functions when compared to the traditional CI recipients. Pitch perception is one of the most basic functions of the auditory system with respect to music appreciation. Hybrid users perform better on these types of tasks when compared to long electrode users but are still significantly poorer-performing than normal hearing listeners (Gfeller et al.,

2007). When provided with lyrics to easily recognizable American songs, Hybrid users were able to identify the songs correctly 65-100% of the time, similar to normal hearing listeners. When the lyrics were removed and only the melody was presented, Hybrid patients did less well (50% correct) but still much better than traditional long electrode users (<10% correct) (Gfeller et al., 2006).

The clinical trials of A + E patients are still in their early years; therefore the issue of long-term success rates still deserves attention. A recent study retrospectively analyzed low frequency hearing stability over time. These patients met criteria for hybrid implantation at the beginning of the study period (Yao et al., 2006). Adults demonstrated stable low frequency thresholds (changing only 1 dB per year over periods as long as 25 years), however for children the rate of hearing loss was generally larger and much more variable. The stability of low-frequency thresholds in actual A + E patients over long periods of time remains to be determined.

4. Technical issues

The goals and theories behind the development of techniques to preserve residual hearing preservation following cochlear implantation encompass more than merely inserting a standard length electrode into the cochlea under modified technique.

The loss of residual acoustic hearing during implantation is multifactorial. Electrode design, surgical technique and host responses to insertional trauma all likely contribute to postoperative hearing change and ultimately patient outcomes.

The diameter, stiffness, and length of standard intracochlear electrodes may induce substantial intracochlear damage. Histological evaluation of the cochlea after insertion of an electrode in human cadaver temporal bones demonstrated a wide range of damage to inner ear structures, including the basilar membrane, osseus spiral lamina and cochlear hair cells (Fayad et al., 1991; Eshraghi et al., 2003). Electrode position and structural damage to the cochlea can be quantified in cadaveric studies using the scale described by Eshraghi and Van De Water (2006) (Table 1). Using this scale and objective electrophysiological testing of the hearing threshold (i.e., DPOAEs and ABRs) in animal models of cochlear implant electrode trauma, experience has shown that most of the causes of postoperative hearing loss after cochlear implantation can be minimized by electrode design and optimized surgical technique (Eshraghi et al., 2003; Balkany et al., 2002).

Grade 1: No observable macroscopic trauma
Grade 2: Elevation of basilar membrane
Grade 3: Dislocation of electrode to scala vestibuli
Grade 4: Fracture of osseous spiral lamina or modiolus, or tear in tissues of stria vascularis / spiral ligament complex

Table 1. Grading system: Cochlear trauma postelectrode array implantation. (Modified from: Eshraghi et al., Comparative study of cochlear damage with three perimodiolar electrode design. Laryngoscope 2003;113:415-419)

4.1 Electrode features

Taking into consideration the frequency-specific nature of the cochlea, partial insertion of standard length electrodes (Nucleus CI22M, CI24M and Nucleus 24 Contour, the Med-EL Combi 40+ and the Advance Bionics HiFocus II) was originally considered in an effort to preserve acoustic hearing in the low tones. All standard electrode arrays are designed to be inserted to a depth exceeding 1 complete turn of the cochlea from base to apex, or 360° (Fig. 2). Reports in the literature have shown the ability to preserve some residual hearing even when a standard electrode array is fully inserted into the scala tympani (Hodges et al., 1997; Balkany et al., 2006). However, passing a standard length electrode beyond the basal turn of the cochlea can result in damage to the organ of Corti due to migration of the electrode through the basilar membrane. Therefore, it is difficult to consistently maintain speech discrimination in addition to pure tones when electrodes are passed beyond the basal turn (Balkany et al., 2006).

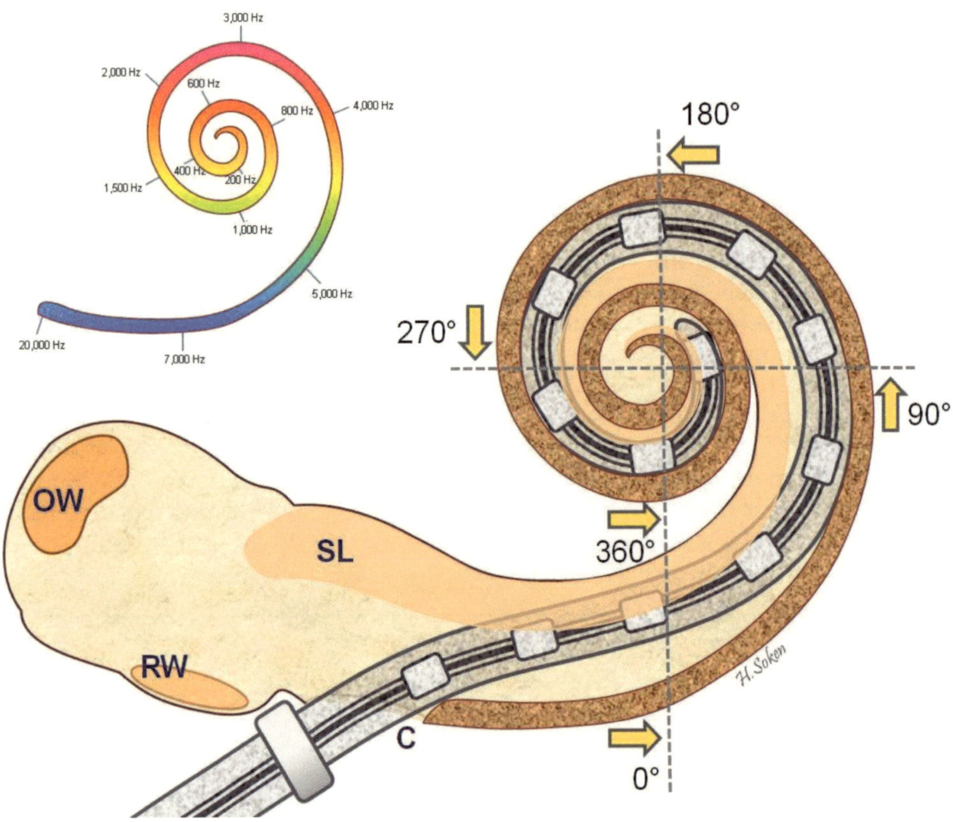

Fig. 2. Insertion depth, and frequency map of the cochlea. SL=Spiral Lamina, OW=Oval Window, RW=Round Window, C=Cochleostomy

In 1995, the University of Iowa CI research team began development of a shortened electrode array based on the Nucleus CI-24 implant in collaboration with the Cochlear Corporation. The first design, "Hybrid S8" has a reduced diameter of 6mm x 0.2 mm x 0.4

mm electrode with six channels. Later, the Iowa/Nucleus Hybrid (short-electrode) device was then lengthened to 10 mm, with the electrodes placed at the distal 6 mm, the Hybrid S12 (Fig. 3). Unique features of the Hybrid electrode include a Dacron collar to limit the intracochlear placement to 10 mm and a titanium marker to orient the electrode contacts toward the modiolus. The ideal insertion depth is approximately 195° of the basal turn of the cochlea (Roland et al., 2008).

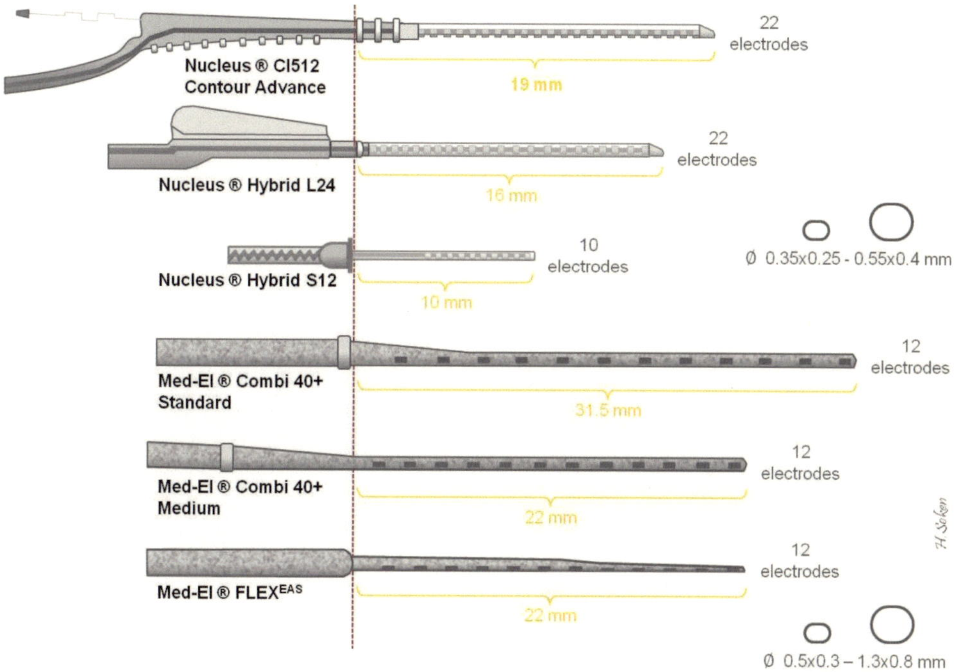

Fig. 3. Examples of various CI electrode arrays.

Another short electrode has been developed in conjunction with the Cochlear Corporation, the Hybrid L24, which is 16 mm length and contains 22 electrodes. The optimal insertion is through 250° of the basal turn of the cochlea. This longer electrode would still preserve residual hearing in the apical portions of the cochlea, but if the low frequency hearing is lost the Hybrid L can be used as a traditional electric-processing only device as it has 22 electrodes, similar to a standard electrode (Fig. 3).

In 2004, Med-El Corporation launched a new atraumatic prototype electrode carrier FLEX^{EAS} in an attempt to minimize the forces generated during insertion and thereby to increase the rate of residual hearing preservation to allow for E + A hearing. Their standard length electrode, the Combi 40+, has a goal insertion length of 31 mm. The shortened electrode, the M, is 22 mm in length and the electrode includes a significantly reduced diameter of the distal portion of the electrode with a flexible tip (Fig. 3). This FLEX^{EAS} electrode can be used for both cochleostomy and round window insertion techniques (Hochmair et al., 2006). Human temporal bone studies confirmed the intended mechanical properties for safe and atraumatic insertion (Adunka et al., 2004).

5. Surgical technique

5.1 Surgical approach

As in all cochlear implant surgeries, an antromastoidectomy is performed, followed by a posterior tympanotomy to visualize the round window niche. The facial recess must be opened to allow complete visualization of the round window. The incudal buttress is preserved and care is taken to leave the ossicular chain intact and untouched. The bed for the receiver/stimulator is prepared before entry into the middle ear. In most temporal bones, the round window cannot be directly viewed until its bony overhang has been properly removed. The round window niche is saucerized with a 1.5 mm diamond burr to expose the round window membrane fully.

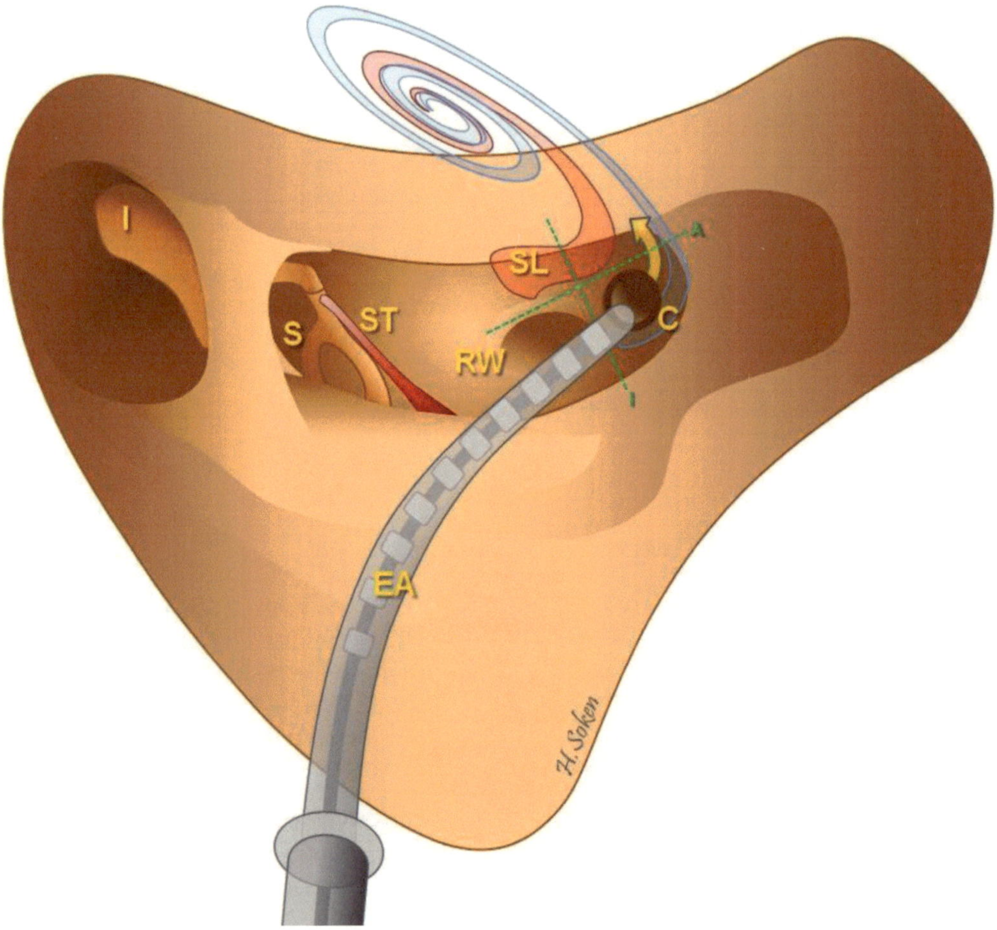

Fig. 4. Cochleostomy anteroinferior to the round window (green dotted lines) and introduction of the electrode array into the scala tympani. The electrode must be directed parallel to the posterior canal wall to ensure the electrode is directed into the basal turn of the cochlea (yellow arrow). C=Cochleostomy, EA=Electrode Array, I=Incus, RW=Round Window, S=Stapes, SL=Spiral Lamina, ST=Stapedial Tendon.

The position and technique of creating the cochleostomy is critical to preserving residual hearing. To standardize the placement of the cochleostomy, it is placed in the anterior inferior quadrant of a box created by drawing a line at the superior margin of the round window and one that crosses perpendicular at the inferior aspect of the round window. Creation of the cochleostomy is begun in the inferior portion of the quadrant, slowly saucerizing the otic capsule bone with a 1.5 mm diamond bur. This position allows a "straight" path into the basal turn of the scala tympani and avoids the osseous spiral lamina when entering the scala tympani (Fig. 4). The cochleostomy hole is drilled so that the "blue-line" of the endosteum will be visible. If the cochleostomy is too far superior, adjacent to the spiral ligament, a whitish color will be evident. A 0.5 mm diamond bur is used to penetrate the final layer of bone and the cochleostomy drilling is done at a slow speed.

Care is taken to use sufficient irrigation to avoid heating the cochlea. Contact with the bone over the facial nerve by the revolving drill shaft must be avoided, since this will heat the bone and may result in a thermal injury to the facial nerve itself. Entry into the scala tympani should not occur until bleeding is controlled and bone dust has been removed from the field.

Several other steps occur prior to cochlear entry. To assist immediate and complete sealing of the cochleostomy hole, a 1.5 x 1.5 mm graft of the temporalis fascia is created and then perforated centrally. The electrode is then passed through this perforation. When implanting the Hybrid S12 it helps to secure the electrode within the mastoid. This is accomplished by drilling a pair of 1 mm holes in the cortical overhang of the tegmen mastoideum. A 4-0 nylon suture is then passed through these holes and the electrode is passed through the loop. The suture is then tied down laterally to secure the electrode. This suture helps to stabilize the orientation of the electrode contacts toward the modioulus and ensures that the electrode is secure within the scala tympani.

5.2 Electrode insertion

Immediately prior to electrode insertion, the surgeon should check that all preliminary steps have been completed. The endosteum is incised using a 0.2 mm right-angle hook to open the scala tympani. The diameter of the cochleostomy varies from 0.5-1.5 mm depending on the electrode used. Some surgeons advocate placing a trapezoid silicon sheath in the posterior tympanotomy and mastoid to guide the insertion of the electrode and to limit contamination of the electrode with blood or bone dust. To facilitate electrode insertion, the surface may be coated with surgical lubricant such as hyaluronic acid. Some surgeons place a drop of crystalline triamcinolone solution (Volon A®) in the cochleostomy hole and then seal the cochleostomy with a drop of hyaluronic acid (Healon®) to prevent the corticosteroid solution from being flushed away.

The time the cochlea remains exposed should be minimized. Once the cochlea is opened, the electrode is then inserted gently and slowly into the scala tympani. Regardless of the type of electrode, it's important that the electrode parallel the posterior canal wall to ensure the electrode is directed into the basal turn of the cochlea (Fig. 4). The tip of the electrode is guided into the cochleostomy using a smooth forceps; at no point is the electrode lead circumferentially grasped or forcefully pushed into the cochlea. To minimize intrascalar pressure waves and to allow a compensational outflow of perilymphatic fluid, the electrode insertion is carried out slowly, over a period of approximately 1-2 minutes. During the insertion of the electrode, the residual cochlear function may be monitored via evoked auditory brainstem response (ABR) if a waveform is present. The surgeon must pause during the insertion to allow for the ABR data to be collected. If changes in the ABR are noted, the insertion proceeds at a slower rate.

The electrode is advanced to the fascia "washer" to ensure a tight seal, and the tegmen mastoideum suture is secured. Sealing of the cochleostomy site and the electrode fixation also can be achieved with injection of fibrin glue (Beriplast®). Because of the desire to preserve residual hearing, the middle ear is not packed with muscle or fascia. The mastoid periostium should then be closed completely over the receiver/stimulator and the electrode. The skin and soft tissues are then closed in the standard fashion.

5.3 Cochleostomy versus round window insertion

During the early years (prior to Lehnhardt et al.'s description of a soft surgery technique in 1993) of cochlear implantation emphasis was on implanting a safe and reliable electrode array into the bony cochlear channel. Entrance was obtained via the round window (as the reliable landmark) but relatively stiff multichannel electrode designs and the hook region of the cochlea led to difficult insertions and injury to the osseous spiral lamina. This bony structure transmits the peripheral auditory nerve fibers. Damage to this delicate bone could then negatively impact a patient's ability to perceive sound provided by the CI. As a result, the round window technique originally used in cochlear implantation was abandoned because of concerns that the angle of insertion lead to trauma of the osseous spiral lamina. It was then proposed that by drilling the promontory bone, one could reliably gain access to the intracochlear lumen. This procedure has been generally known as the cochleostomy. The classic cochleostomy approach has become popular among most otologists as it provides reliable access to the scale tympani of the cochlea.

Briggs et al. (2005) studied 27 temporal bones and described the complex anatomy of the hook region of the cochlea, especially in relation to the optimal placement of the cochleostomy for electrode insertion during hearing preservation surgery. They recommended that the cochleostomy be performed directly inferior to the round window membrane through the crista fenestra (the ridge of bone immediately inferior of the round window membrane) to minimize intracochlear damage during electrode insertion.

However, with the creation of softer, more flexible electrode arrays some authors have revisited the concept of a round window insertion technique. Adunka et al. (2004) described a method of cochlear implantation using the round window membrane insertion technique in eight human fresh temporal bones. Using the standard Combi 40+ and the FLEX^{EAS} electrode, manufactured by Med-El, they implanted these electrodes through the round window membrane. Using the electrode insertion trauma (EIT) grading system (Table 1), they found that the round window insertion was less traumatic, especially in the basal parts of the cochlea, compared with the cochleostomy approach.

There are proponents of both approaches (Roland et al., 2008; Adunka et al., 2004; Gantz et al., 2005; Skarzynski et al., 2007; Wright & Roland, 2005). However, it should be noted that the angle of insertion for round window electrode insertion is not anatomically straightforward and should only be considered for patients who have laterally facing round window membrane.

A bony cochleostomy is appropriate for most patients and can be fashioned to receive the different commercially available electrodes. The Cochlear Corporation Hybrid S12 and L24 are designed to be inserted through a bony cochleostomy. The Med-El FLEX^{EAS} can be inserted through either a cochleostomy or a round window insertion.

6. Post-implantation hearing loss: Potential causes & therapy

Despite advances in both surgical techniques and new less traumatic electrode designs some patients still lose some or all of their residual hearing after implantation.

A recent study in rats characterized the hearing loss following EIT. Eshrahgi et al. (2005) reported an initial hearing loss of 25 to 35 dB sound pressure level (SPL) and then a progressive loss of hearing of an additional 15 dB SPL postimplantation (i.e.; Days 0-7) for all of the frequencies tested (i.e.; 4-32 kHz). Subsequently these investigators confirmed the same pattern of hearing loss due to EIT in a guinea pig model (Eshraghi et al., 2006). The cochleae of control guinea pigs and implanted guinea pigs were removed at 12, 24, and 36 hours after surgery for analysis. Interestingly, they observed changes in nuclear morphology (i.e. nuclear condensation and fragmentation) of the sensory hair cells of the traumatized cochlea at a site distal to the initial site of EIT that are consistent with apoptosis. Furthermore, there was a progressive increase in terminal deoxynucleotide transferase-mediated dUTP nick-end labeling (TUNEL)-labeled hair cell nuclei in the traumatized cochlea over time compared with the contralateral control cochlea, consistent with apoptotic cell death in hair cells remote from the electrode insertion site.

Many additional animal studies confirmed that the insertion of a cochlear implant electrode array causes cellular injury on a molecular level that cannot be correlated to the degree of direct physical trauma. With these observations, grade 0 physical trauma is now considered as no observable macroscopic damage, but with the possibility of damage on a molecular level that results in EIT-induced hearing loss (Table 1).

6.1 Mechanism of cell death

Auditory hair cells may die via necrosis, necrosis-like programmed cell death (PCD), apoptosis, or any combination of these mechanisms in response to a variety of insults (eshraghi et al., 2006; Do et al., 2004). The insertion of a cochlear implant electrode array into the scala tympani can directly kill residual hair cells via necrosis. It can also lead to oxidative stress within the damaged tissues of the cochlea resulting in the apoptosis of hair cells and subsequent loss of hearing. Necrosis is a passive consequence of an overwhelming injury to a cell and is marked by nuclear swelling and lysis of the affected cell. The lysis of the cell results in exposure of the intracellular contents to the extracellular environment and provokes an inflammatory response. The inflammatory response itself may cause further localized tissue destruction as inflammatory cells are recruited to the injured site.

In contrast to necrotic cell death, apoptosis (type 1 PCD) and necrosis-like programmed cell death (type 2 PCD) are associated with an active cell death process and involve a series of biochemical intracellular signaling events that occur in response to injury (Fig. 5). After an insult, PCD protects the organism by removing cells that have sustained sufficient damage to become potentially harmful to the integrity of a tissue or organ. The cytoplasm and nuclear chromatin of the injured cell condense; ribosomes and mitochondria aggregate; and the cell begins to die by forming cellular fragments called apoptotic bodies. While there is blebbing in the plasma membrane, its integrity is largely retained so that, unlike necrosis, and an inflammatory response is not initiated. The biochemical cascade within an apoptotic cell involves the orderly fragmentation of DNA. These fragments, called nick-ends, offer multiple sites for labeling with chemicals during preparation of tissue for examination by microscopy. For example, TUNEL allows for the objective identification of cells dying by apoptosis.

Apoptosis is a tightly controlled process within the cell. Members of the Bcl-2 family of pro (e.g., Bax and Bid) and antiapoptotic (e.g., Bcl-2 and Bcl-X_L) proteins, cytochrome c and some of the members of the family of caspase proteases all regulate entry into PCD (Hertz et

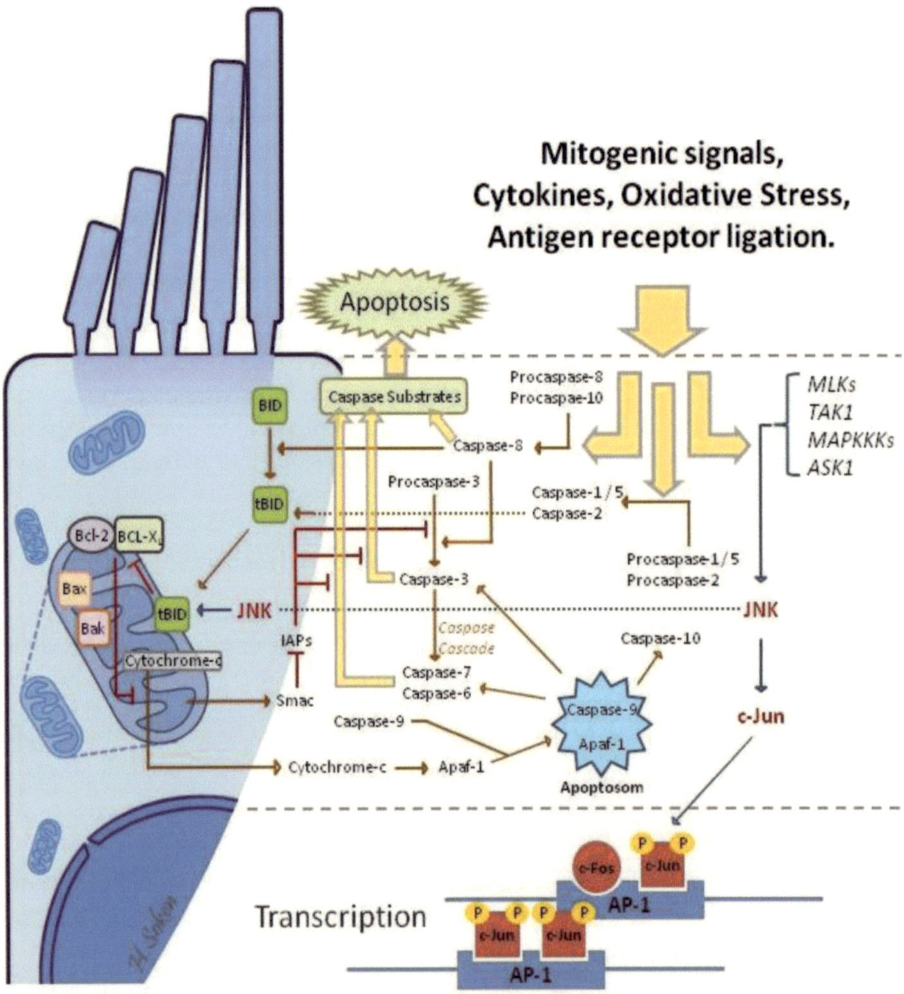

Fig. 5. Overview of caspase pathway and signal transduction cascades involved in apoptosis.

al., 2005; Kim et al., 2005). Caspases are a family of aspartate-specific cysteine proteases, which exist as latent intracellular zymogens (Van De Water et al., 2004). Effector caspases, once activated, selectively cleave distinct intracellular substrates that lead to the dismantling of a cell's architecture, DNA, signaling apparatus, and restorative repair mechanisms. The sequence of caspase activation shows that distinct cascades are activated depending on the specific pathology, conditions employed, and the cell type. At present, caspases 8, 9, and 3 are known to be involved in the apoptosis of physically damaged hair cells (Nicotera et al., 2003), caspases 5, 6, 7 and 10 are suggested to participate in the apoptosis of hair cells in response to physical trauma (Do et al., 2004; Van De Water et al., 2004) (Fig. 5). The underlying events include loss of mitochondrial transmembrane potential, release of cytochrome c from the damaged mitochondria into the cytoplasm, formation of an apoptosome, sequential activation of activator and then effector procaspases, and a subsequent increase in lipid peroxidation of cellular membranes.

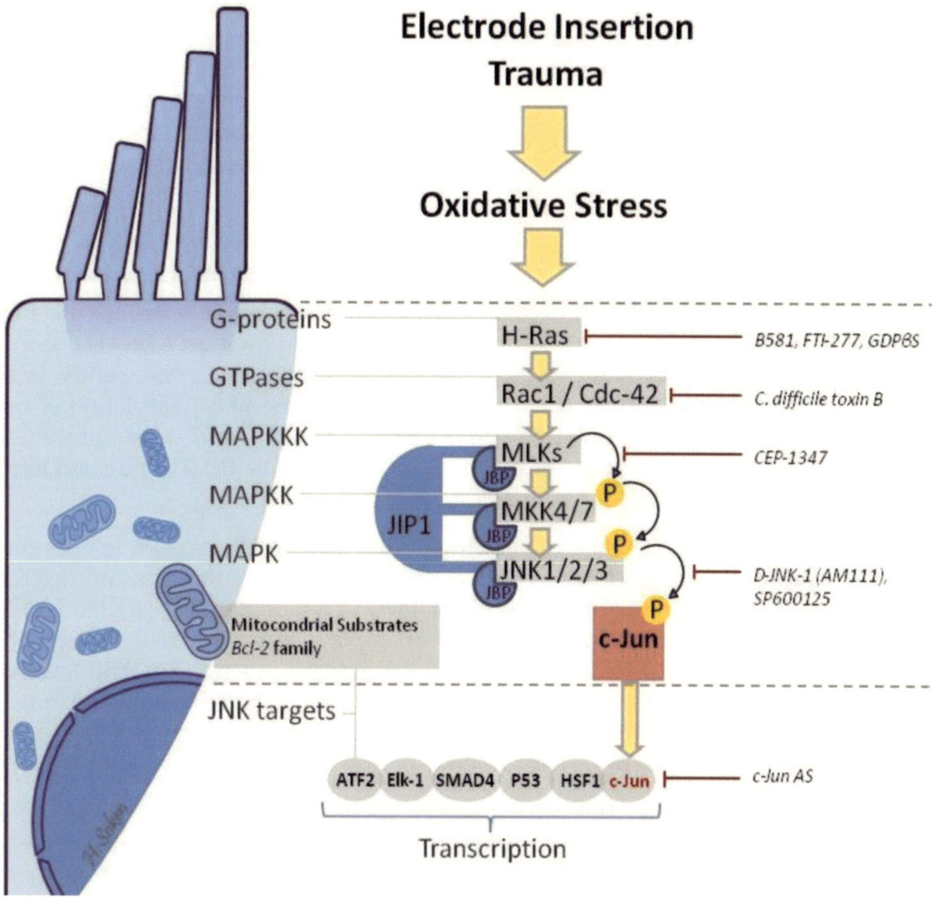

Fig. 6. The MAPK/JNK cell death signal cascade and the site of activation of many pharmacologic inhibitors that have been demonstrated either to block or partially to block different points within this signaling pathway. The mechanism of activation by which D-JNK-1 blocks the actions of JNK, with c-Jun being used as the example of a major downstream target.

Another proposed molecular pathway for cellular insult to apoptosis is via the activation and expression of immediate early genes, such as *c-jun* (Atkins et al., 1996). Jun:Jun homodimers and Jun:Fos heterodimers are major components of the activator protein-1 (AP-1) transcription complex (Fig. 6). Strong c-Jun/AP-1 activation is found in apoptotic cells during the process of naturally occurring (programmed) cell death in the developing rat brain (Ferrer et al., 1996). The phosphorylation cascade necessary for c-Jun activation has also been established. In response to a variety of cell injuries, c-Jun N-terminal kinase (JNK) phosphorylates c-Jun, stimulating its ability to activate transcription of target genes. JNK is a member of the MAP kinase family and is itself regulated by a phosphorylation via a kinase cascade (Kyriakis & Avruch, 1996; Derijard et al., 1995) (Fig. 6). This JNK/c-Jun cell death pathway contributes to the loss of hair cells and auditory neurons in response to oxidative stress (Pirvola et al., 2000; Scarpidis et al., 2003; Wang et al., 2003).

6.2 Pharmaceutical approaches and drug treatment

To maximize hearing preservation after electrode insertion and to enhance the performance of the cochlear implant, direct delivery of pharmacological agents to the inner ear is under active investigation. The invasive nature of cochlear implant electrode insertion itself provides both an opportunity for direct local drug delivery and a platform for the development of a delivery device, e.g., syringes, osmotic pumps, cochlear prosthesis-based delivery and other newer devices have been employed.

6.2.1 c-Jun N-terminal Kinase (JNK) inhibitors

To prevent apoptosis of injured auditory hair cells, one strategy involves the use of a highly effective peptide JNK inhibitor (D-JNKI-1). D-JNKI-1 (also known as AM 111) is a cell-permeable peptide which acts by interrupting the MAPK/JNK signal cascade at the level of the three JNK molecular isoforms. This inhibition prevents the phosphorylation of c-Jun, and thus disrupts the formation of an AP-1 transcription factor. D-JNK-1 also prevents the JNKs from disrupting the activity of antiapoptotic members of the Bcl-2 family and inhibits activation of other JNK targets (e.g., ATF-2) (Figs. 5, 6).

A previous study using D-JNK-1 has demonstrated that this inhibitory peptide can prevent loss of both hearing capacity and hair cells in animals challenged with exposure to either a damaging level of sound trauma or to an ototoxic level of aminoglycoside antibiotic (Wang et al., 2003). Using guinea pig models of cochlear implant trauma Van de Water, et al., showed that treatment with D-JNK-1 prevented the progressive increase in ABR thresholds and decrease in DPOAE amplitudes that occur after electrode insertion trauma (Eshraghi et al., 2006). In another study, Barkdull et al. (2007) confirmed the efficacy of D-JNKI-1 in preventing hearing loss caused by inflammation.

D-JNKI-1, represent promising potential therapeutics for the prevention of hearing loss during electrode insertion in partial hearing patients. In sum, the delayed progressive component of EIT- hearing loss may be mitigated by treating the cochlea immediately after insertion with a JNK inhibitor. Further research in this area is ongoing.

6.2.2 Caspase inhibitor therapy

Among antiapoptotic agents, the general caspase inhibitor z-VAD-FMK (carbobenzoxy-valyl-alanyl-aspartyl-[O-methyl]-fluoromethylketone) is also currently under investigation.

Z-VAD-FMK is a cell-permanent pan-caspase inhibitor that irreversibly binds to the catalytic site of caspase proteases thus inhibiting apoptosis. To be effective, Z-VAD-FMK should be added at the same time that apoptosis is induced (Wang et al., 2004).

Animal experiments have shown caspase inhibition by Z-VAD-FMK can rescue hair cells from the lethal effects of aminoglycosides or cis-platinum (Wang et al., 2004; Matsui et al., 2003). Do et al. (2004) found in their mouse model of implantation trauma that the use of cell death inhibitors (e.g., pancaspase inhibitor Z-VAD-FMK and specific inhibitors to caspase 3, 5, and 6) significantly protected the hearing in response to hydraulic trauma.

6.2.3 Mild hypothermia therapy

Necrosis is generally thought to occur rapidly and therefore is thought to be very difficult to reverse with most otoprotection treatments, e.g. z-VAD-fmk or JNK inhibitors. Reasonable approaches to the prevention of trauma induced necrosis of hair cells would be to either prevent the insult from occurring (e.g. modified surgical approach) (Eshraghi et al., 2003) or to slow the metabolic response of a cell to injury as can be accomplished by the application of protective hypothermia (Balkany et al., 2005).

Hypothermia has been shown to have a protective effect in the brain following a traumatic injury (Busto et al., 1987; Dietrich et al., 1994; Kil et al., 1996). The beneficial effect of hypothermia on neuronal injury has been attributed to a variety of mechanisms. These include a reduction in metabolic rate, reduced tissue oxygen consumption, decreased metabolic acidosis, a suppression of calcium influx into neurons, diminished nitric oxide production, and a reduction in the level of glutamate excitotoxicity (Hyodo et al., 2001).

Hypothermia has also been demonstrated to reduce brain damage following ischemia by limiting the extent of oxidative stress (Zhao et al., 1996). More recently, it was reported that hypothermia could protect against noise-induced hearing threshold elevation in mice (Henry, 2003). In a recent study, it has been shown that mild hypothermia can reduce the immediate component of trauma-induced hearing loss and prevent the progressive component of loss of auditory function following cochlear electrode insertion in the rat model of cochlear implantation trauma-induced hearing loss (Balkany et al., 2005).

6.2.4 Glucocorticoid therapy

Glucocorticoid receptors are expressed in the inner ear. In the adult rat cochlea, they are expressed in the stria vascularis, the organ of Corti and the spiral ganglion neurons. At the cellular level glucocorticoids provide a wide spectrum of cytoprotective activities, including antioxidant and homeostatic effects. *In vitro* experiments have shown that steroids have a protective effect on cultured hair cells. Further, tumor necrosis factor α, an important inflammatory mediator, is released after injury of the cochlea and induces the loss of auditory hair cells; an effect which is inhibited by dexamethasone. Experiments performed on guinea pigs showed that local treatment of the cochlea with dexamethasone reduces EIT-induced hearing loss (James et al., 2008).

A number of groups have investigated the use of steroids using a variety of delivery methodologies (e.g., elution from the electrode carrier, intracochlear injection prior to electrode insertion, delivery through a gel-filled reservoir in the electrode carrier], demonstrating efficacy in the protection of hearing after mild to moderate levels of trauma (James et al., 2008; Eshraghi et al., 2007; Ye et al., 2007; Vivero et al., 2008). Thus, glucocorticoids represent another class of potential therapeutical compounds to mitigate hearing loss following cochlear implantation.

7. Conclusion

Preservation of residual hearing provides significant audiologic advantages and enhances overall performance in patients receiving cochlear implants; preservation of residual hearing should be a goal of all future CI surgeries. This requires intimate knowledge of cochlear microanatomy and careful microsurgical techniques to limit intracochlear damage. In addition, emerging otoprotective therapeutic strategies may help maintain residual auditory function after implantation. Taken together, these microsurgical and therapeutic strategies should lead to improved outcomes for cochlear implant recipients.

8. References

Adunka O, Unkelbach MH, Mack M, et al. (2004). Cochlear implantation via the round window membrane minimizes trauma to cochlear structures: a histologically controlled insertion study. Acta Otolaryngol. Vol.124, No.7, pp. 807-812

Atkins PT, Liu PK, Hsu CY. (1996). Immediate early gene expression in response to cerebral ischemia, friend or foe? Stroke. Vol.27, pp. 1682-7

Balkany T, Eshraghi AA, Yang N. (2002). Modiolar proximity of three new perimodiolar cochlear implant electrodes. Acta Otolaryngol. Vol.122, pp. 363-369

Balkany TJ, Connell SS, Hodges AV, et al. (2006). Conservation of residual acoustic hearing after cochlear implantation. Otol Neurotol. Vol.27, No.8, pp. 1083-8

Balkany TJ, Eshraghi AA, He J, Polak M, Mou C, Dietrich WD, Van De Water TR. (2005). Mild hypothermia protects auditory function during cochlear implant surgery. Laryngoscope. Vol.115, pp. 1543-1547

Barkdull GC, Hondarrague Y, Meyer T, Harris JP, Keithley EM. (2007). AM-111 reduces hearing loss in a guinea pig model of acute labyrinthitis. Laryngoscope. Vol.117, No.12, pp. 2174-2182

Briggs R, Tykocinski M, Stidham K, Roberson JB. (2005). Cochleostomy site: implication for electrode placement and hearing preservation. Acta Otolaryngol. Vol.125, No.8, pp. 870-876

Busto R, Dietrich WD, Globus MY-T, et al. (1987). Small differences in intra-ischemic brain temperature critically determine the extent of ischemic neuronal injury. J Cereb Blood Flow Metab. Vol.7, pp. 729-738.

Ching T, Dillon H, Byrne D. (1998). Speech recognition of hearing-impaired listeners: Predictions from audibility and the limited role of high-frequency amplification. Journal of the Acoustical Society of America. Vol.103, No.2, pp. 1128-1140

Cohen NL, Roland JT, Fishman A. (2002). Surgical technique for the Nucleus Contour cochlear implant. Ear Hear. Vol.23, pp. 59-66

Derijard B, Raingeand J, Barrett T, et al. (1995). Independent human MAP-kinase signal transduction pathways defined by MEK and MKK isoforms. Science. Vol.267, pp. 682-5

Dietrich WD, Alonso O, Busto R, et al. (1994). Post-traumatic brain hypothermia reduces histopathological damage following concussive brain injury in the rat. Acta Neuropathol. Vol.87, pp. 250-258

Do K, Baker K, Praetorius M, Staecker H. (2004). A mouse model of implantation trauma. Internat Cong Ser. Vol.1273, pp. 167-170

Eshraghi AA, Polak M, He J, et al. (2005). The pattern of hearing loss in a rat model of cochlear implantation trauma. Otol Neurotol. Vol.26, pp. 442-447

Eshraghi AA, Van De Water TR. (2006). Cochlear function, physical trauma, oxidative stress, induction of apoptosis and therapeutic strategies. Anat Rec. Vol.288A, pp. 473-481

Eshraghi AA, Wang J, Adil E, He J, Zine A, Bublik M, Bonny C, Puel JL, Balkany TJ, Van De Water TR. (2007). Blocking c-Jun-Nterminal kinase signaling can prevent hearing loss induced by both electrode insertion trauma and neomycin ototoxicity. Hear Res. Vol.226, pp. 168-177

Eshraghi AA, YangNW, Balkany TJ. (2003). Comparative study of cochlear damage with three perimodiolar electrode designs. Laryngoscope. Vol.113, pp. 415-419

Fayad J, Linthicum FR Jr, Otto SR, et al. (1996). Cochlear implants: histopathologic findings related to performance in 16 human temporal bones. Ann Otol Rhinol Laryngol. Vol.100, pp. 807-811

Ferrer I, Seguı J, Olive M. (1996). Strong c-Jun immunoreactivity is associated with apoptotic cell death in human tumors of the central nervous system. Neurosci Lett. Vol.214, pp. 49-52

Gantz BJ, Hansen MR, Turner CW, et al. (2009). Hybrid 10 Clinical trial. Audiol Neurotol. Vol.14(suppl 1), pp. 32-38

Gantz BJ, Turner CW, Gfeller KE, et al. (2005). Preservation of hearing in cochlear implant surgery: Advantages of combined electrical and acoustic speech processing. Laryngoscope. Vol.115, No.5, pp. 796-802

Gantz BJ, Turner CW, Gfeller KE. (2006). Acoustic plus electric speech processing: preliminary results of a multicenter clinical trial of the Iowa/Nucleus Hybrid implant. Audiol Neurootol. Vol.11(Suppl 1), pp. 63-68

Gantz BJ, Turner CW. (2003). Combining acoustic and electric hearing. Laryngoscope. Vol.113, pp. 1726-1730

Gfeller KE, Olszewski C, Turner CW, et al. (2006). Music perception with cochlear implants and residual hearing. Audiol Neurotol. Vol.11(suppl 1), pp. 12-15

Gfeller KE, Turner CW, Oleson J, et al. (2007). Accuracy of cochlear implant recipients on pitch perception, melody recognition, and speech reception in noise. Ear Hear. Vol.28, No.3, pp. 412-423

Gstoettner WK, Helbig S, Maier N, et al. (2006). Ipsilateral electric acoustic stimulation of the auditory system: results of long-term hearing preservation. Audiol Neurotol. Vol.11(Suppl 1), pp. 49-56

Gstoettner WK, Helbig S, Maier N, Kiefer J, Radeloff A, Adunka OF. (2006). Ipsilateral electric acoustic stimulation of the auditory system: results of long-term hearing preservation. Audiol Neurootol. Vol.11(Suppl 1), pp. 49-56

Gstoettner WK, van de Heyning P, O'Connor AF, et al. (2008). Electric acoustic stimulation of the auditory system: results of a multi-centre investigation. Acta Otolaryngol. Vol.128, No.9, pp. 968-975

Henry KR. (2003). Hyperthermia exacerbates and hypothermia protects from noise-induced threshold elevation of the cochlear nerve envelope response in C57BL/J mouse. Hear Res. Vol.179, pp. 88-96

Hertz CA, Torres V, Quest AFG. (2005). Beyond apoptosis: non-apoptotic cell death in physiology and disease. Biochem Cell Biol. Vol.83, pp. 579-588

Hochmair I, Nopp P, Jolly C, et al. (2006). Med-El cochlear implants: State of the art and a glimpse into the future. Trends in Amplification. Vol.10, No.4, pp. 201-220

Hodges AV, Schloffman J, Balkany T. (1997). Conservation of residual hearing with cochlear implantation. Am J Otol. Vol.18, No.2, pp. 179-183

Hogan C, Turner CW. (1998). High-frequency amplification: benefits for hearing-impaired listeners. Journal of the Acoustical Society of America. Vol.104, No.1, pp. 432-441

Hyodo J, Hakuba N, Koga K, Watanabe F, Shudou M, Taniguchi M, Gyo K. (2001). Hypothermia reduces glutamate efflux in perilymph following transient cochlear ischemia. Neuroreport. Vol.12, pp. 1983-1987

James DP, Eastwood H, Richardson RT, O'Leary SJ. (2008). Effects of round window dexamethasone on residual hearing in guinea pig mode; of cochlear implantation. Audiol Ear Institute. Vol.13, pp. 86-96

Kiefer J, von Ilberg C, Reimer B, et al. (1998). Results of cochlear implantation in patients with severe to profound hearing loss-implications for the indications. Audiology. Vol.37, pp. 382-95

Kil HY, Zhang J, Piantadosi C. (1996). Brain temperature alters hydroxyl radical production during cerebral ischemia/reperfusion in rats. J Cereb Blood Flow Metab. Vol.16, pp. 100-106

Kim R, Emi M, Tanabe K. (2005). Role of mitochondria as the gardens of cell death. Cancer Chemother Pharmacol. Vol.21, pp. 1-9

Klenzner T, Stecker M, Marangos N, Laszig R. (1999). Extended indications for cochlear implantation. The Freiburg results in patients with residual hearing. HNO. Vol.47, pp. 95-100

Kyriakis JM, Avruch J. (1996). Sounding the alarm: protein kinase cascades activated by stress and inflammation. J Biol Chem. Vol.271, pp. 24313-6

Lehnhardt E. (1993). Intracochlear placement of cochlear implant electrode in soft surgery technique. HNO. Vol.41, pp. 356-359.

Lenarz TA, Stover T, Buechner A, et al. (2009). Hearing conservation surgery using the Hybrid-L electrode. Audiol Neurotol. Vol.14(suppl 1), pp. 22-31

Matsui JI, Haque A, Huss D, Messana EP, Alosi JA, Roberson DW, Cotanche DA, Dickman JD, Warchol ME. (2003). Caspase inhibitors promote vestibular hair cell survival and function after aminoglycoside treatment invivo. J Neurosci. Vol.23, pp. 6111-6122

Nelson P, Jin SH, Carney AE, et al. (2003). Understanding speech in modulated interference: cochlear implant uses and normal-hearing listeners. J Acoust Soc Am. Vol.113, No.2, pp. 961-968

Ni D, Shepherd RK, Seldon HL, et al. (1992). Cochlear pathology following chronic electrical stimulation of the auditory nerve. I: Normal hearing kittens. Hear Res. Vol.62, No.1, pp. 63-81

Nicotera TM, Hu BH, Hendrson D. (2003). The caspase pathway in noise-induced apoptosis of the chinchilla cochlea. J Assoc Res Otolaryngol. Vol.4, pp. 466-477

Pirvola, U., Xing-Qun, L., Virkkala, J., Saarma, M., Murakata, C., Camoratto, A.M., Walton, K.M., Ylikoski, J. (2000). Rescue of hearing, auditory hair cells, and neurons by CEP-1347/KT7515, an inhibitor of c-Jun N-terminal kinase activation. J. Neurosci. Vol.20, pp. 43-50

Reiss LA, Turner CW, Erenberg SR, et al. (2007). Changes in pitch with a cochlear implant over time. JARO. Vol.8, pp. 241-257

Roland JT Jr, Zeitler DM, Jethanamest D, et al. (2008). Evaluation of the short hybrid electrode in human temporal bones. Otol Neurotol. Vol.29, No.4, pp. 482-488

Scarpidis BC, Madnani D, Shoemaker C, et al. (2003). Arrest of apoptosis in auditory neurons: implications for sensorineural preservation in cochlear implantation. Otol Neurotol. Vol.24, pp. 409-417

Skarzynski H, Lorens A, Piotrowska A, et al. (2007). Preservation of low frequency hearing in partial deafness cochlear implantation (PDCI) using the round window surgical approach. Acta Otolaryngol. Vol.127, No.1, pp. 41-48

Turner CW, Cummings KJ. (1999). Speech audibility for high-frequency hearing loss listeners. American Journal of Audiology. Vol.8, pp. 47-56

Turner CW, Gantz BJ, Vidal C, et al. (2004). Speech recognition in noise for cochlear implant listeners: benefits of residual acoustic hearing. J Acoust Soc Am. Vol.115, No.4, pp. 1729-1735

Van De Water TR, Lallemend F, Eshraghi AA, et al. (2004). Caspases, the enemy within, and their role in oxidative stress-induced apoptosis of the inner ear sensory cells. Otol Neurotol. Vol.25, pp. 627-632

Vivero RJ, Joseph DE, Angeli S, He J, Chen S, Eshraghi AA, Balkany TJ, Van de Water TR. (2008). Dexamethasone base conserves hearing from electrode trauma induced hearing loss. Laryngoscope. Vol.118, pp. 2028-2033

von Ilberg C, Kiefer J, Tillein J, et al. (1999). Electric-Acoustic stimulation of the auditory system. New Technology for severe hearing loss. ORL J Otorhinolaryngol Relat Spec. Vol.61, No.6, pp. 334-40

Wang J, Ladrech S, Pujol R, Brabet P, Van De Water TR, Puel JL. (2004). Caspase inhibitors, but not c-Jun NH2-terminal kinase inhibitor treatment, prevent cisplatin induced hearing loss. Cancer Res. Vol.64, pp. 9217-9224

Wang J, Van De Water TR, Bonny C, et al. (2003). A peptide inhibitor of c-Jun N-Terminal Kinase (D-JNKI-1) protects against both aminoglycoside and acoustic trauma-induced auditory hair cell death and hearing loss. J Neurosci. Vol.23, pp. 596-8607

Wright CG, Roland PS. (2005). Temporal bone microdissection for anatomic study of cochlear implant electrodes. Cochlear Implants Int. Vol.6, No.4, pp. 159-168

Xu J, Shepherd RK, Millard RE, et al. (1997). Chronic electrical stimulation of the auditory nerve at high stimulus rates: a physiological and histopathological study. Hear Res. Vol.10(1-2), pp. 1-29

Yao, A., Turner, C.W., Gantz, B.J. (2006). Stability of low-frequency residual hearing in patients who are candidates for combined acoustic plus electric hearing. J. Speech Hear. Res. Vol.49, pp. 1085-1090

Ye Q, Tillein J, Hartmann R, Gstoettner W, Kiefer J. (2007). Application of a corticosteroid (Triamcinolon) protects inner ear function after surgical intervention. Ear Hear. Vol.28, pp. 361-369

Zhao W, Richardson JS, Mombourquette MJ, Weil JA, Ljaz S, Shuaib A. (1996). Neuroprotective effects of hypothermia and U-78517F in cerebral ischemia are due to reducing oxygen-based free radicals: an electron paramagnetic resonance study with gerbils. J Neurosci Res. Vol.45, pp. 282-288

2

Modifications on the Alternative Method for Cochlea Implantation

R.A. Tange
Department of Otorhinolaryngology,
University Center of the University of Utrecht, Utrecht
The Netherlands

1. Introduction

House [1] introduced the classic surgical technique for cochlear implantation. This surgical technique consists of a mastoidectomy and a posterior tympanotomy and this approach is still worldwide the most frequently used technique for cochlear implantation. This classic surgical technique uses a complete mastoidectomy with an attempt to leave a bony overhang posterior and superiorly to capture the proximal electrode lead [2,3]. After the complete mastoidectomy a posterior tympanotomy is performed with special attention to the facial nerve and the chorda tympani. Through the large posterior tympanotomy (intraoperative facial nerve monitoring is mandatory) a cochleostomy can be performed for electrode insertion. The classic technique has proven to be sufficient in the vast majority of cochlear implantations. Still complications concerning the facial nerve can occur due to the fact of drilling within a millimetre of the facial nerve making the posterior tympanotomy [4,5] To avoid negative side effects as a temporary or permanent injury to the facial nerve Kronenberg et al [6],Kiratzidis [7] and later Hausler [8] designed a different approach in which no mastoidectomy was needed to create the pathway towards the cochleostomy. These new cochlear implantation techniques without a mastoidectomy and a posterior tympanotomy seem to be safe and effective procedures. After experienced the classic approach of cochlear implantation our cochlear implant team moved over to the new innovative alternative surgical approach introduced by Joan Kronenburg in 2001. Our first positive experiences with the suprameatal approach and our modifications have been published in 2004 [9]. Our method consists of a number of following steps as shown in the table 1.

Steps in our approach for cochlear implantation	
1	Retroauriculair skin incision : middle ear approach
2	Creating of the suprameatal tunnel towards incus : Making a connection between middle ear and tunnel
3	Second temporal incision to create the well for the cochlear implant device
4	Subcutaneous subperiostal tunnel between two incisions (plastic canula)
5	Imbedding implant in temporal area with guiding the active array (and ball electrode) towards retro auricular incision.
6	Creating cochleostomy through external auditory canal.
7	Insertion of the array via combined approach into the cochlea

Table 1.

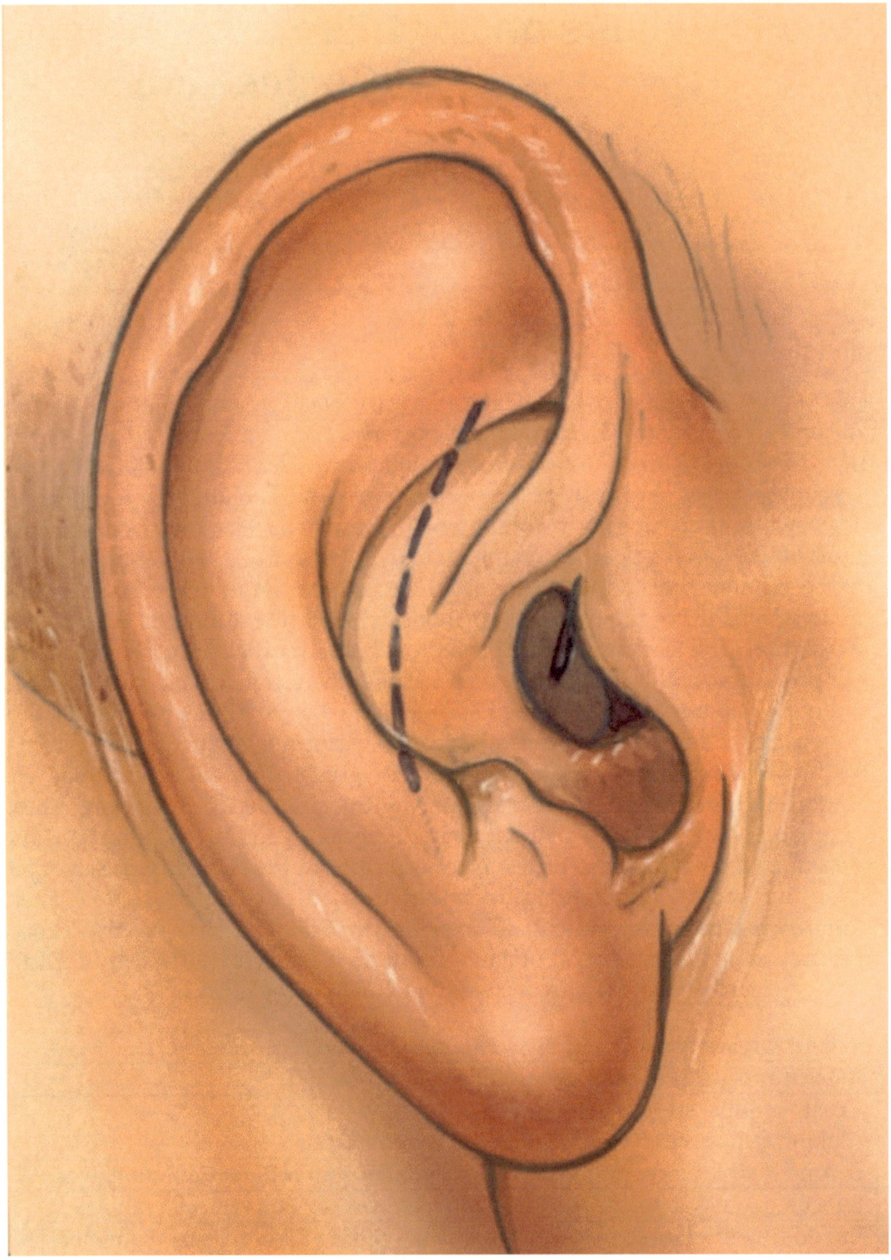

Fig. 1. Small retroauriculair incision (step1)

2. Retroauriculair skin incision: Middle ear approach

All our patients are operated in general anaesthesia. After sterile draping the incisions and the site for the internal processor are marked . After local sub and intra cutaneus injection of adrenalin 1:100.000 the first retroaricular incision (5mm from the tragus fold) of 2 cm is made. The periost is cut in and elevated to explore the introitus of the external ear canal. The skin of the canal is elevated without opening the external ear. The annulus of the eardrum is carefully elevated and special attention is given to the course of the chorda tympani. The middle ear will be inspected then. Important anatomical structures to distinguish are the round window nice and the stapes incus complex. In cases of a curved bony external ear canal sometimes lateral some bony "overhang" need to be removed to facilitate optimal view into the middle ear and to ease the cochleostomy in a later phase of the surgery. The position of the cochleostomy is located by the point of junction of a line drawn anteriorly from the middle of the round window niche intersecting a line drawn inferiorly from the oval window niche. The middle ear area is now filled with a sterile sponge to prevent entering bone dust in the middle ear and to open the middle ear approach.

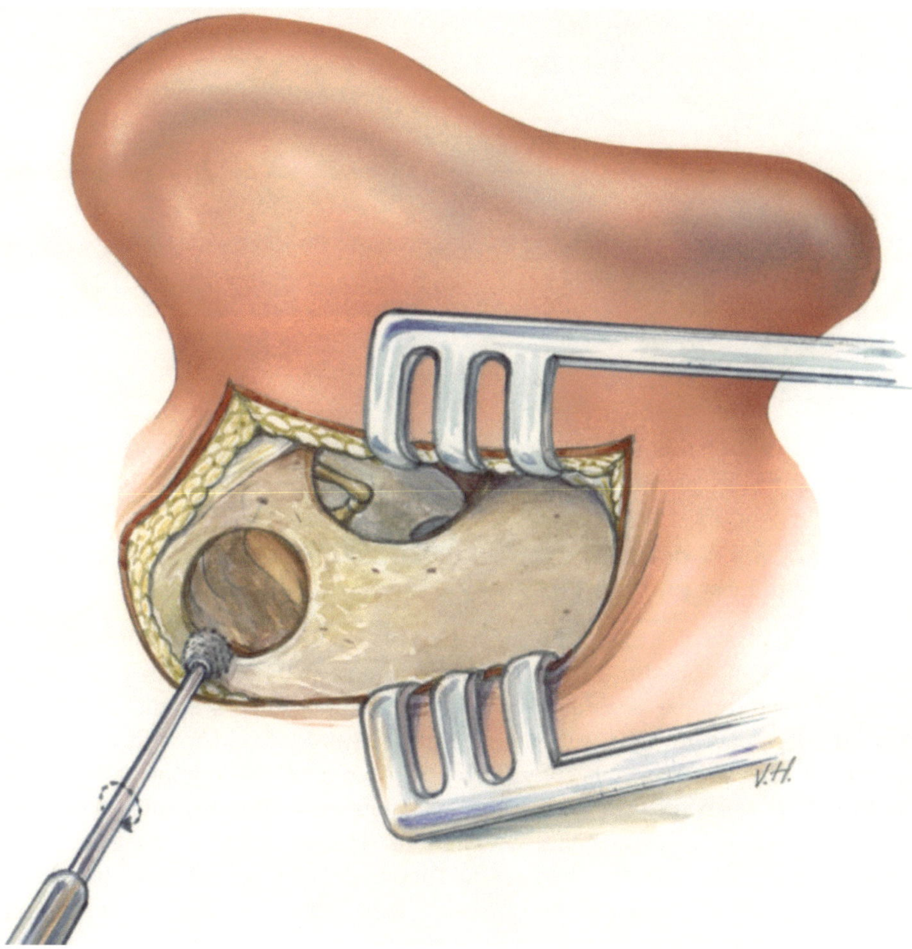

Fig. 2. Middle ear approach by retroauriculair incision (step1)

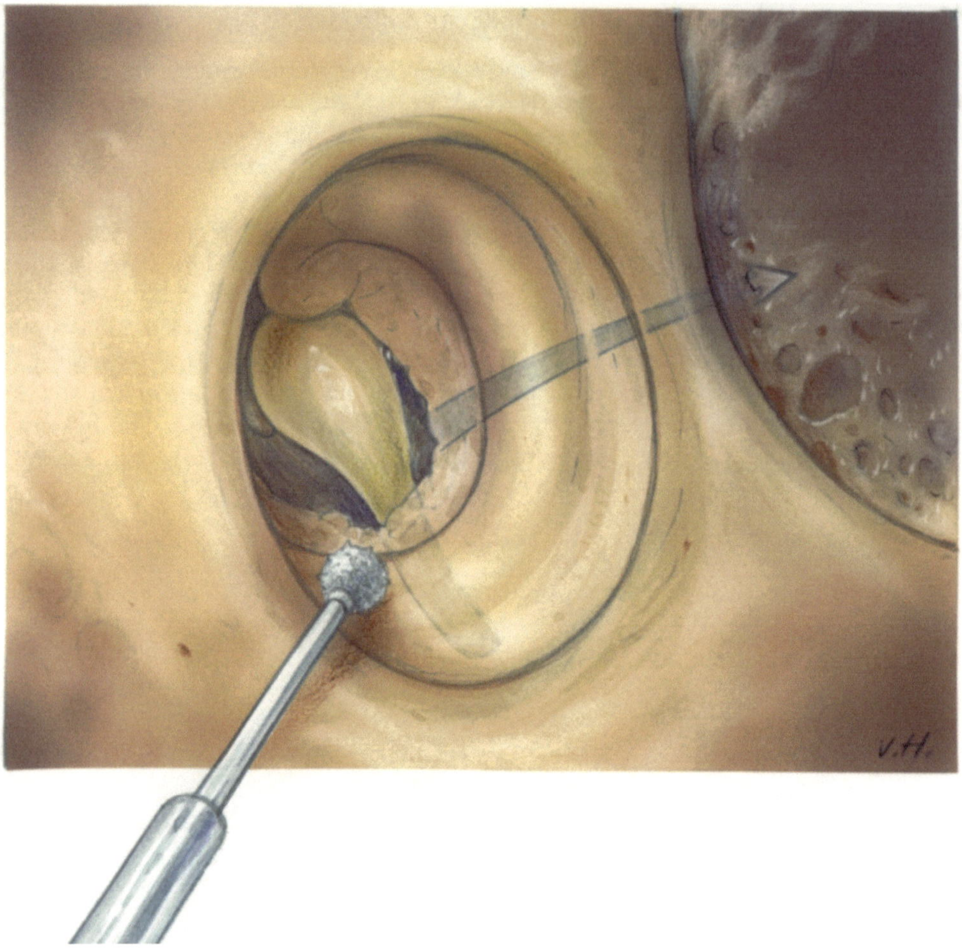

Fig. 3. Creating of the suprameatal tunnel towards incus : Making a connection between middle ear and tunnel (step 2)

3. Creating of the suprameatal tunnel towards incus: Making a connection between middle ear and tunnel

In the following phase of our approach a small tunnel is drilled from the suprameatal spine towards the body of the incus. Preoperatively thorough analyzing op the preoperative CT-scans of the operating ear is obligator. Axial and coronal images predict the state of the mastoid and the space for the creation of the suprameatal tunnel. According the scans one can decide whether to perform the alternative approach for cochlear implantation or not. On the other hand it is of course always possible to change from our alternative technique to the classical approach in cases anatomical variations. In our series we have only changed towards the classical method in two cases. The small bony tunnel canal is drilled from behind the suprameatal spine to the posterior attic. When the pneumatized mastoid is opened with a sharp 5 mm drill the next orientation point is the horizontal semicircular bony canal near the short process of the incus. A limited posterior atticotympanotomy is performed to visualize the short process if the incus. The space between the lateral edge of the short process of the incus and the canal wall is now opened and must be enlarged by drilling with the diamond burrs (1.5 - 2 mm). The long process of the incus becomes visible and in most of the cases the incudo-stapedial joint can be observed. Introducing the gentle curved pick needle through the created opening between incus and canal wall the pathway for the array towards the cochlea in the middle ear is tested. Using this approach there is no danger for the facial nerve and the chorda tympani. When we decide that the this supra tympanotomy approach is sufficient for the introduction of the array a second sterile sponge is placed in the created tunnel. The retro auricular incision is closed with one temporary suture.

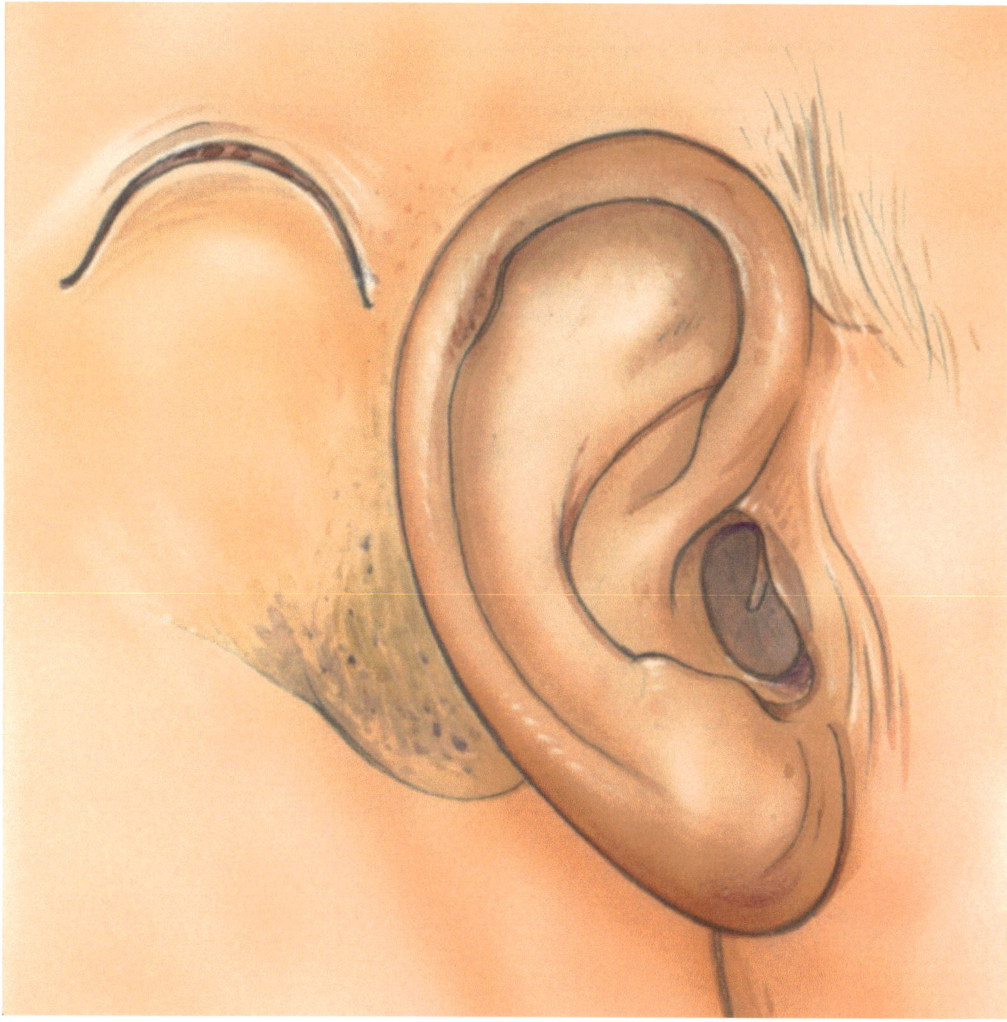

Fig. 4. Second temporal incision to create the well for the cochlear implant device (step 3)

4. Second temporal incision to create the well for the cochlear implant device

Different from the classic method of implantation and the methods describes by Kronenberg Kiratzidis and other we do not extent the retro auricular skin incision superoposteriorly to expose the temporomastoid region for the drilling of the well for the device. To keep the natural tension of the skin and the periost of the temporomastoid region we make a small semicircular skin incision with a diameter of about 2.5-3 cm at the site where the well for the device is planned. When the skin and the subcutaneous tissue is elevated the periost covering the temporal bone is incised with an opposite semicircular periost incision. With this modification the two incisions will not be in the same level and the skin/periost tension over the implanted device is distributed equally this way. According the size of the cochlear implants used the well can be created through the second skin incision. Because of the semicircular shape of the incision optimal room is created for the implantation of the device without losing much tension of the skin and periost. Tie-down holes are not necesssary using our procedure. The tension of the skin and periost keep the implant safe in the well of the temporal bone. When the well is created a subperiost tunnel in created between the "well incision" and the retro auricular incision. A sterile plastic canula with a diameter of about 3 mm is inserted in this sub periostal tunnel.

At this moment the cochlear implant device is unpacked and introduced into the "well incision" after making sub periost room for the magnet. The array (and the ball electrode) are introduced into the plastic canula. This canula is then gently pulled towards the retro auricular incision presenting the array (and the ball electrode) near the suprameatal tunnel. The "well incision" is now sutured in two layers.

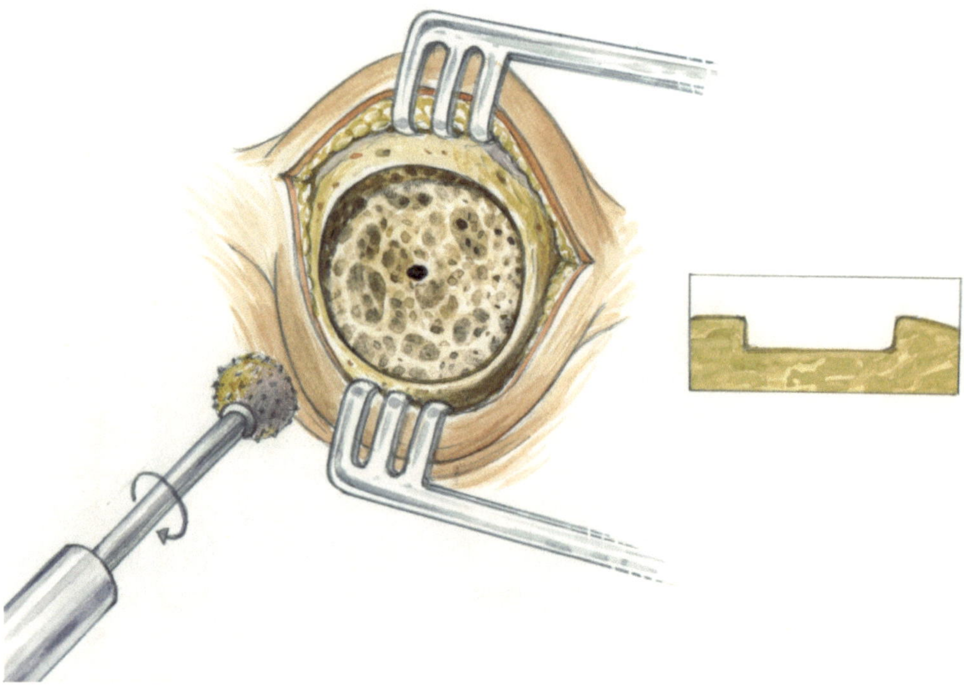

Fig. 5. Creation of the well for the cochlear implant device (step 3)

5. Creating cochleostomy through external auditory canal

Having the array near to the cochlea the time has arrived to create the cochleostomy. The two protecting sponges are removed and the suprameatal tunnel and middle ea are cleaned. At the point where a junction of a line drawn anteriorly from the middle of the round window niche intersecting a line drawn inferiorly from the oval window niche a cochleostomy is created through the external ear canal. With a 1.5 diamond burr, the bone of the promontory is drilled away to a dept of approximately 1.5 mm until the endosteum of the scala tympani is visualized. Then a 1-mm bur is used to complete the bony removal, with an attempt to leave the endosteum intact until all bone work is done. With a sharp pick the endosteum is incised and the sharp bony edges of the cochleostomy are removed. The undersurface of the basilar membrane is now visible and lumen of the scala tympani is open to insert the array of the cochlear implant. It is important to attempt to limit the amount of bone dust into the cochlea to prevent new bone formation in the inner ear.

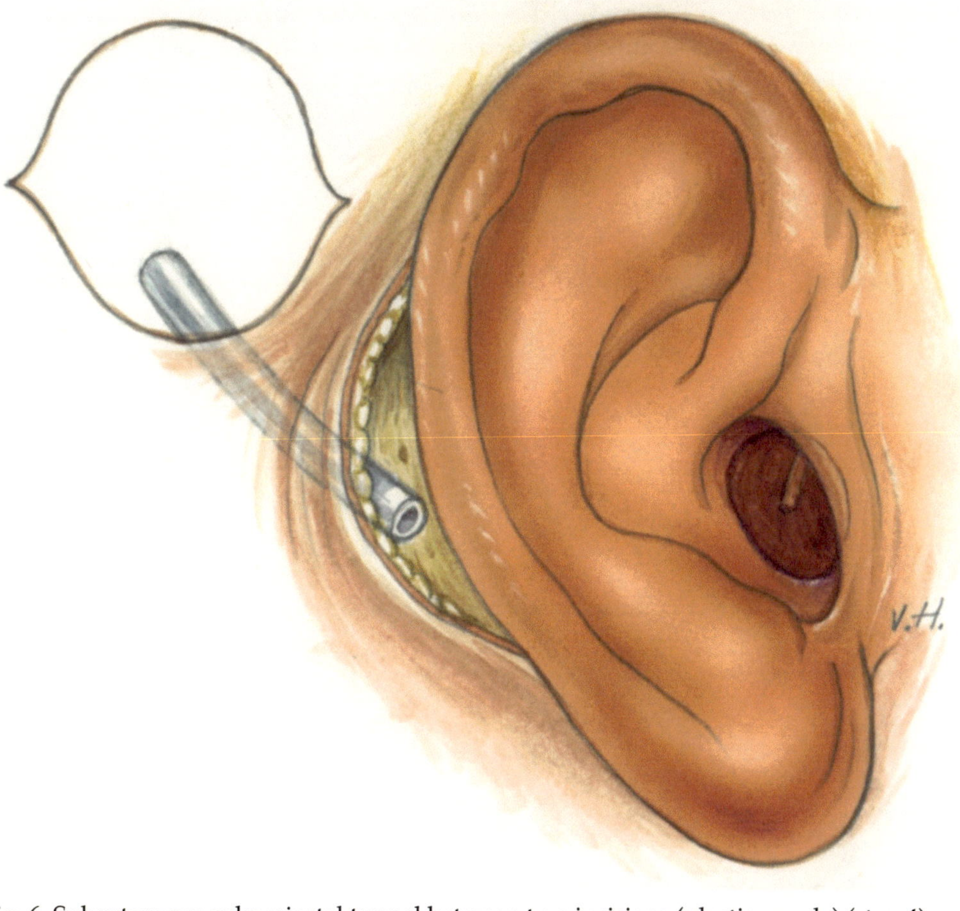

Fig. 6. Subcutaneous subperiostal tunnel between two incisions (plastic canula) (step 4)

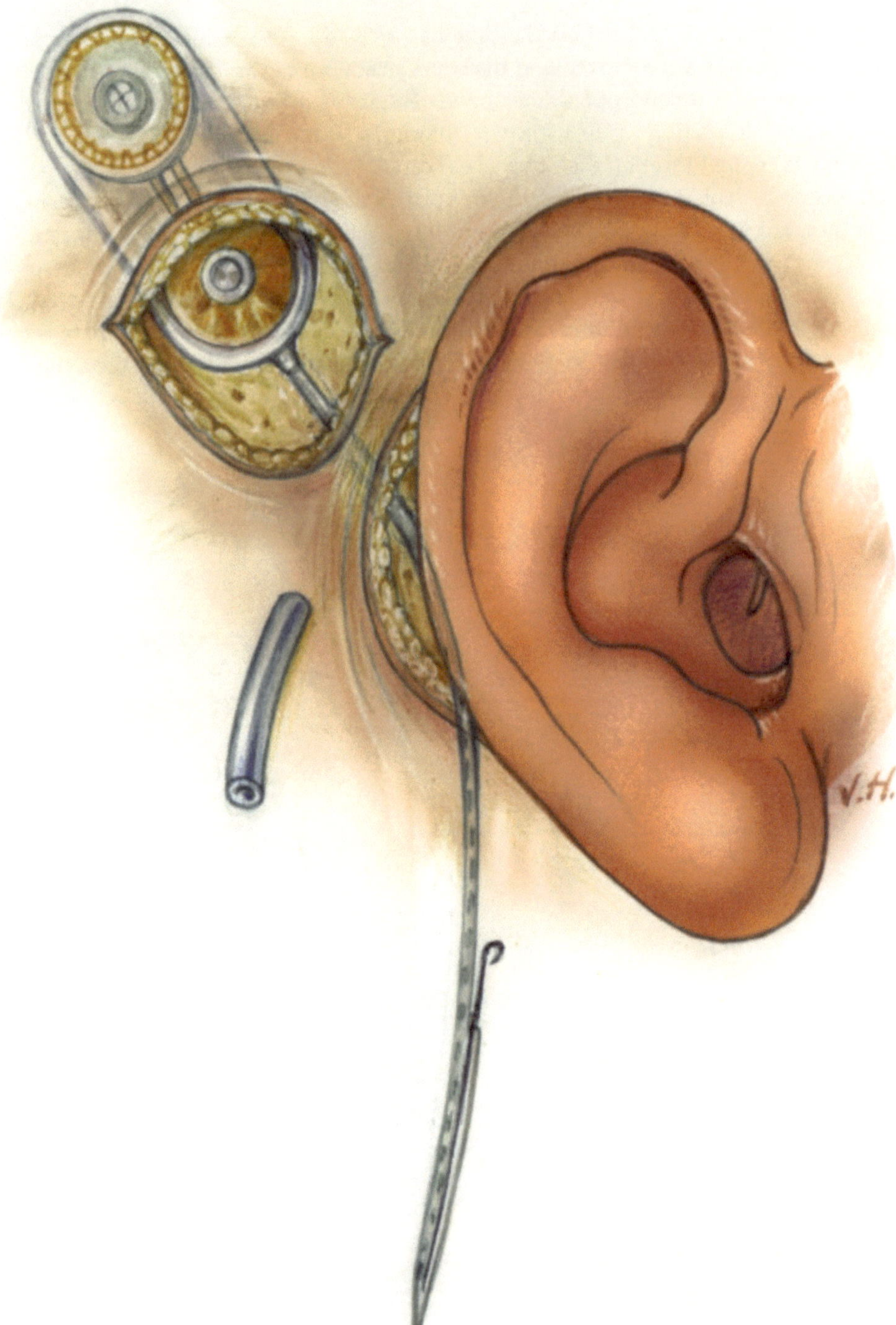

Fig. 7. Imbedding implant in temporal area with guiding the active array (and ball electrode) towards retro auricular incision. (step 5)

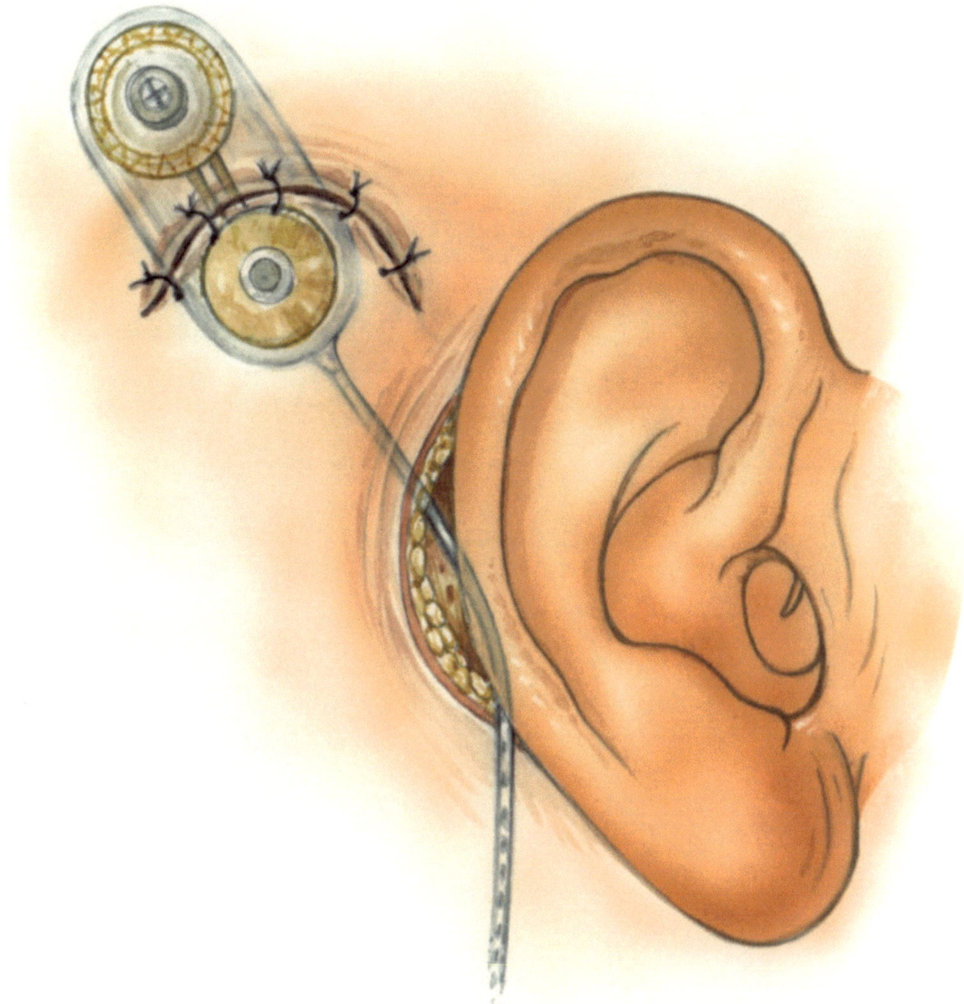

Fig. 8. Closure of the 2nd temporal incision (step 5)

6. Insertion of the array via combined approach into the cochlea

After the creation of the cochleostomy the electrode insertion can be performed. Using instruments as a micro-jeweller forceps, insertion claw, suction tip or angled pick the electrode is guided through the suprameatal tunnel towards incus. The tip of the electrode is than introduced into middle ear along the long process of the incus. Via the external ear canal the tip of the electrode is now visible and can be guided towards the cochleostomy. Prior to the insertion we use a drop of lubricant hyaloron acid (Healon) to ease the insertion of the electrode. The electrode is now gently inserted into the cochlea advancing the array 1 to 2 mm at the time. Halfway the insertion (white mark Nucleus device) the stylet of the

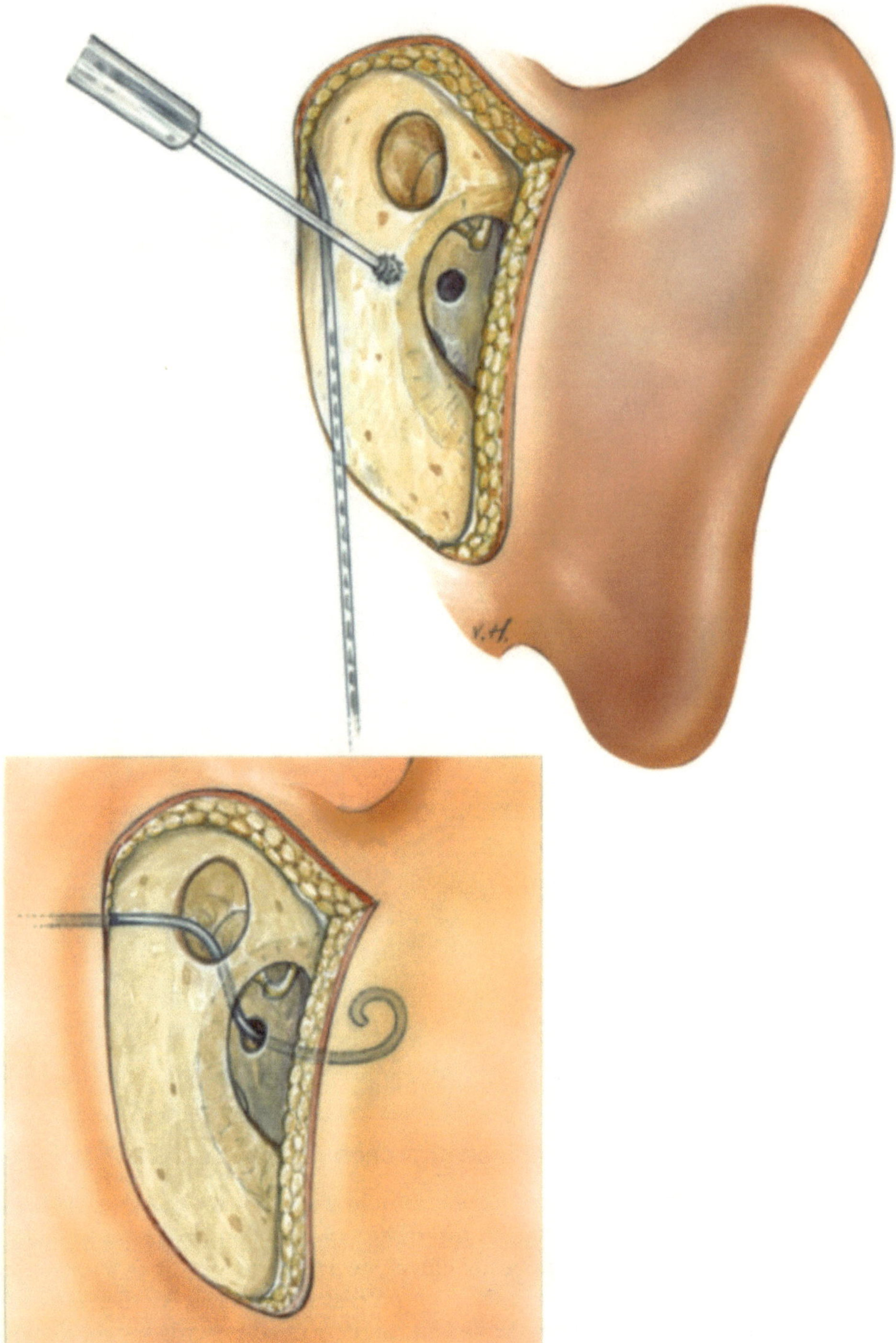

Fig. 9. Creating cochleostomy through external auditory canal and insertion of the array via combined approach into the cochlea. (step 6 &7)

array is gently removed while the array is pushed off-stylet in to the cochlea. Using the insertion claws a total insertion is pursued and will be possible in almost all the cases. Sometimes some tiny pieces of fascia can be placed around the electrode at the cochleostomy area. When the implantation of the electrode into the cochlea is performed the array is fixed in the opening of suprameatal tunnel by local bone dust. The retroauriculaire incision is now carefully sutured in two layers and a dressing of the external ear canal is placed through the external meatus. At this point the implanted device is tested by electrophysiological or neural response measurements. A transmitter coil in a sterile endosheath is placed on the magnet area of the implant. Electrode impedances are measured and other electrically tests like neural response telemetry (NRT/NRI) can be performed depending the device used. These tests are important to assure that the implant is functioning properly and that the patient receives an auditory stimulus and responds appropriately. In our centre, the 3D-RX, a way of three dimensional rotational imaging with a mobilized C arm in the OR is now the standard procedure for illustrating the electrode position in the cochlea right after implantation. This method is described recently by Carelsen et al [9] When all the electrophysiological or neural response measurements are in favour of a good functioning implant and patient responses are adequate together with normal imaging of the array in the cochlea the surgery is ended.

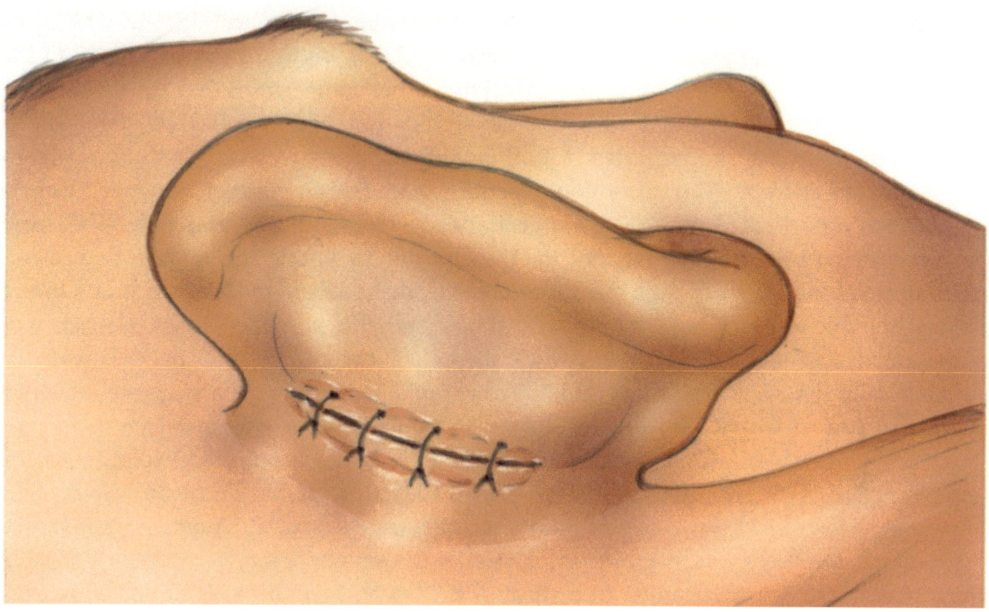

Fig. 10. Closure of the small retroauriculair incision

7. The data of our approach for cochlea implantation

We started our cochlear implant programme in 2003 and, to date, 260 patients have received their cochlear implant according the suprameatal method. Initially, we started our cochlear implant programme using the classic method with mastoidectomy and posterior tympanotomy approach. But soon we altered our cochlear implant strategy in favour of the new innovative alternative surgical approach. The mean age of the 260 patients implanted was 39.6 years (1.0-82.3 years) and the mean duration of deafness was 26.3 years (0.3-66.0 years). The main etiology of the deafness of our cochlear implant group was a congenital hearing (31.4 %) and a progressive sensorineural hearing ((24.8%). Other causes of deafness were meningitis (13.3 %) and otosclerosis (6.7%). Prelingual deafness and postingual deafness accounted for 51.0 % and 49.0 % respectively. Four different types of cochlear implants have been used for implantation; the Nucleus®24Countour™ , the Nucleus®24Countour™ Advance with Softip ™ , Advanced Bionics® HiFocus Helix and Medel Sonata® Ti100. We recorded the duration of surgery for all cochlear implantations. The mean duration of cochlear implantation was 111.7 minutes. The shortest procedure accounted for 57 minutes; the longest duration of surgery was 261 minutes which was a consequence of difficult insertion of the electrode due to otosclerosis of the cochlea. With respect to the duration of surgery we excluded the time of audiological measurements after implantation. Studying the data of last years there is no tendency of declination of the duration time of the surgery. The mean time of surgery stays constant during the study period which means there is no learning curve with respect to duration of the surgery. Maximum time of surgery in two procedures was prolonged in 2004 and 2006. In both procedures the insertion of the electrode was extremely difficult due to otosclerosis of the cochlea and secondly by a low-lying middle fossa dura. Complication of our approach can be divided into minor and major complications. The minor complication rate was 23 per cent. These complications consisted out of tinnitus (7.2%), vertigo postoperatively (5.2%), eardrum perforation (1.3%), haematoma (1.3%) and other some causes (3.8 %). We did have one case (otosclerosis) of mild facial nerve stimulation which could be managed by switching off a number of electrodes. All minor complications were successfully overcome by conservative therapy. The major complications were five in number. The overall major complication rate was 3 %. All complications developed postoperatively. The major complications consisted of extrusion of the implant due to wound infection in two cases, a fausse route of the electrode [11], a misdirected electrode in severe otosclerosis and a case of explantation due to psychiatrically illness and pain sensations. All five cases of major were re-implanted and ended up successfully thereafter except for the patient with the psychiatrically illness. She still has all kind of complaints in spite of a perfect functioning device and perfect wound healing. In our series we had one case of a device failure (the speech recognition declined one year after implantation) which required explantation and re-implantation. Concerning the hearing gain achieved with the cochlear implants the average gain for the whole group of adults was almost 84 % CVC. Average preoperative CVC was 12 %. Of the whole group implanted only two non users of the hearing device which makes 99,5 % happy users. In a study [12] on the postoperative status of the mastoid cavity after cochlear implantation with our mastoid saving surgical method we compared pre- and postoperative protocolair prepared CT-scans of the mastoid cavity of 79 patients. In 76 cases no abnormalities were observed in the mastoid of the operated ear for cochlear implantation. In two cases of otosclerosis swollen mucosa was observed without any clinical relevance. In one case (a child) opicafication of the whole mastoid and middle ear was observed without destruction of the structures of the mastoid. We concluded with others[13] from these data that the delicate structures of the mastoid cavity can be kept intact using a mastoid saving surgical approach.

8. In conclusion

Our alternative approach for cochlea implantation has like the methods introduced by Kronenberg and others been proven a reliable alternative approach for cochlear implantation. It is a functional approach leaving the delicate structures of the pneumatized mastoid intact. An important fact of this innovative approach is the safety for the facial nerve. It is almost impossible to injure the facial nerve or the chorda tympani with this approach. Bilateral simultaneous cochlear implantation using the alternative approach is possible and recommended to reduce the extra surgery time. Because of our two small incisions approach to fix the processor the creation of tie-down holes are not necessary anymore which reduces the extra risk of infection of the implant. In our opinion it is of great importance to use the combined approach in cases of anatomical changes of this area as in severe cochlear otosclerosis. An other great advantage of the suprameatal approach with all its variations is the possibility to switch over when needed to the classic surgical approach introduced may years ago.

9. References

[1] House W.F. Cochlear implants. Ann.Otol.Rhinol. Laryngol. 1976;8 (suppl.27) : 2-7

[2] Clark G.M.A. : A surgical approach for a cochlear implant : An anatomical study. J.Laryngol.Otol. 1975 ; 89/1 : 9-115

[3] Goycolea M.V., Papparella M.M., Muchow D. Mastoidectomy tympanotomy approach for cochlear implantation. Laryngoscope 1987; 97 : 766-771

[4] Cohen N.L., Hoffman R.A. Complications of cochlear implant surgery in adults and children. Ann. Otol.Rhinol. Laryngol. 1991; 100 :708-711

[5] Kempf H-G. Tempel S. Johann K. Lenarz Th. Complications in cochlear implant surgery. Laryngo- Rhino- Otologie. 1999. Vol 78(10) : 529-537

[6] Kronenberg J. Migirov L. Dagan T. Suprameatal approach: New surgical approach for cochlear implantation. Journal of Laryngology & Otology. 2001. Vol 115(4): 283-285

[7] Kiratzidis T. "Veria operation" : Cochlear Implantation without a mastoidectomy and a poaterior tympanotomy – a new surgical technique. In : Kim C.S.,Chang S.O.,Lim D. (eds): Updates in Cochlear Implantations. Ad.Otorhinolaryngol. Basel Karger 2000 vol 57 pp 127-130

[8] Hausler R. Cochlear implantation without mastoidectomy: The pericanal electrode insertion technique. Acta Oto-Laryngologica. Vol 122(7) (pp 715-719), 2002.

[9] Tange R.A. Grolman W. Mastoid saving surgical approach (MASSA) and our experience with a new electrode with softip for cochlear implantation Journ Ind.Soc.Otol. Vol 2 nr 1&2 2004 29-32

[10] Carelsen B, Grolman W, Tange RA, Streekstra GJ, van Kemenade P, Jansen RJ, Freling NJ, White M, Maat B, Fokkens WJ. Cochlear implant electrode array insertion monitoring with intra-operative 3D rotational X-ray. Clin Otolaryngol. 2007 Feb;32(1):46-50.

[11] Tange R.A. Grolman W., Maat A. Intracochlear misdirection implantation of a cochlear implant. Acta Otolaryngol (Scand.) 2006 126:6 : 650-652

[12] Tange R.A.,Grolman W. Het mastoid na CI implantatie met de mastoid-sparende benadering . Ned.Tijdschr. KNO-Heelk 2007 ; 13(4) 22-223

[13] Kronenberg J.,Migirov L.The role of mastoidectomy in cochlear implant surgery. Acta Oto-Laryngologica. 2003 Vol 123(2) ; 219-222.

Section 2

Speech Processing Strategies

3

Wavelet Based Speech Strategy in Cochlear Implant

Gulden Kokturk
Dokuz Eylul University
Turkey

1. Introduction

A significant percentage of the populations in developed countries encounter hearing impairment. Cochlear Implant was developed to increase the hearing capacity of these people. In recent years, adults and children have benefited from the usage of Cochlear Implant and the users were positively affected by the improvement of implant techniques. Although these devices allow for increased performance, a significant gap still remains in speech recognition between Cochlear Implant user and people, who possess normal listening capabilities.

The Cochlear implant prosthesis, works with direct stimulation of the auditory nerve cells of deaf people, whose recipient cells in their cochlea were destroyed (House&Berliner, 1982; House&Urban, 1979; Christiansen&Leigh, 2002; Loeb, 1990; Parkins&Anderson, 1983; Wilson, 1993). The system basically consists of the following sections; microphone, speech processor, transmitter, receiver and electrode array. Mainly, implant stimulation systems, signal processing strategies and techniques in increasing the suitability of the instrument to various patients were the improved upon this prosthesis. However, new developments in this area also exist on the configuration of hearing function, especially signal processing strategies.

Speech processing techniques are very important in increasing the users' hearing potential (Eddington, 1980; Wilson et al., 1991; Dormon et al., 1997; Moore&Teagle, 2002). A variety of strategies were developed in the recent years with the aim to improve the hearing abilities of deaf people and take these abilities closer to those of people with natural hearing. Of these, various speech processing strategies were developed for multi-channel cochlear implants (Derbel et al., 1994; Cheikhrouhou et al., 2004; Gopalakrishna et al., 2010; Millar et al., 1984). These strategies can be classified mainly in three parts; waveform strategies, feature extraction strategies and hybrid strategy (N-of-M strategy).

Wavelet method is a basic method that is used for noise filtering, compression and analysis of nonstationary signals and images. The wavelet transform is an appropriate method for semistationary signals and provides a good resolution in both time and frequency. Several studies were carried out on the use of the wavelet transform for speech processing. The wavelet transform gives better results than traditional methods in improving speech. The wavelet packet transform is a type of the discrete wavelet transform that allows for subband analysis in the second decomposition without any constraints. Basically, the wavelet packet transform adapts to the frequency axis and allows decomposition. This particular decomposition is implemented with the optimization criteria. Studies show that the filter banks used in the sound strategies of cochlear implants are parallel to the filter banks used in the wavelet transform. This indicates that the wavelet transform is a method that can be used in Cochlear implants. However, the author could not find any distinctive study on the analysis of speech using the wavelet packet transform for speech processing.

In this study, a new strategy, which uses the wavelet packet transform in obtaining the sequence of the electrode array to be stimulated, is proposed. Thus the stimulated electrode array is based upon but would be different from the N-of-M Strategy. An experimental study was performed and analyzed using Turkish words. The words were selected and grouped based on Turkish sound knowledge, and were recorded in the silent rooms of Ege University, Department of Otology. The experimental subjects listened to the words for both the N-of-M strategy and the proposed strategy, thus comparative results were obtained. Better intelligibility results were attained by the usage of the proposed strategy.

2. Strategies for cochlear implants

Multi-channel implants provide electrical stimulation in the cochlea using an array of electrodes. An electrode array is used so that different auditory nerve fibers can be stimulated at different places in the cochlea. Electrodes respond for each frequency of the signal and hair cells. The ones near the base of the cochlea are stimulated with high frequency signals while electrodes near the apex are stimulated with low frequency signals.

The various signal processing strategies developed for multi-channel cochlea can be examined under two main categories: waveform strategies and feature-extraction strategies. These strategies extract the speech information from the speech signal and redeliver it to the electrods. The waveform strategies use some type of waveform (in analog or pulsatile form) derived by filtering the speech signal into different frequency bands. The feature extraction strategies use some type of spectral features, such as formants, derived by feature extraction algorithms.

There are various parameters that present the acoustic signal information to the electrodes in these signal processing strategies. The first parameter is the number of electrodes used for stimulus that decides the frequency resolution. Mostly, it is used as 16-22 electrodes for stimulation. This also depends on receivers of the individual cochlear implant relating to neuron population distribution. The second parameter is the electrode configuration. Different configurations are controled since the electric current distributes electrodes symmetrically. The most important parameter is the amplitude of the electric current which is constructed using some envelope detection algorithms from the filtered waveform. It is controlled by the loudness level of the stimulation that could be comprehended. The electric current amplitude includes spectral information generated from the time varying current amplitude levels on each electrode and on different electrodes stimulated in the same cycle.

The main strategies are discussed below.

2.1 Compressed analog approach

The strategy of compressed analog approach has been developed mainly by Symbion Company (Edington, 1980). In this system, first, the audio signal is compressed using the automatic gain control unit. Later the signal is filtered with four side by side frequency bands at the center frequencies of 0.5, 1, 2 and 3.4 kHz. Then, the filtered waveforms are changed into stimulation format and sent to four electrodes that were placed into the cochlea by surgical intervention (Dorman et al., 1989).

The compressed analog approach gives useful spectral information to the electrodes. But the channel interaction causes problems in the compressed analog approach. Since the stimulation is analog, the stimulus is transmitted continuously to the four electrodes at the same time. The simultaneous stimulation causes channel interaction and can negatively affect the performance of the device.

2.2 Continuous interleaved sampling

The continuous interleaved sampling approach was developed by researchers of the Research Triangle Institute (Wilson et al., 1991). In this strategy, the signal is sent through the electrode not by stimulation but by interleaved strokes. Here, the amplitude of the pulse is derived from the envelope of bandpass filter. Later, this resulting envelope is compressed and used for modulation of two-phase pulses. The patient's hearing unit is electronically excited. Non-linear compression function (i.e. logarithmic function) is used to ensure that the envelope output is suitable for the patient's dynamic range. A block diagram of the continuous interleaved strategy is shown in Figure 1.

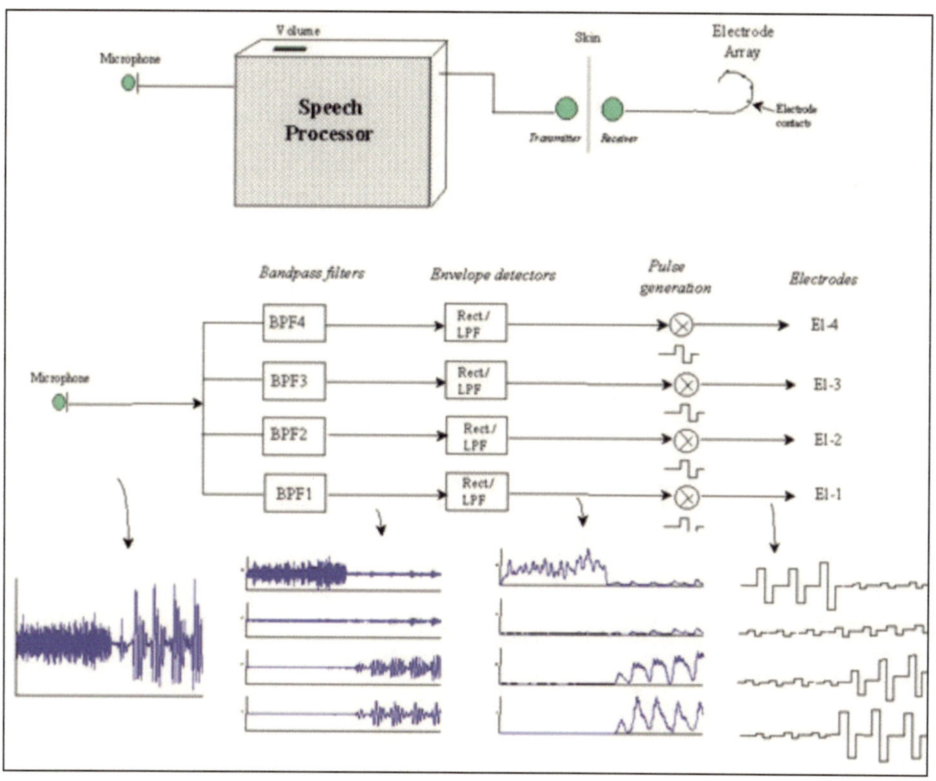

Fig. 1. Detailed block diagram of continuous interleaved sampling speech strategy in cochlear implant (Loizou, 1998)

2.3 N-of-M (N-M) speech processing

In N-M strategy, the audio signal is divided into m frequency bands; and the processor selects n number of the highest-energy envelope outputs (see in Figure 2). Only the electrodes corresponding to the selected n outputs are stimulated at each cycle (Nogueira et al., 2006). For example; in a strategy of 22-6, only 6 of the 22 channel outputs are selected, thus only these 6 selected channels are stimulated. N-M strategy is a hybrid strategy since it also includes feature representation. A general block diagram showing the feature inference for N-M system is given in Figure 3.

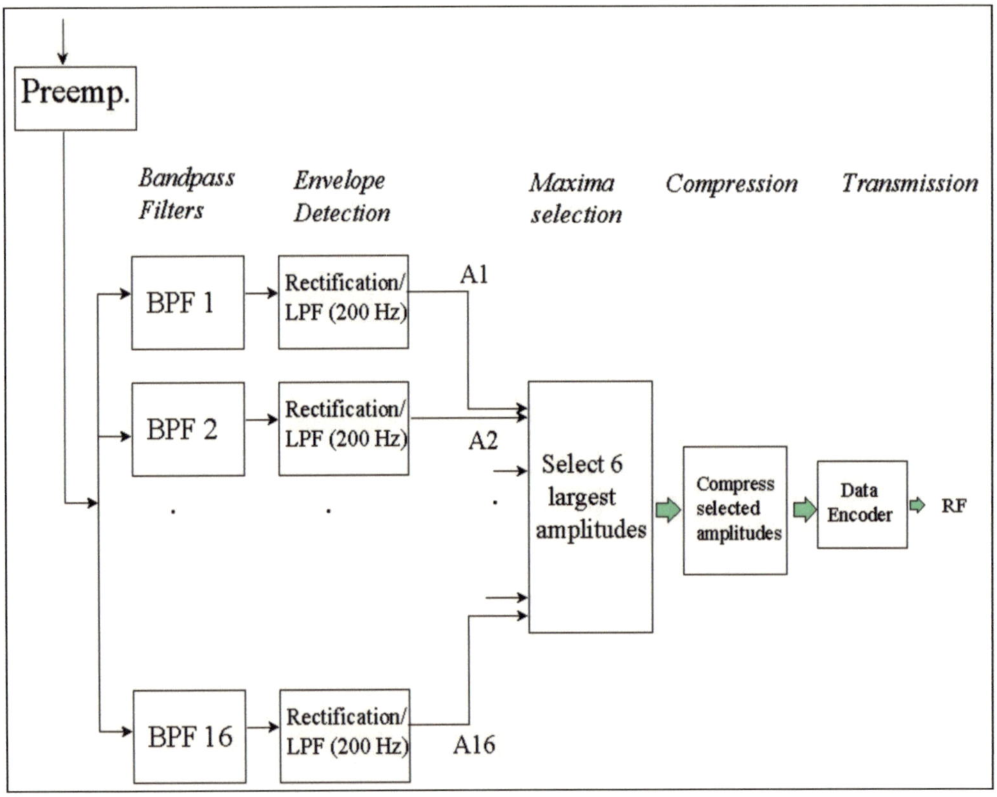

Fig. 2. Detailed block diagram of N-M speech strategy in Cochlear implant (Loizou, 1998)

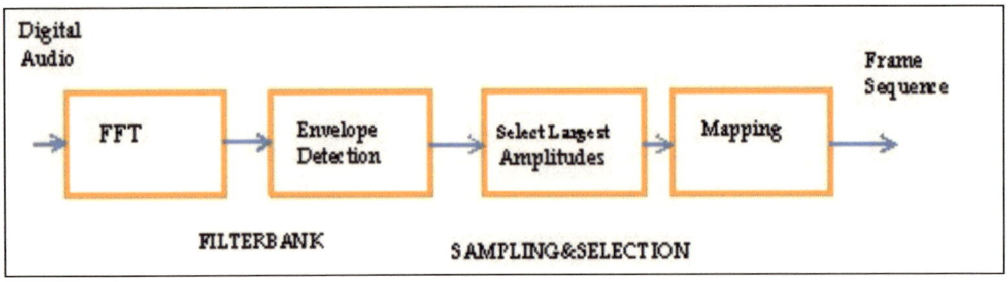

Fig. 3. General block diagram showing the feature inference of N-M speech strategy in Cochlear implant (Loizou, 1998)

3. Wavelet transform

A time signal can be evaluated by a series of coefficients, based on an analysis function. For example, a signal can be transformed from time domain to frequency domain. The oldest and best known method for this is the Fourier transform. Joseph Fourier developed his method that represents signal contents by using basis functions in 1807. Based on this work the wavelet theory was developed by Alfred Haar in 1909. In 1930's, Paul Levy improved Haar basis function using scale varying. In 1981, a transformation method of decomposing a signal into wavelet coefficients and reconstructing the original signal form these coefficients was found by Jean Morlet and Alex Grossman. And Stephane Mallat and Yves Meyer derived multiresolution decomposition using wavelets. Later, Ingrid Daubechies developed a new wavelet analysis method to construct her own family of wavelets using the multiresolution theory. The set of wavelet orthonormal basis function based on Daubechies' work is the milestone of wavelet applications today. With these developments, theoretical investigations of wavelet analysis began to accrue. (Merry, 2005).

Generally, the Fourier transform is an efficient transform for stationary and pseudo stationary signals. But this technique is not suitable for the nonstationary signals such as noisy and aperiodic signals. These signals can be analyzed using local transformation methods; the short time Fourier transform, time-frequency distributions and wavelets. All these techniques analyzed the signal using the correlation between original signal and analysis function.

Wavelet transform can be classified as; continuous wavelet transform, discrete wavelet transform and fast wavelet transform (Holschneider, 1989, Mallat, 1998; Meyer, 1992). The wavelet transform applied to a wide range of use, subjects including signal and image processing, and biomedical signal processing. The most important advantage of the wavelet transform is that it allows for the local analysis of the signal. Also, wavelet analysis reveals such as discontinuities, corruptions etc. in a signal.

A a wavelet function, ψ(t) is a small wave. In wavelet function, the wavelet must be zero as soon as possible while still having oscillatory. Therefore, it includes different frequencies to

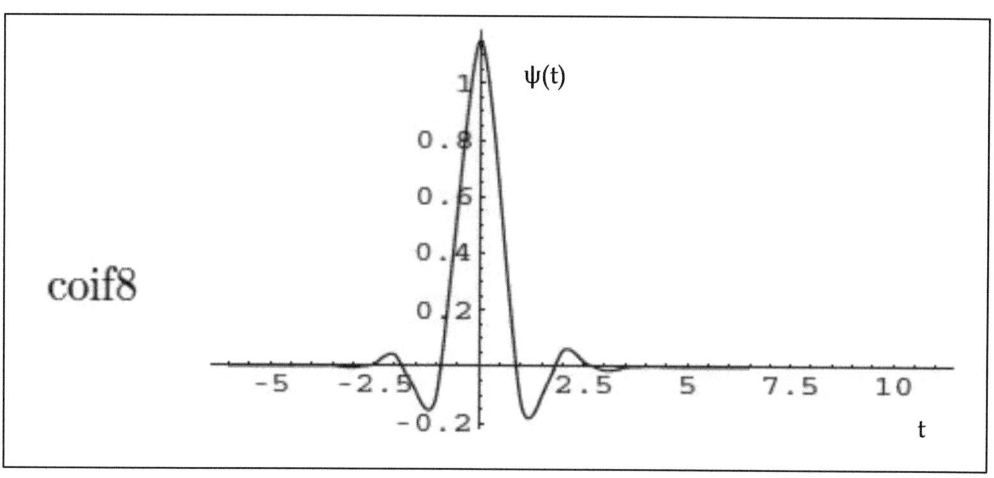

Fig. 4. An example wavelet, Coiflet wavelet

be analyzed. An example of a possible wavelet known as Coiflet wavelet function is shown in Figure 4. (Misiti et al., 2000).

The wavelet basis is a grid decomposition of the phase plane which is shown in Figure 5 (Pereyra&Mohlenkampy, 2004).

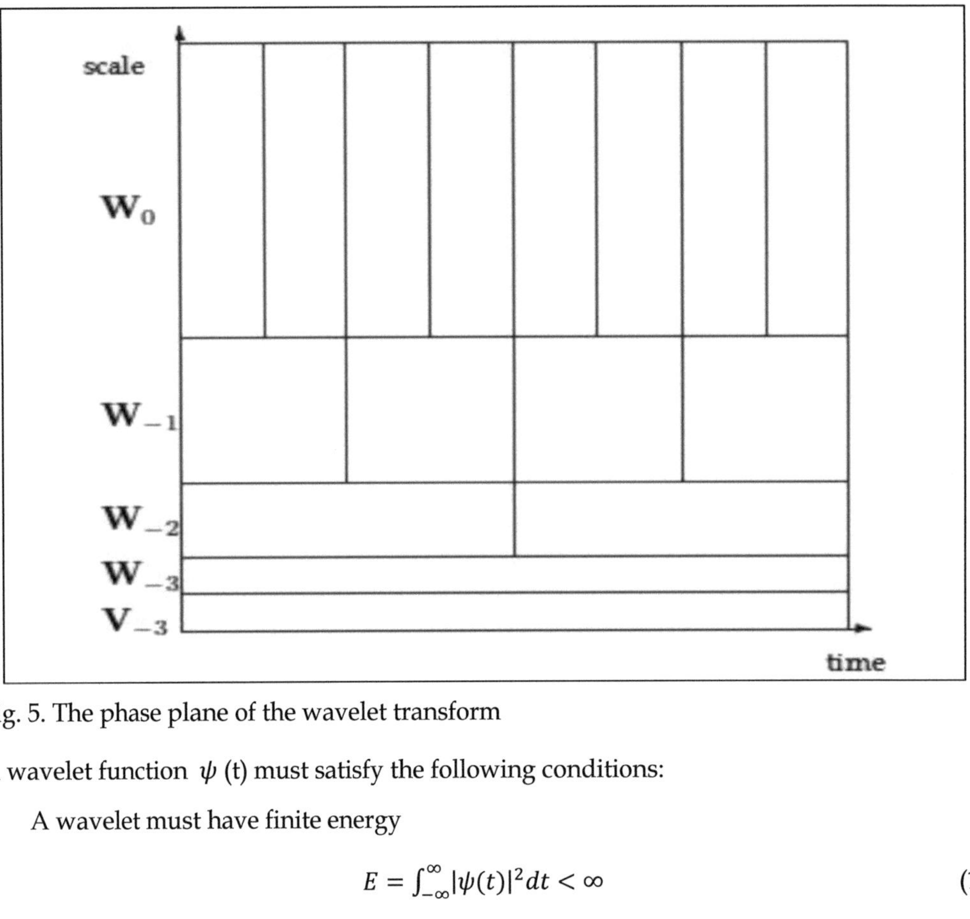

Fig. 5. The phase plane of the wavelet transform

A wavelet function ψ (t) must satisfy the following conditions:

1. A wavelet must have finite energy

$$E = \int_{-\infty}^{\infty} |\psi(t)|^2 dt < \infty \tag{1}$$

where E is the energy of the wavelet function. This means that the energy of the analyzing function is equal to the integrated square magnitude of ψ (t) and it must have a finite value.

If $\hat{\psi}(\omega)$ is the Fourier transform of ψ (t), then the following condition must satisfy the so called the admissibility condition.

$$C_\psi = \int_0^{\infty} \frac{|\hat{\psi}(\omega)|^2}{\omega} d\omega < \infty \tag{2}$$

This condition indicates that the wavelet has no zero frequency components. The mean of wavelet must equal zero. This is known as the admissibility condition.

2. The Fourier transform of C_ψ must both be real for complex wavelets and must vanish for negative frequencies (Daubechies, 1992; Rioul&Vetterli, 1991; Pereyra &Mohlenkampy, 2004).

3.1 Continuous wavelet transform

As a family of functions, wavelets can be reconstructed from translation and dilation of a single wavelet ψ (t). Here, b is the translation parameter and a is the scale parameter. It is called the mother wavelet and is defined as

$$\psi_{a,b} = \frac{1}{\sqrt{|a|}}\psi\left(\frac{t-b}{a}\right), \qquad a, b \in \mathbb{R}, \quad a \neq 0 \tag{3}$$

The integral transformation of $\psi_{a,b}$ is given by (Polikar, 1999)

$$X_{WT}(a,b) = \int_{-\infty}^{\infty} f(t)\, \psi_{a,b}^{*}(t)dt \tag{4}$$

where b is translation parameter, a is dilation parameter and * indicates the complex conjugate which is used in a complex wavelet. This equation $X_{WT}(a,b)$ is called a continuous wavelet transform of f(t). The energy of the signal is normalized by dividing wavelet coefficients with $1/\sqrt{|a|}$ at each scale. This enables the wavelets to have the same energy for each scale. When scale parameter is changed at each scale, the center frequency of wavelet and the window length are also changed. Therefore scale is used instead of frequency for the wavelet analysis. The translation parameter identifies the location of the wavelet function in time. Change in translation parameter shows shifted wavelet over the signal. In time-scale domain, the rows are filled for constant scale and varying translation. Similarly, the columns are filled for constant translation and varying scale. The coefficients $X_{WT}(a,b)$ are called wavelet coefficients and are associated with a scale in frequency domain and a time in time domain.

The inverse continuous wavelet transform can also be defined as

$$f(t) = \frac{1}{C_{\psi}^{2}}\int_{-\infty}^{\infty}\int_{-\infty}^{\infty} X_{WT}(a,b)\frac{1}{a^2}\psi\left(\frac{t-b}{a}\right) dbda \tag{5}$$

Note that the admissibility constant C must adhere to the second wavelet condition.

A wavelet function has a center frequency and it changes inversely to this frequency. Small scale change indicates that high frequencies corresponding to the scale include detailed information of the signal. In contrast, a large scale corresponds to a low frequency and gives coarser information of the signal. In wavelet transform, Heisenberg inequality must be satisfied. Therefore the bandwidth of time and scale $\Delta t \Delta \omega$ is constant and bounded. When the scale is decreased the time resolution Δt will increase. This indicates that the frequency resolution $\Delta \omega$ is proportional to the frequency ω. Consequently, the wavelet transform has a constant relative frequency resolution (Debnath, 2002).

The continuous wavelet transform is a linear transformation like the Fourier transform. It accomplishes the discrete values of scale and translate parameters. The resulting coefficients are called wavelet series. Later, the discretization of coefficients can be done arbitrarily, but reconstruction is required.

3.2 Discrete wavelet transform

There are two ways to introduce the discrete wavelet. One is the discretization of the continuous wavelet transform and the other is through multiresolution analysis.

In many applications, the data is represented by a finite sequence, so it is important to analyze the discrete form of the continuous wavelet transform. From a mathematical view, a continuous notation of two continuous parameters a and b can be converted into the discrete form. Then, two positive constants a_0 and b_0 are defined as (Strang&Nguyen, 1997).

$$\psi_{m,n} = a_0^{-m/2}\psi(a_0^{-m}x - nb_0), \qquad m,n \in \mathbb{Z} \tag{6}$$

It is noted that the discrete wavelet transform can be derived directly from the corresponding continuous version by using $a = a_0^m$ and b= $nb_0a_0^m$. Therefore, the discrete wavelet transform gives a function of a finite set of the wavelet coefficients in the time-scale domain that was indexed m and n.

The aim of the multiresolution analysis is to represent a signal as a limit of consecutive approximations. These correspond to different levels of resolutions. In multiresolution analysis, the orthogonal wavelet bases are constructed using a definite set of rules, where a multiresolution analysis is a sequence of closed space V_j if the following conditions hold.

1. $\{0\} \subset \cdots \subset V_1 \subset V_0 \subset V_{-1} \subset \cdots L^2(\mathbb{R})$
2. $f(t) \in V_j \Leftrightarrow f(2^J t) \in V_{j-1}$
3. $f(t) \in V_0 \Leftrightarrow f(t-k) \in V_0$
4. There exists a scaling function $\phi \in V_0$ such that $\{\phi(t\text{-}k)\}_{k\in Z}$ is an orthonormal basis of V_0.

The function ϕ is called the scaling function. If V_j is a multiresolution in $L^2(\mathbb{R})$ and V_0 is the closed subspace, then ϕ produces the multiresolution analysis. Therefore the scaling function is used to approximate the signal up to a particular level of detail.

A family of scaling function can be constructed via shifts and power of two stretches given by the mother scaling function.

$$\phi_{j,k} = 2^{-j/2}\phi(2^{-j}t - k) \qquad j,k \in \mathbb{Z} \tag{7}$$

As with scaling function, wavelet is defined as

$$\psi_{j,k} = 2^{-j/2}\psi(2^{-j}t - k) \qquad j,k \in \mathbb{Z} \tag{8}$$

In multiresolution analysis, $\phi(t)$ is a lowpass filter and $\psi(t)$ is a highpass filter. $\psi(t)$ provides localization in time and frequency.

The discrete wavelet transform was first given by Mallat. For detailed information, the reader is also referred to Mallat (Mallat, 1989).

3.3 Fast wavelet transform

The fast wavelet transform is a method to compute the discrete wavelet transform just like the fast Fourier transform which computes the discrete Fourier transform.

In the discrete Fourier transform, the transform can be made fast because the transformation is represented as a product of sparse elementary matrices. Hovewer, the transformation matrix is orthogonal and its inverse is equal to its transpose. This matrix is made orthogonal by choosing the unit vectors as basis in time domain and the exponential terms as basis in the frequency domain. If the fast wavelet transform is generated from the discrete wavelet transform, Similar observation holds. The detailed information can be found in Mallat's book (Mallat, 1998).

4. Wavelet packet transform

The wavelet packet transform is based on the traditional discrete wavelet transform in terms of both approach and analysis of detail coefficients. With this method, better resolution can be obtained for both time and frequency depending on the contents of the data. It was first proposed by Coifman, Meyer and Wickerhauser (Coifman et al., 1992).

The wavelet transform is signal-dependent since the decomposition of the signal is performed by taking the best set of functions from the basis. The basis is determined by selecting the second filter bank tree structure, from which conversion coefficients are obtained (Coifman&Wickerhauser, 1990, 1992). Therefore, application of the separation process is simple in terms of ease of calculation.

The wavelet packet analysis for a time series can be summarized as follows (Mallat, 1989).

A space V_j of a multiresolution analysis in $L^2(\mathbb{R})$ is analyzed in a lower resolution space W_{j+1} and a detail space W_{j+1} of is added. Dividing the orthogonal basis $\{\emptyset_j(t\text{-}2^{j_n})\}_{n\epsilon Z}$ to the new orthogonal basis constitutes $\{\emptyset_{j+1}(t\text{-}2^{j+1_n})\}_{n\epsilon Z}$ of V_j and $\{\psi_{j+1}(t\text{-}2^{j+1_n})\}_{n\epsilon Z}$ of W_{j+1}

The decompositions of ϕ_{j+1} and ψ_{j+1} are denoted by a pair of conjugate mirror filters, $h[n]$ and g[n]. The relation between $h[n]$ and $g[n]$ is given as (Herley&Vetterly, 1994)

Any node of the binary tree is labeled by (j, k), where $j\text{-}L \geq 0$, j is the depth of the node on the tree, and k is the number of nodes. A space W_j^k allowing an orthonormal basis $\{\psi_j^k(t - 2^{j_n})\}_{n\epsilon Z}$ is associated to each node (j, k) when going down the tree. At the root, it has $W_L^0 = V_L$ and $\psi_L^0 = \phi_L$. The wavelet packet orthogonal bases at the nodes are defined by

$$\psi_{j+1}^{2k}(t) = \textstyle\sum_{n=-\infty}^{+\infty} h[n]\psi_j^k(t - 2^{j_n}) \tag{9}$$

$$\psi_{j+1}^{2k+1}(t) = \textstyle\sum_{n=-\infty}^{+\infty} g[n]\psi_j^k(t - 2^{j_n}) \tag{10}$$

According to this, the filter functions are derived as

$$h[n] = \langle \psi_{j+1}^{2k+1}(t), \psi_j^k(t - 2^{j_n}) \rangle \tag{11}$$

and

$$g[n] = \langle \psi_{j+1}^{2k+1}(t), \psi_j^k(t - 2^{j_n}) \rangle \tag{12}$$

where $\{\psi_j^k(t\text{-}2^{j_n})\}_{n\epsilon Z}$ is orthonormal.

Because of the filtering operation in the wavelet spaces, the phase space can participate in various ways. Any choice of decompositions gives the wavelet packet decomposition. This procedure is given in Figure 6 and phase plane is shown in Figure 7.

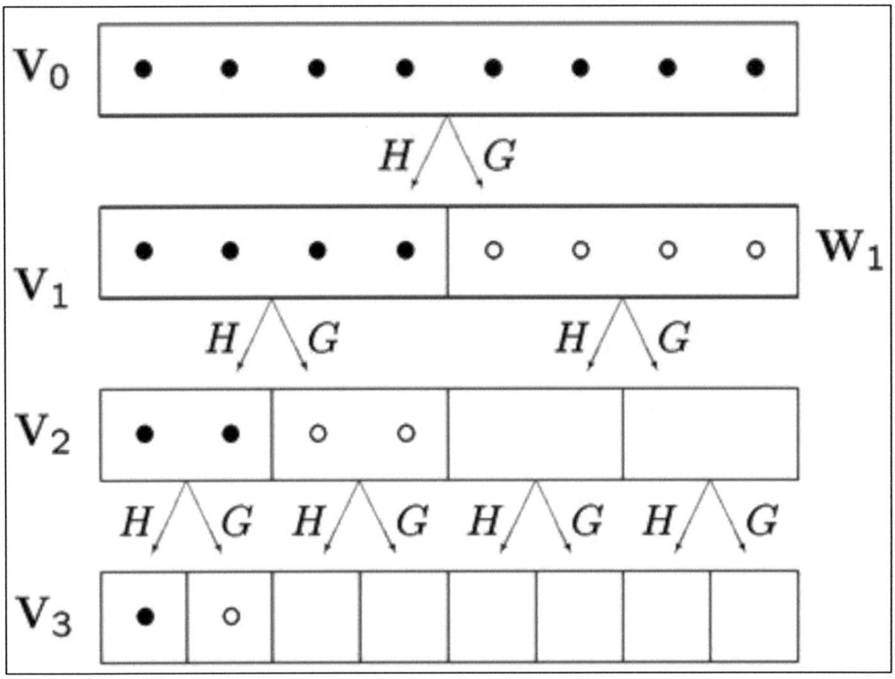

Fig. 6. General structure of the wavelet packet transform

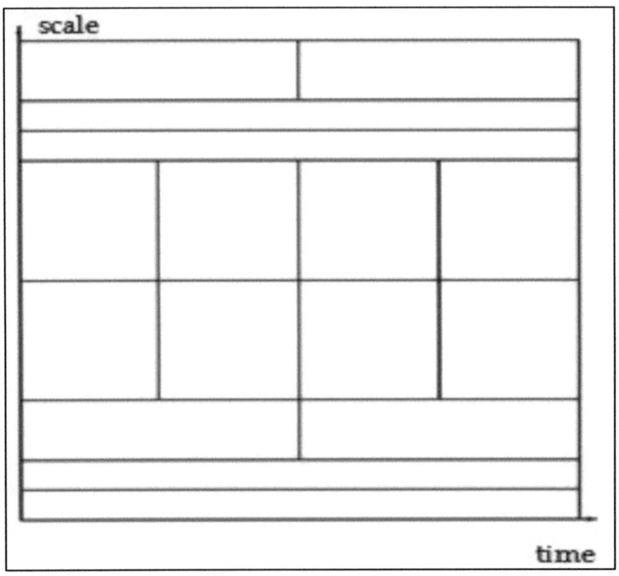

Fig. 7. The phase plane of the wavelet packet transform

From the first rule of the multiresolution analysis, the recursive splitting determines a binary tree of the wavelet packet spaces, which are defined as

$$W_{j+1}^{2k} \oplus W_{j+1}^{2k+1} = W_j^k \tag{13}$$

Consequently, coefficients of decomposition and reconstruction are

$$D_{j+1}^{2k}[t] = d_j^k * \tilde{h}[2t] \tag{14}$$

$$d_{j+1}^{2k+1}[t] = d_j^k * \tilde{g}[2t] \tag{15}$$

$$d_j^k[t] = \tilde{d}_{j+1}^{2k} * h[2t] + \tilde{d}_{j+1}^{2k+1} * g[2t] \tag{16}$$

To sub sampling of the convolution of d_j^k with $\tilde{h}$ and $\tilde{g}$, the coefficients must be obtained. By the iteration of these equations, all the branches of the tree are computed by the wavelet packet coefficients. This is given in Figure 8 and Figure 9.

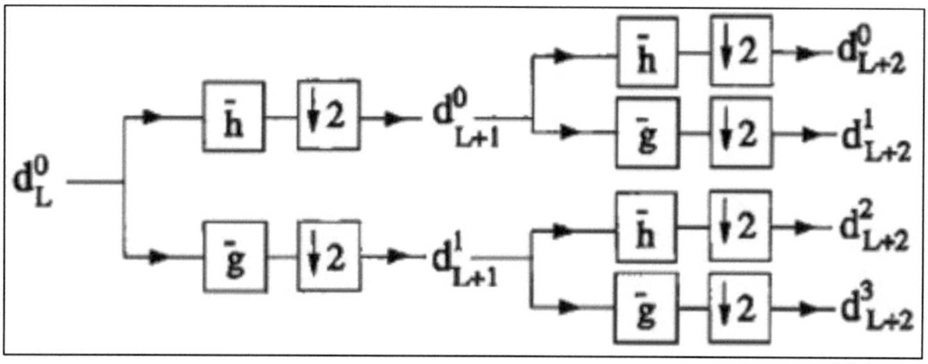

Fig. 8. Two level wavelet packet decomposition with down sampling

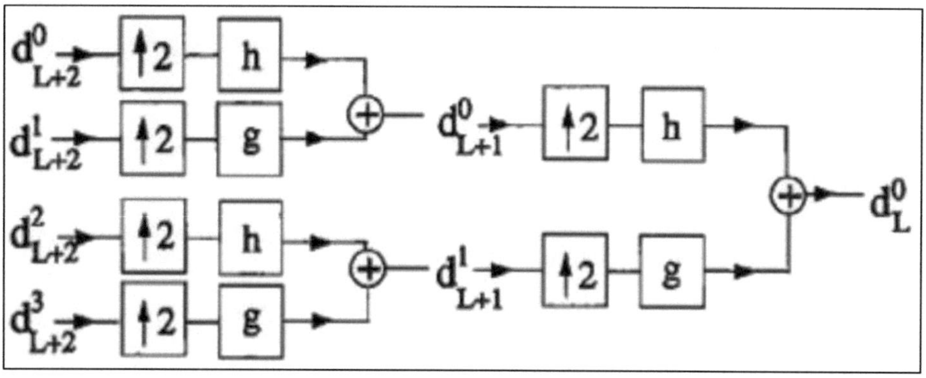

Fig. 9. Two level wavelet packet reconstruction with up sampling

Best tree function is a one- or two-dimensional wavelet packet analysis function that computes the optimal sub tree of an initial tree with respect to an entropy type criterion (Coifman&Wickerhauser, 1992). The resulting tree may be much smaller than the initial one. Following the organization of the wavelet packets library, it is natural to count the decompositions issued from a given orthogonal wavelet. A signal of length N = 2L can be expanded in α different ways, where α is the number of binary sub trees of a complete binary tree of depth L, where $a \geq 2^{N/2}$. This number may be very large, and since explicit enumeration is generally intractable, it is interesting to find an optimal decomposition with respect to a convenient criterion, computable by an efficient algorithm (Donoho, 1995; Guo et al., 2000; Johnstone, 1997).

The difference between the discrete wavelet transform and the wavelet packet transform is in the decomposition of detail space. The wavelet packet transform decomposes not only the approximation space but also the detail space. This means that it can separate frequency band uniformly. Figure 10 and Figure 11 show 2-level analysis and synthesis part of the discrete wavelet transform for comparison.

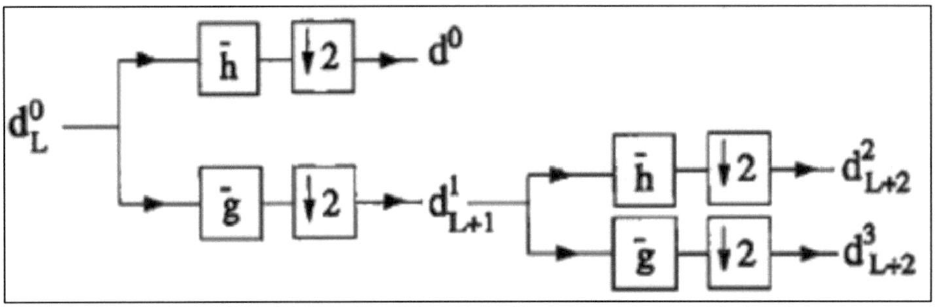

Fig. 10. Two level analysis part of the discrete wavelet transform

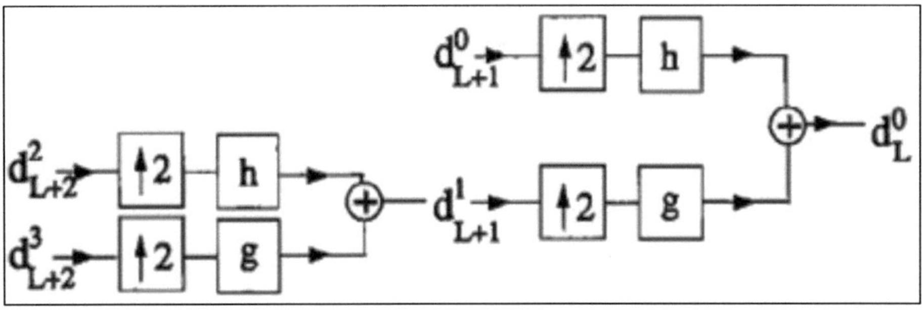

Fig. 11. Two level synthesis part of the discrete wavelet transform

5. Wavelet based speech strategy

The proposed speech processing strategy is based on wavelet packet transform. The strategy consists of five basic parts. Since the basis for the selection of electrode is frequency selection, it is improved by the use of the wavelet packet transform. The main wavelet function is experimentally selected as Daubechies 10. It is analyzed till level 8. Hanning window is used, to prevent short-term changes of the signal in windowing. A block diagram showing the proposed strategy is given in Figure 12. The channel outputs of the matching function is determined by finding the best tree in the matching block. The matching function shows the relationship between electrodes and output nodes of the wavelet packet transform. In this study the number of electrodes used to stimulate the cochlea is 22. The frequency position function is used to calculate channel frequency bands for cochlea. The selection of electrodes is the same as that of N-of-M model. 6 electrodes are selected for 22 channel electrodes. Only these 6 electrodes, with the highest amplitude, are analyzed using the wavelet packet transform.

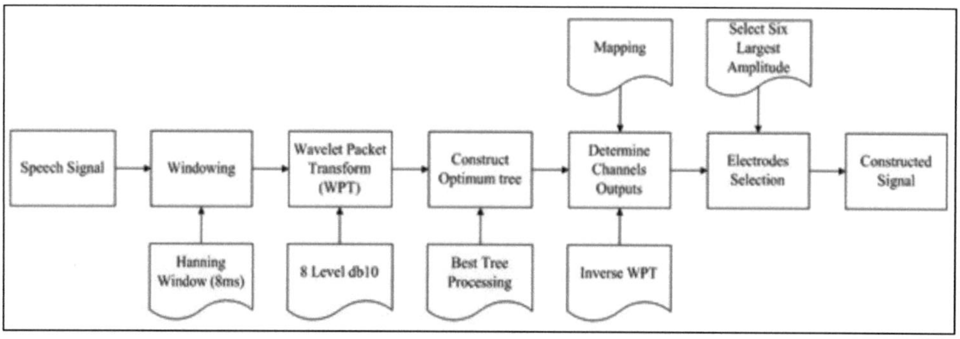

Fig. 12. Block diagram of the new speech processing method

In the new speech processing method, the best tree is determined from a block, which is structured to eliminate noise and unwanted elements of the sound signal. Thus the new output electrodes are determined with less error than those of N-of-M strategy. Moreover better transmittance is obtained by minimizing the interference between neighboring channels.

The channel outputs of the matching function is determined by finding the best tree in the matching block. The used matching function is described as

$$E_k = M \cdot C_{i,j} \tag{17}$$

Here, E_k shows the electrode output, and M shows the matching function. $C_{i,j}$ is the wavelet coefficients. The matching function shows the relationship between electrodes and output nodes of the wavelet packet transform.

In this study, 22 electrodes are used for stimulation and the frequency position function of

$$f = A \cdot 10^{ax} - k \tag{18}$$

is used to calculate channel frequency bands for cochlea (Greenwood, 1990). Here; f shows the frequency in Hz unit, while x describes the length ratio of base from 0 to 1. 'A' and 'a' are constant and their values are 156,4 and 2,1 respectively. The selection of electrodes is the same as that of N-M model. In this study, 6 electrodes are selected from 22 channel electrodes and only these 6 electrodes, which have the highest amplitude, are analyzed using the wavelet packet transform.

The proposed new strategy is essentially based on N-M strategy. The input waveform is given in Figure 13. In addition, the output waveforms for the proposed strategy and the N-M strategy are given in Figure 14 and Figure 15, showing that the input and output waveforms are very similar.

As shown from the graphs, traditional N-M strategy removes some high frequency components that are between 25 ms and 75 ms at wideband spectrogram, high frequency components are very important for intelligibility and consonant recognition such as 's', 'ş', 'f', and such. New method keeps high frequency components using the wavelet packet transform because the wavelet packet transform analyses high frequency components as well as low frequency components. Another effect is mother wavelet selection; and experimentally Daubechies 10 is found to be more effective in high frequency analysis.

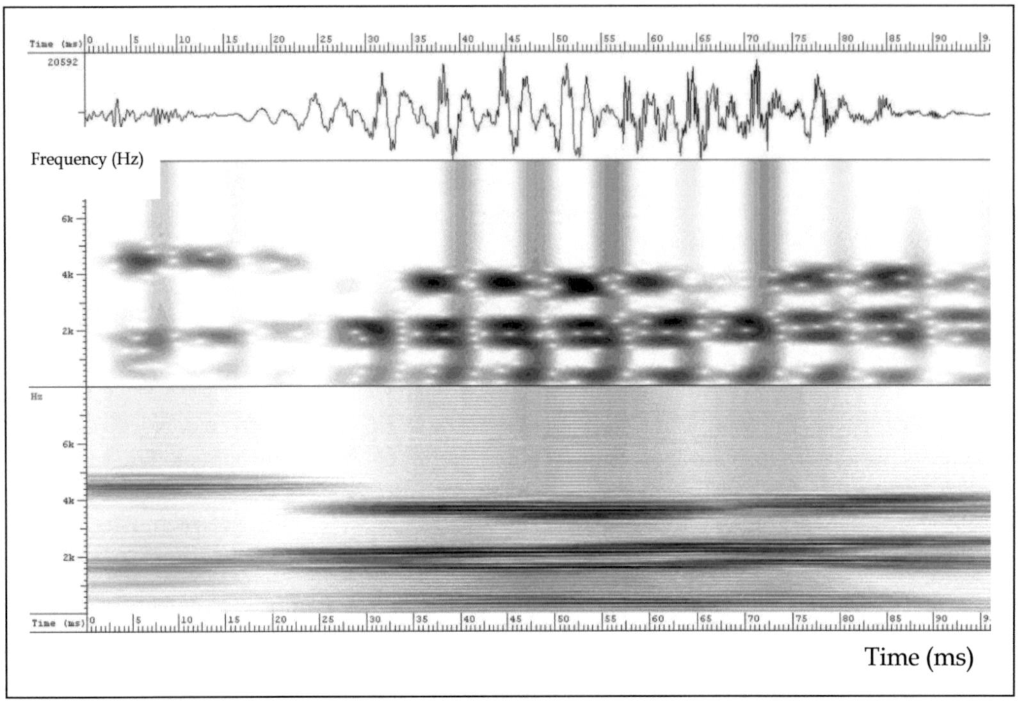

Fig. 13. Wide-band and narrow-band spectrum of the input signal

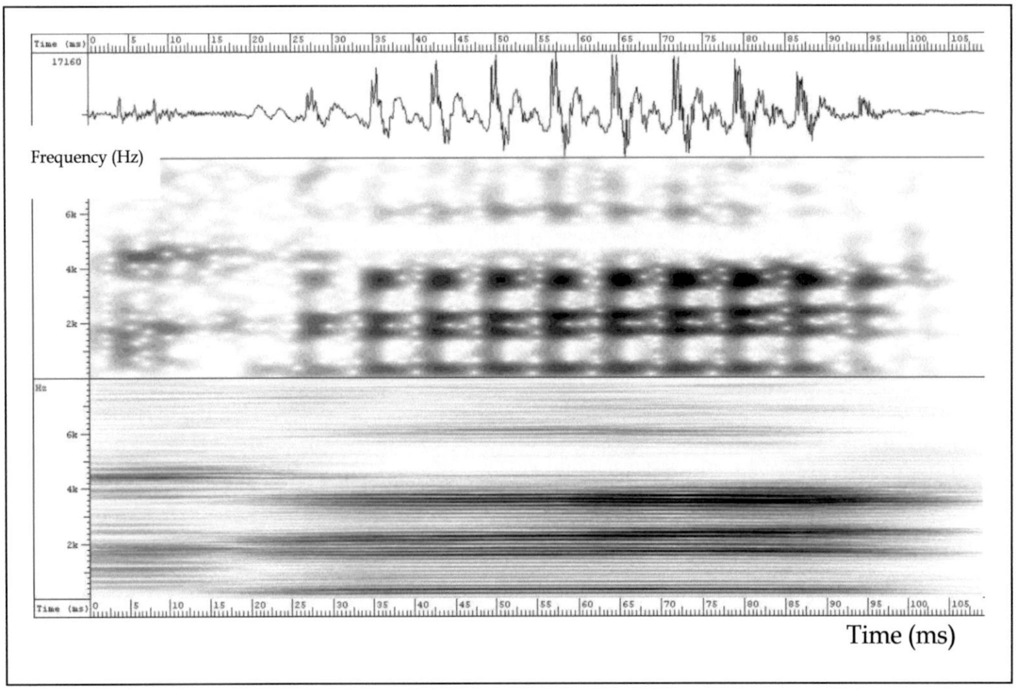

Fig. 14. Wide-band and narrow-band spectrum of the output signal for the proposed speech processing method

'Determine optimum tree' block eliminates noise and unnecessary components in speech signal. Therefore, it obtains better result than N-M strategy for electrode selection. New strategy output channels are more accurate than N-M strategy and conduces to reduce interaction between neighbour channels.

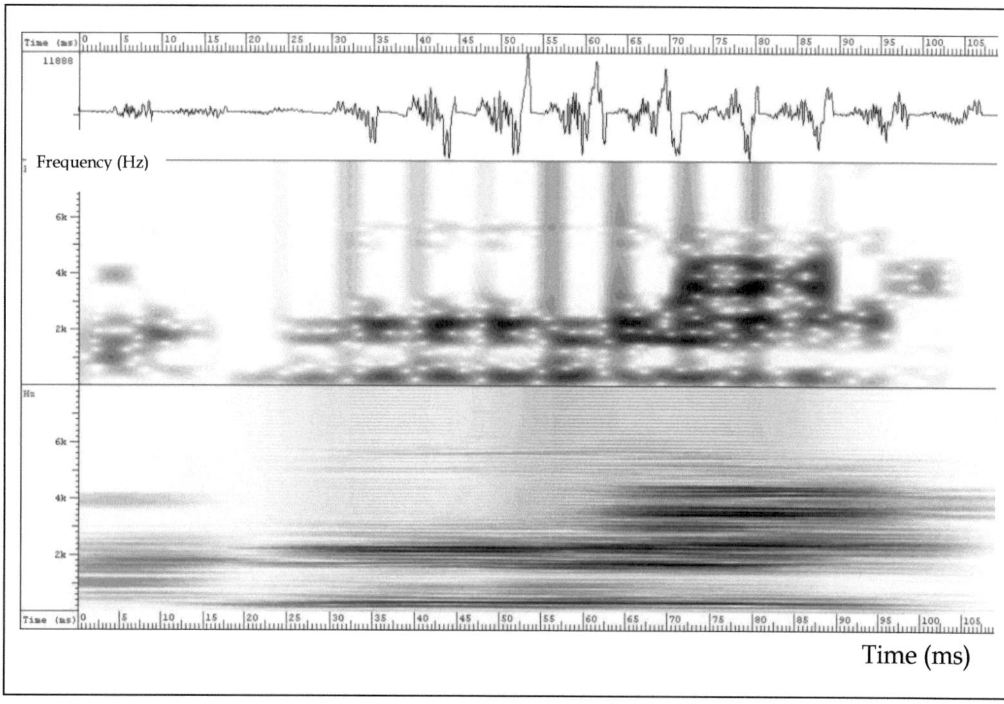

Fig. 15. Wide-band and narrow-band spectrum of the output signal for the N-M strategy

6. Experimental study

The experimental study was carried out on 20 healthy subjects between the ages of 23 and 30. The main language of all the subjects is Turkish and they have obtained air conduction thresholds better than 20 dB at octave frequencies ranging from 250 to 6000 Hz bilaterally. Since the subjects would listen to the words in both algorithms and the possibility exists that the subjects could memorize the given words and their order, separate word lists were arranged for the new strategy, and the N-of-M strategy. The arrangements were attained consultation with a Turkish Language specialist and by referring to The Turkish Language Dictionary by Turkish Language Association. All words were balanced in terms of speech knowledge and degree of difficulty at both of the lists. The usage frequencies of vowels and consonants in the lists were determined according to Turkish grammar. In addition, the lists were recorded in the silent rooms of Ege University, the Department of Otology, and the doctors of the Department approved the reader's sound levels.

The test subjects listened to the lists from a microphone that was directly connected to their heads. While listening, they were asked to write the words they heard and leave a space for the words they could not comprehend within a table format in the listening order. The intelligibility percentage is calculated as follows.

$$\text{Intelligibility} = \frac{\text{Number of correct words}}{\text{Number of all the words on the list}} \times 100 \quad (19)$$

The results of intelligibility test are given in Table 1 for both the N-of-M Strategy and the Proposed Speech Processing Strategy. The intelligibility percent of the proposed wavelet packet transform based strategy is higher than that of N-of-M strategy. The average percentages of intelligibility according to gender are also given in Figure 16.

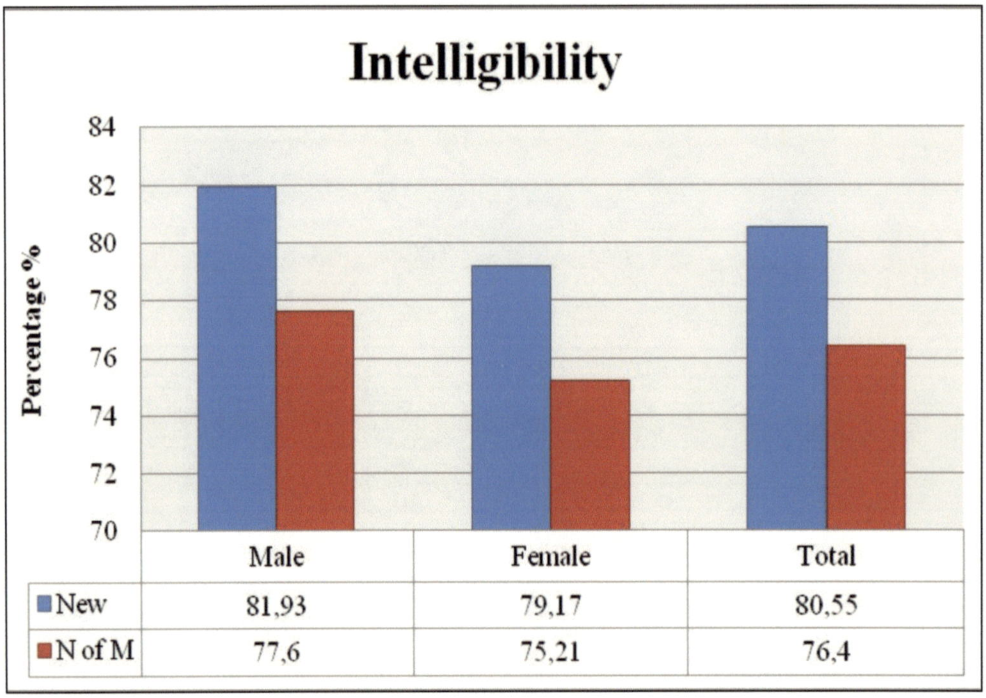

Fig. 16. Graphical representation of the intelligibility test results

	Gender	Age interval	**Number of test subjects**	Intelligibility (%)
New/Proposed	Male	23-29	8	81,93
	Female	23-33	12	79,17
	Total	23-33	20	80,55
N-M	Male	23-29	8	77,60
	Female	23-33	12	75,21
	Total	23-33	20	76,40

Table 1. Intelligibility test results for both the N-M strategy and the proposed strategy

To test the noise resistance of the proposed strategy, SNR improvement test was applied to the system. This test was performed by adding 5 dB of pink noise, F-16 noise, Volvo noise and factory noise respectively to the recorded data. All the added noise is real noise recorded as indicated by their names. Later, both the proposed method and the N-of-M method were separately applied to this data. The results were evaluated by looking at the SNR given in Figure 17. Consequently, the proposed method gives better results for each type of added noise.

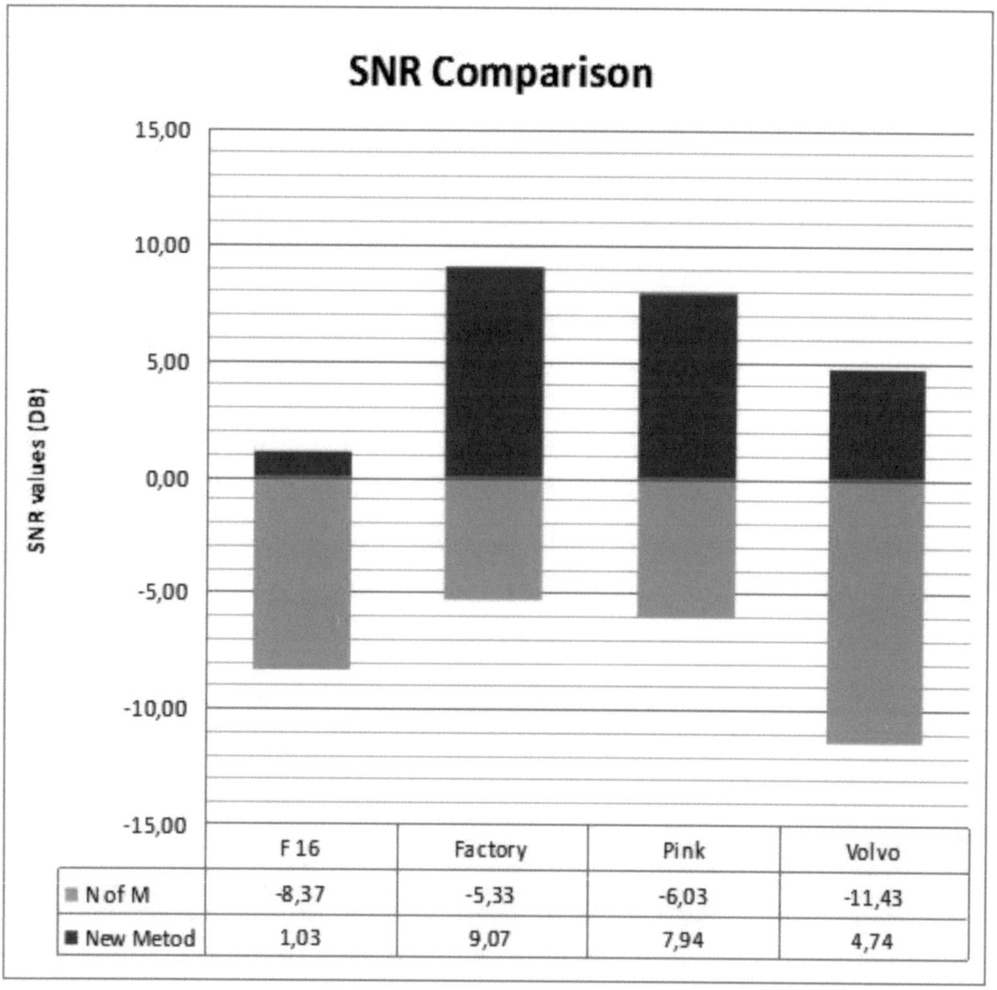

Fig. 17. SNR for different types of noise

7. Conclusion

In this study, a new speech processing strategy, based on the wavelet packet transform, is proposed for Cochlear implant applications. The foundation of the system lies in, first, obtaining the highest-energy coefficients, and then stimulating the linked electrodes and therefore improving the deaf patient's hearing ability.

The core of the system is based on the wavelet packet transform and it also uses the energy of the wavelet coefficients. By the application of various tests, the effect of intelligibility and noise resistance for the suggested speech processing method was investigated. Then, a new electrode selection algorithm, which depends on wavelet entropy distribution, was presented. The proposed electrode selection increases the noise performance and intelligibility. Additionally, the performance of the proposed method is better than the traditional and recently published methods.

In this study, the system was tested in terms of intelligibility; besides, SNR results were compared with those of the N-of-M Strategy. As a result, the proposed method was observed to increase performance in terms of intelligibility.

In the part of the wavelet packet transform, the determination of the optimum tree using the best tree functions is a significant part of this study because this part eliminates noise and unnecessary components from the speech signal. It also helps to improve intelligibility of speech in noisy environments.

During the live experiments session, people with normal hearing are used and also all results are based on only normal-hearing people. A further study on patients who use cochlear implant would give more accurate results for intelligibility.

For future works, hybrid mother wavelet in wavelet decomposition process is recommended. In this hybrid model, Daubechies family can be used for low-pass filter decomposition and Symlet family for high-pass filter decomposition. Moreover, the mother wavelet for deciding the choice of wavelet family can be selected according to speech signal characteristics in real time. This might give better results for speech intelligibility. Additionally, the bionic wavelet instead of the wavelet packet transform can be suggested in entire speech processing (Yuan, 2003).

8. Acknowledgment

We would like to specially thank the Department of Otology in Ege University and Yahya Ozturk for their assistance in this work.

9. References

Cheikhrouhou I., Atitallah R. B., Ouni K., Hamida A. B., Mamoudi N., Ellouze N. (2004). Speech analysis using wavelet transforms dedicated to cochlear prosthesis stimulation strategy, *Int. Sym. On Control, Communication and Signal Processing*, pp. 639-642

Christiansen J. B., Leigh I. W. (2002). *Cochlear implants in children: Ethics and choices*, Washington, Gallaudet University Press

Coifman R. R., Meyer Y., Wickerhauser M. V. (1992). Wavelet Analysis and Signal Processing

Coifman R. R., Wickerhauser M. V. (1990). *Best adapted wave packet bases, Numerical Algorithm*, Research Group, Dept. of Mathematics, Yale University, NewHaven, Connecticut

Coifman R. R., Wickerhauser M. V. (1992). Entropy based algorithms for best basis selection, *IEEE Trans. on Information Theory*, vol. 38, part 2

Daubechies I. (1992). *Ten Lectures on Wavelets*, Society for Industrial and Applied Mathematics, ISBN 0-89871-274-2

Debnath L. (2002). Wavelet Transforms and Their Applications, Birhauser

Deller J. R., Proakis J. G., Hansen J. H. L. (1994). *Discrete-time processing of speech signals*, New York, Macmillan Publishing Company

Derbel A., Ghorbel M., Samet M., Ben Hamida A. (2009). Implementation of strategy based on auditory model based wavelet transform speech processing on DSP dedicated to cochlear prosthesis, *Int. Sym. On Comp. Intelligence and Intelligent Informatics*, pp. 143-148

Dorman M., Hannley M., Dankowski K., Smith L., McCandless G. (1989). Word recognation by 50 patients fitted the Symbion multichannel cochlear implant, *Ear and Hearing*, vol. 10, no. 1

Dorman M., Loizou P., Rainey D. (1997). Speech intelligibility as a function of the number of channels of stimulation for signal processors using sine-wave and noise-band outputs, *Journal of the Acoustical Society of America*, vol. 102, pp. 2403-2411

Donoho L. (1995). Denosing by soft thresholding, *IEEE Trans. on Information Theory*, vol. 41, no. 3, pp. 613-627

Eddington D. (1980). Speech discrimination in deaf subjects with cochlear implants, *J. Acoust. Soc. Am.*, vol. 68, no. 3, pp. 885-891, 1980

Greenwood D. D. (1990). A cochlear frequency-position function for several species-29 years later, *J. Acoust. Soc. Am.*, vol. 87, no. 6, pp. 2593-2605

Gopalakrishna V., Kehtarnavaz N., Loizou P. C. (2010). A recursive wavelet-based strategy for real time cochlear implant speech processing on PDA platforms, *IEEE Trans. On Biomedical Eng.*, vol. 57, no. 8, pp. 2053-2063

Guo D., Zhu W. H., Gao Z. M., Zhang J. Q. (2000). A study of wavelet thresholding denoising, *IEEE International conference on signal processing*, vol.1, pp. 329-332

Herley C., Vetterly M. (1994). Orthonormal time varying filterbanks and wavelet packets, *IEEE Trans. on Signal Processing*, vol. 41, no. 10

Holschneider M. (1989). Wavelet, time frequency methods and phase space, *First International conference on wavelet*, Springer-Verlag

House W., Urban J. (1973). Long term results of electrode implantation and electronic stimulation of the cochlea in man, *Annals of Otology, Rhinology and Laryngology*, vol. 82, pp. 504-517

House W., Berliner K. (1982). Cochlear implants: Progress and perspectives, *Annals of Otology, Rhinology and Laryngology*, pp. 1-124

Johnstone I. M. (1997). Wavelet threshold estimators for data with correlated noise, *J. Royal Statistical Society*, vol. 59, no. 2, pp. 319-351

Loeb G. (1990). Cochlear prosthetics, *Annual Review in Neuroscience*, vol. 13, pp. 357-371

Loizou P. (1998) Mimicking the human ear, *IEEE Signal Processing Magazine*, vol. 15, no. 5, pp. 101-130, 1998

Mallat S. (1998). *A wavelet tour of signal processing*, New York, Academic Press

Mallat S. (1989). A theory for multiresolution signal decomposition, *IEEE Trans. on Pattern Anal. Machine Intell.*, vol. 11, pp. 674-693

Merry R. J. E.(2005) Wavelet Theory and Applications A literature study, Eindhoven Un. of Tech., Dept. of Mechanical Engineering, Control Systems Technology Group, Eindhoven, June 7, 02.05.2008 Available from http://www.narcis.nl/publication/RecordID/oai:library.tue.nl:612762

Meyer Y. (1992). *Wavelets and Operators*, Cambridge University

Millar J., Tong Y., Clark G. (1984). Speech processing for cochlear implant prostheses, *Journal of Speech and Hearing Research*, vol. 27, pp. 280-296

Misiti M., Misiti Y., Oppenheim G., Poggi J. M. (2000) *Wavelets Toolbox Users Guide*, The MathWorks, Wavelet Toolbox

Moore J. A., Teagle H. F. B. (2002). An introduction to cochlear implant technology, activation, and programming Language, Speech, and Hearing Services in Schools, pp.153-161

Nogueira W., Giese A., Edler B., Buchner A. (2006). Wavelet Packet Filterbank for Speech Processing Strategies in Cochlear Implants, *ICASSP*

Parkins C., Anderson S. (Eds.) (1983). Cochlear prostheses, *An international symposium New York*, New York Academy of Sciences

Pereyra M. C., Mohlenkampy M. J. (2004). Wavelets, their friends, and what they can do for you, June 20, Department of Mathematics and Statistics, MSC03 2150, Un. of New Mexico, Albuquerque NM 87131-0001 USA, 23.08.2005, Available from http://www.math.unm.edu/crisp

Polikar R. (1999). The wavelet tutorial, 06.06.2000, Available from http://users.rowan.edu/ polikar/WAVELETS/WTtutorial.html

Quatieri (2001). *Discrete-Time Speech Signal Processing*, Principles and Practice. PrenticeHall

Saeed V. V. (2000). *Advanced Signal Processing and Noise Reduction*, 2nd Edition, John Wiley and Sons

Rioul O., Vetterli M. (1991). Wavelets and signal processing, *IEEE SP Magazine*, pages 14–38, October 1991

Sheikhzadeh H., Abutalebi H. R. (2001). An improved wavelet-based speech enhancement system, *Eurospeech*, pp. 1855-1858

Strang G., Nguyen T. (1997). *Wavelets and Filter Banks*, Wellesley-Cambridge Press, second edition, ISBN 0-9614088-7-1

Wilson B. S., Finley C. C., Lawson D. T., Wolford R. D., Eddington D. K., Rabinowitz W. M. (1991). Better speech recognition with cochlear implants, *Nature*, 352, pp. 236-238

Wilson B., (R. Tyler, ed.) (1993). *Signal processing in Cochlear Implants: Audiological Foundations*, pp. 35-86, Singular Publishing Group, Inc.

Yuan X. (2003). *Auditory Model-based Bionic Wavelet Transform*, Speech and Signal Processing Lab., Milwaukee, Wisconsin

4

Strategies to Improve Music Perception in Cochlear Implantees

Joshua Kuang-Chao Chen[1,2], Catherine McMahon[3] and Lieber Po-Hung Li[1,2,4,*]

[1]*Department of Otolaryngology, Cheng Hsin General Hospital*
[2]*Faculty of Medicine, School of Medicine, National Yang-Ming University*
[3]*Center for Language Sciences, Macquarie University*
[4]*Integrated Brain Research Laboratory, Taipei Veterans General Hospital*
[1,2,4]*Taiwan*
[3]*Australia*

1. Introduction

Cochlear implants have been an effective device for the management of patients with total or profound hearing loss over the past few decades. Significant improvements in speech and language can be observed in implantees following rehabilitation. In spite of remarkable linguistic perception, however, it is difficult for these patients to enjoy music although we did see some "superstars" for music performance in our patients. This article aimed to clarify current opinions on the strategies to improve music perception ability in this population of subjects. In part I, we included one of our previous work (Chen et al., 2010) talking about the effect of music training on pitch perception in prelingually deafened children with a cochlear implant. In part II, other factors related to the improvement of music perception in cochlear implantees were discussed, including residual hearing, bimodal hearing, and coding strategies. Evidences from results of our researches and from literature review will both be presented.

2. Part I: Music training improves pitch perception in prelingually deafened children with cochlear implants

2.1 Introduction

Cochlear implants have been an effective device for the management of deaf children over the past few decades. Significant improvements in speech and language can be observed in implanted children following rehabilitation. In spite of remarkable linguistic perception, however, it is difficult for these children to enjoy music (Galvin et al., 2007; McDermott, 2004). Essential attributes of music include rhythm, timbre, and pitch. Previous studies have shown that perception of rhythm is easier than timbre and pitch for cochlear implant users (Gfeller & Lansing, 1991). Recognition of timbre depends, at least partly, on the

---

* Corresponding Author

discrimination of pitch in terms of fundamental frequency (Gfeller et al., 2002). The ability to differentiate pitch thus plays an important role in perception of music for implanted children. Fundamental traits of pitch acoustically transmitted to the auditory pathway of cochlear implantees via the apparatus are much less precise than those of normal-hearing subjects (Sucher & McDermott, 2007). Built-in restrictions for pitch perception in contemporary systems of cochlear implants arise from the electrical model of temporospatial stimulation, which in turn leads to a finite spectral resolution (McDermott, 2004). Efforts have been made to improve pitch resolution of cochlear implants for tonal languages and music perception (Busby & Plant, 2005; Firszt et al., 2007; Hamzavi & Arnoldner, 2006). However, the conclusions have been indecisive.

Neural correlates crucial for music processing have been demonstrated in cochlear implantees in an electroencephalographic study (Koelsch et al., 2004). Furthermore, magnetoencephalographic evidence of auditory plasticity has been noted in sudden deafness (Li, 2003, 2006). This plasticity facilitates tone perception in cochlear implantees, which can be mirrored by the progressive optimization of neuromagnetic responses evoked by auditory stimuli after implantation (Pantev et al., 2006). Considering limitations of cochlear implant processing strategies for pitch differentiation, education might have a major effect on improvement of music processing by inducing plastic changes in the central auditory pathway of cochlear implantees (Pantev et al., 1998). In fact, musical training has been found to be associated with improved pitch appraisal abilities in normal-hearing subjects, and comparatively poor music performance in cochlear implantees might be ascribed in part to an inadequate exposure to music (Sucher & McDermott, 2007). However, few studies exist on music performance in implanted children, and the effect of training on music perception in prelingually deafened children with cochlear implants has not been addressed. In the present study, twenty-seven prelingually deafened children with monaural cochlear implant were recruited to investigate whether or not musical education improved pitch perception. Thirteen subjects received structured training on music before and/or after implantation. Music perception was evaluated by using a test-set of pitch differentiation. To mirror real-world auditory environments, pure tones were presented using a tuned piano. Effect of age, gender, pitch-interval size, age of implantation, and type of cochlear implant were also addressed.

2.2 Patients and methods

2.2.1 Subjects

Twenty-seven subjects with congenital/prelingual deafness of profound degree (eighteen males and nine females; 5~14y/o, mean=6.7) were studied (Table 1). No other neurological deficits were identified. Thirteen subjects used Nucleus24 (Cochlear™, Australia)(left=6, right=7), thirteen subjects used Clarion (Advanced Bionics™, USA)(left=7, right=6), and one subject used Med-El (MED-EL™, Austria) cochlear implant system (right). Elapsed time for the evaluation of pitch perception after cochlear implantation ranged from 10 to 69 months (mean=29). Thirteen subjects attended the same style of structured music classes at YAMAHA Music School (2~36 months, mean=13.2). The programs included training of listening, singing, score-reading, and instruments-playing. They attended classes with normal-hearing children. Subject 4 and 5 have had musical education before the implantation. The study conformed to the Declaration of Helsinki. Written informed consent was obtained from parents with a protocol approved by Institutional Ethics Committee of Cheng-Hsin General Hospital.

		Age	Age*		DuM	DuC		Correct rate (%)					
No	Gender	(yr)	(mo)	Device	(mo)	(mo)	HA	O	P	A	A>5	D	D>5
1	F	6	20	Clarion	0	48	y	45.3	37.1	45.7	40.0	48.6	46.7
2	M	5	42	Clarion	3	17	y	56.1	60.0	41.9	46.7	64.8	80.0
3	M	6	36	Nucleus	12	33	y	44.6	42.9	55.2	76.7	26.7	40.0
4	M	10	78	Nucleus	36	11	y	60.7	48.6	52.4	53.3	70.5	76.7
5	F	10	64	Nucleus	30	22	y	88.2	94.3	91.4	93.3	80.0	93.3
6	F	6	53	Nucleus	0	10	y	36.4	40.0	31.4	30.0	41.9	36.7
7	M	8	57	Clarion	0	34	y	50.5	65.7	55.2	53.3	41.0	46.7
8	M	6	36	Nucleus	0	33	n	48.2	5.7	52.4	66.7	52.4	50.0
9	M	6	54	Clarion	24	26	y	55.7	57.1	71.4	73.3	41.0	33.3
10	M	5	17	Nucleus	0	46	y	46.9	40.0	43.8	53.3	51.4	43.3
11	F	6	58	Nucleus	3	13	y	46.2	42.9	41.9	46.7	55.2	33.3
12	F	7	29	Nucleus	6	55	y	52.1	94.3	28.6	73.3	67.6	10.0
13	M	8	22	Nucleus	0	69	y	52.5	45.7	43.8	50.0	61.0	63.3
14	F	5	37	Nucleus	0	19	n	17.4	25.7	20.0	26.7	8.6	20.0
15	F	6	48	Nucleus	0	23	y	69.2	68.6	67.6	83.3	67.6	66.7
16	F	5	32	Nucleus	0	24	y	38.7	97.1	27.6	33.3	34.3	30.0
17	M	8	65	Clarion	0	25	y	56.1	94.3	68.6	76.7	33.3	26.7
18	M	5	30	Med El	0	31	y	55.4	62.9	55.2	70.0	50.5	50.0
19	M	6	37	Nucleus	2	31	y	56.1	88.6	61.0	63.3	44.8	33.3
20	M	8	68	Clarion	14	36	n	37.4	42.9	37.1	36.7	38.1	30.0
21	M	6	45	Clarion	0	33	y	46.2	20.0	41.9	36.7	56.2	66.7
22	M	6	36	Clarion	14	16	y	68.2	82.9	72.4	80.0	54.3	73.3
23	M	14	163	Clarion	0	17	y	89.2	97.1	95.2	93.3	79.0	90.0
24	F	5	53	Clarion	6	15	n	9.5	17.1	9.5	23.3	5.7	0.0
25	M	5	34	Clarion	0	30	n	50.2	5.7	30.5	30.0	81.0	83.3
26	M	5	32	Clarion	20	35	y	92.5	100.0	91.4	93.3	90.5	93.3
27	M	8	86	Clarion	2	22	y	36.4	0.0	41.0	40.0	41.9	40.0

No, participant number; Age, y/o; Age*, age at implantation; Device, type of cochlear implant; DuM, duration of musical training (months); DuC, duration of cochlear implant use (months); HA, use of hearing aid in the other ear; Correct rate, percentage of correct response for pitch-interval differentiation; O, overall correct rate; P, correct rate for prime pitch interval; A, correct rate for ascending interval; A>5, correct rate for ascending interval over 5 semitones; D, correct rate for descending interval; D>5, correct rate for descending interval over 5 semitones.

Table 1. General data for all participants.

2.2.2 Experiment paradigm

Experiments were conducted in an acoustically-shielded room using a tuned piano (YAMAHA™, Japan). Subjects sat upright with eyes open, facing away from the piano at a distance of about 1 meter, and were instructed to attend to the auditory stimuli during experiments. A modification of a two-alternative forced choice task was used. Each test-stimulus consisted of two sequential piano tones, ranging from C (256 Hz) to B (495 Hz). To avoid the possible effect of intensity variation on the test, the loudness was monitored on site by a sound-pressure meter and was maintained within 70±6 dB SPL for loudness matching of different pitch tones. The first note was any of the following: C, D (294 Hz), E (330 Hz), F (349 Hz), G (392 Hz), A (440 Hz) or B. Once the first note was determined, the second note was presented randomly from C to B. The interval of two notes was thus between prime degree (two same notes, e.g."C-C") and major-seventh degree (eleven semitones, e.g."C-B"), either ascending or descending in direction. A total of 49 (7x7) tone-pairs were delivered to a subject in one experiment. The task was divided into two stages depending on the response. Each time after presentation of the stimuli, the subject would be asked whether the two notes were the same (i.e.,prime degree) or not. When the two notes were the same, the answer was recorded as correct or incorrect. When the two notes were different and the answer was incorrect, the answer was recorded as incorrect. When the two notes were different and the answer was correct, the subject would then be asked if the second tone was higher or lower than the first tone, and this subsequent answer was recorded as correct or incorrect. There was no feedback to subjects on their answers. Each tone-pair was presented five times. To avoid the effect of random guessing of the results, the answer needed to be correctly answered at least three times (≥60% correct) for a single tone-pair recognition response to be recorded as correct. The correct rate for each subject was obtained by averaging the number of correct responses across the number of total tone pairs (49). The programming of speech processors for each subject varied, based on the speech intelligibility programs optimal for respective users.

2.2.3 Data analysis

Statistical analysis was performed using the software of SAS8.1 (SAS Institute Inc., USA). Performance of pitch perception in terms of correct rate was grouped into six sets for statistical analysis: overall, prime degree, ascending interval, ascending interval larger than perfect-fourth degree (five semitones, e.g."C-F"), descending interval, and descending interval larger than perfect-fourth degree. Differences in the performance of pitch perception by pitch-interval size were analyzed using analysis of variance. Differences of correct rate for pitch perception (cutoff value=50%) in terms of age were evaluated by dividing subjects into two groups: subjects >6 and subjects ≤6 y/o. Gender and age differences in overall task performance of pitch perception were evaluated using t-test. Correlations between pitch perception and period of musical training, age of implantation, or type of cochlear implant were evaluated using simple correlation analysis for three conditions respectively: all subjects, subjects divided into two groups by age (>6 and ≤6 y/o), and subjects divided into two groups by duration of cochlear implant use (>18 and ≤18 months). Threshold for statistical significance was set at $P < 0.05$.

2.3 Results

2.3.1 Differences of correct rate for pitch perception by pitch-interval size, gender, and age

Overall, the correct rate for pitch perception varied between 9.5% and 92.5% (Table 1). Fifteen subjects (13 male and 2 female, mean age=7.3 y/o) accomplished the test with a correct rate ≥50% (i.e., chance level). When subjects were divided by gender/age, boys/subjects >6 y/o tended to accomplish the test with a correct rate ≥50% than girls/subjects ≤6 y/o, respectively. The mean correct rate of overall task performance was better for boys (56%)/subjects >6 y/o (58%) than for girls (45%)/subjects ≤6 y/o (49%), respectively, although the difference was insignificant (p=0.237 for gender, p=0.243 for age; Table 2). There were no differences in the performance of pitch perception between various conditions of pitch-interval size (F(5,156)=0.342, p=0.887; Figure 1).

	Total		Gender				Age			
Pitch Interval			Boy		Girl		> 6 yrs		≦ 6 yrs	
	≧50%	<50%	≧50%	<50%	≧50%	<50%	≧50%	<50%	≧50%	<50%
O	15	12	13	5	3	6	7	2	8	10
P	13	14	9	9	4	5	5	4	8	10
A	13	14	11	7	2	7	5	4	8	10
A>5	16	11	13	5	3	6	7	2	9	9
D	15	12	11	7	4	5	5	4	10	8
D>5	12	15	10	8	2	7	4	5	8	10

Age, y/o; Correct rate at cutoff value of 50% for pitch perception; O, overall correct rate; P, correct rate for prime pitch interval; A, correct rate for ascending interval; A>5, correct rate for ascending interval over 5 semitones; D, correct rate for descending interval; D>5, correct rate for descending interval over 5 semitones.

Table 2. Differences in correct rate for pitch perception (cutoff value=50%) by gender and age.

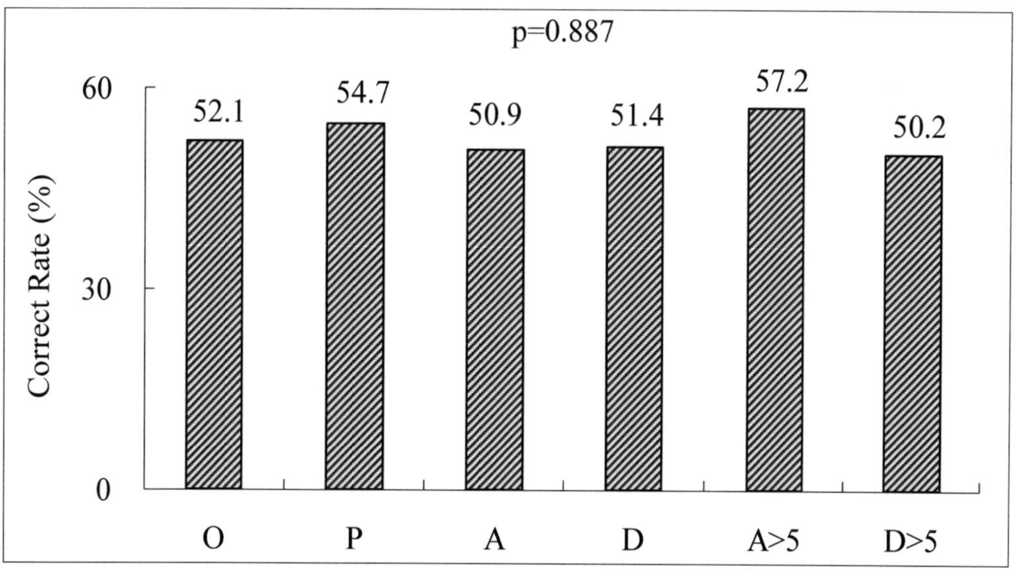

Fig. 1. Differences of correct rate for pitch perception by pitch-interval size. There were no differences in the performance of pitch perception between various conditions of pitch-interval size (F(5,156) = 0.342, p=0.887). O, overall correct rate; P, correct rate for prime pitch interval; A, correct rate for ascending interval; A>5, correct rate for ascending interval over 5 semitones; D, correct rate for descending interval; D>5, correct rate for descending interval over 5 semitones.

2.3.2 Correlation between pitch perception and period of musical training, age of implantation, or type of cochlear implant (Table 3, 4a~d)

For all subjects combined, the duration of musical training positively correlated with the correct rate of overall (r^2=0.389, p=0.045) and ascending pitch-interval (r^2=0.402, p=0.038) perception. There is no correlation between pitch perception and the age of implantation or type of cochlear implant.

To assess the effect of age on the significance of correlation, additional analysis was conducted with children separated by age >6 and ≤6 y/o (i.e., preschool). For children >6 y/o, there is no correlation between pitch perception and duration of musical training, age of implantation, or type of cochlear implant. For children ≤6 y/o, the duration of musical training strongly correlated with correct rate of ascending pitch-interval (r^2=0.618, p=0.006) and ascending pitch-interval over 5 semitones (r^2=0.584, p=0.011) perception; there is no correlation between pitch perception and age of implantation or type of cochlear implant.

	O		P		A		A>5		D		D>5	
Variable	r^2	*p*	r^2	*p*	r^2	*p*	r^2	*p*	r^2	*p*	r^2	*p*
DuM(mo)	0.389	0.045†	0.238	0.232	0.402	0.038†	0.366	0.061	0.271	0.172	0.303	0.124
Device	0.046	0.818	-0.085	0.675	0.111	0.581	-0.099	0.624	0.026	0.897	0.149	0.459
Age*	0.293	0.138	0.146	0.466	0.381	0.050	0.229	0.251	0.154	0.445	0.226	0.257

Threshold for statistical significance using simple correlation analysis was set at P < 0.05 (denoted as †). r^2, correlation coefficient; DuM, duration of musical training (months); Device, type of cochlear implant; Age*, age at implantation; O, overall correct rate; P, correct rate for prime pitch interval; A, correct rate for ascending interval; A>5, correct rate for ascending interval over 5 semitones; D, correct rate for descending interval; D>5, correct rate for descending interval over 5 semitones.

Table 3. Correlation between variables and correct rate of pitch perception.

Since some patients >6 y/o have had a longer period of music training, additional analysis was conducted with children separated by duration of cochlear implant use >18 and ≤18

	O		P		A		A>5		D		D>5	
Variable	r^2	*p*	r^2	*p*	r^2	*p*	r^2	*p*	r^2	*p*	r^2	*p*
DuM(mo)	0.293	0.445	0.012	0.975	0.145	0.710	0.074	0.850	0.459	0.214	0.442	0.234
Device	-0.261	0.497	-0.169	0.664	0.120	0.758	-0.183	0.637	-0.660	0.053	-0.253	0.511
Age*	0.493	0.178	0.115	0.768	0.635	0.066	0.358	0.344	0.252	0.513	0.492	0.178

Correlation between variables and correct rate of pitch perception (> 6 years old, n=9).

	O		P		A		A>5		D		D>5	
Variable	r^2	*p*	r^2	*p*	r^2	*p*	r^2	*p*	r^2	*p*	r^2	*p*
DuM(mo)	0.435	0.071	0.382	0.118	0.618	0.006†	0.584	0.011†	0.098	0.698	0.151	0.550
Device	0.132	0.602	-0.101	0.691	0.070	0.783	-0.110	0.663	0.231	0.357	0.338	0.170
Age*	-0.189	0.453	-0.122	0.631	-0.126	0.619	-0.117	0.645	-0.176	0.486	-0.254	0.310

Correlation between variables and correct rate of pitch perception (≤ 6 years old, n=18).

For description, see Table 3.

Table 4a. and 4b. Correlation between variables and correct rate of pitch perception adjusted for age (> 6 or ≤ 6 years old).

Variable	O		P		A		A>5		D		D>5	
	r^2	p	r^2	p	r^2	p	r^2	p	r^2	p	r^2	p
DuM(mo)	0.564	0.010†	0.353	0.127	0.625	0.003†	0.549	0.012†	0.295	0.207	0.305	0.191
Device	-0.005	0.983	-0.201	0.396	0.071	0.767	-0.240	0.308	0.064	0.787	0.114	0.632
Age*	0.020	0.932	-0.051	0.832	0.238	0.312	0.064	0.787	-0.163	0.492	-0.043	0.859

Correlation between variables and correct rate of pitch perception (Duration of cochlear implant use > 18 months, n=20).

Variable	O		P		A		A>5		D		D>5	
	r^2	p	r^2	p	r^2	p	r^2	p	r^2	p	r^2	p
DuM(mo)	0.133	0.776	-0.057	0.903	0.072	0.878	0.078	0.868	0.216	0.642	0.265	0.566
Device	0.169	0.717	0.402	0.371	0.246	0.594	0.369	0.415	-0.109	0.816	0.194	0.677
Age*	0.595	0.159	0.539	0.212	0.657	0.109	0.603	0.152	0.500	0.253	0.421	0.346

Correlation between variables and correct rate of pitch perception (Duration of cochlear implant use ≤ 18 months, n=7).

For description, see Table 3.

Table 4c. and 4d. Correlation between variables and correct rate of pitch perception adjusted for duration of cochlear implant use (> 18 or ≤ 18 months).

months to assess the effect of implant use duration on the significance of correlation. For children with duration of implant use >18 months, the duration of musical training significantly correlated with correct rate of overall (r^2=0.564, p=0.010) and ascending pitch-interval (r^2=0.625, p=0.003) perception; there is no correlation between pitch perception and age of implantation or type of cochlear implant. For children with duration of implant use ≤18 months, there is no correlation between pitch perception and duration of musical training, age of implantation, or type of cochlear implant.

2.4 Discussion

2.4.1 Insignificant effect of pitch-interval size on pitch perception

In the present study, the size of the pitch interval did not considerably affect the performance of pitch perception in subjects of prelingually deafened children with a cochlear implant (Figure 1, Table 1). For the pitch perception of descending interval >5 semitones, however, the correct rate was lower than for that of descending interval ≤5 semitones. This finding was paradoxical since it's reasonable to infer that a larger pitch interval is easier to perceive correctly than a smaller one. It might imply a general intricacy in pitch perception of descending interval for cochlear implant users of all age, since scores of "falling" melodic contour perception was much lower than those of "rising" one (even lower than chance level) for adult cochlear implantees in one previous study (Galvin et al., 2007; McDermott, 2004).

Various factors have been reported to affect the pitch perception in implanted children. The insignificant effect of pitch-interval size on the differentiation tasks in the present study could be ascribed partly to the channel-setting of sound frequency and/or tone perception changes caused by cochlear implants (Nardo et al., 2007; Reiss et al., 2007).

Obvious disparity could occur between frequencies assigned to electrodes and those actually perceived by cochlear recipients possibly related to the channel-setting of frequency during mapping (Nardo et al., 2007). After appropriate mapping, pitch perception via cochlear implants might still have great spectral variations for years, which can echo the extent of damage of peripheral innervations patterns in the early stage and plasticity-dependent modifications in the later stage of implant use (Reiss et al., 2007). In fact, effect of musical training was much more significant for pitch perception of ascending interval >5 semitones in children with duration of cochlear implant use >18 months. Our results showed that a duration ≤18 months of cochlear implant use might not be long enough for the plasticity-dependent adaptation of aforementioned disparity to happen (Table 4c~d).

Another possibility for better results with smaller intervals might be the use of loudness- instead of pitch-cues for tone discrimination. It has been shown that a musical note at the center of a frequency band for one electrode may be louder than that at edge of the frequency band (Singh et al., 2009). Besides, a musical note at the edge of the band may activate two electrodes instead of one (Donaldson et al., 2005). The way these different musical intervals align with the frequency ranges allocated to each electrode (i.e., MAPs) potentially provide additional cues for tones discrimination. However, it has been revealed that electrode activation differences did not influence recognition performance with low- (104–262Hz) and middle-frequency (207–523Hz) melodies (Singh et al., 2009). Since the frequency range in our study lies between 256 and 495Hz, electrode activation differences did not seem to be a confounding factor in our study.

One more plausible explanation is the abnormal frequency-coding resolution resulting from the disorganization of tonotopic maps in the auditory cortices of those prelingually deafened children. Topographically arranged representations of frequency-tuning maps (i.e.,tonotopy) have been known to exist in the auditory system (Huffman & Cramer, 2007). The orderly maps of tonotopy start at the cochlea and continue through to the auditory cortex. Mechanisms underlying the development of tonotopic maps remained unknown. In previous studies, however, deprivation of auditory input due to cochlear ablation and/or misexpression of essential proteins in the auditory pathway in neonatal birds and mammals have been shown to affect the normal development of tonotopic maps (Harrison et al., 1998; Huffman & Cramer, 2007; Yu et al., 2007; Zhang et al., 2005). This might in turn lead to a diminished capacity of the auditory system to decode the acoustic information in terms of frequency resolution (Harrison et al., 1998; Huffman & Cramer, 2007; Yu et al., 2007), which could underpin our finding of the insignificant effect for pitch-interval size on the differentiation tasks.

2.4.2 Musical training improving pitch perception

One major and novel finding in this study is that the duration of musical training correlates with music perception in subjects of prelingually deafened children with a cochlear implant. That is, higher scores for the performance of pitch perception positively correlated with a longer duration of musical training in implanted children. Furthermore, the performance for the perception of ascending interval was significantly enhanced after the musical training (Table 3).

Our finding was in line with a previous study, in which structured training was suggested to have positive correlation with recognition and appraisal of the timbre of musical instruments by postlingually deafened cochlear implant recipients (Gfeller et al., 2002). After twelve weeks of training, those implant recipients assigned to the training group showed significant improvement in timbre recognition and appraisal compared to the control group. The effect of training in music perception of prelingual cochlear implantees, however, was not addressed in the aforementioned study. As far as we know, our present research is the first study ever reporting such finding of enhanced music perception by musical training in prelingually deafened children with cochlear implants.

Mechanisms underlying the enhanced performance of pitch perception after musical training in those prelingually deafened children with cochlear implants remained unclear. One possibility is the modification of disorganized tonotopy through auditory plasticity in the central auditory pathway of our subjects. The reinstatement of afferent input via cochlear implantation could consequently launch a cascade of plastic changes in the auditory system. Such reorganization, probably coupled with essential changes in neurotransmission or neuromodulation, might assist in reducing further deterioration in the nervous system resulting from cessation of electrical input due to cochlear damage (Durham et al., 2000; Illing & Reisch, 2006). This might reverse the disrupted tonotopic maps toward a relatively "normal" organization (Guiraud et al., 2007), which in turn may lead to a better development of frequency tuning in the auditory cortices. In normal-hearing children, improved music perception via music education has been revealed by increased auditory evoked fields, possibly due to a greater number and/or synchronous activity of neurons (Pantev et al., 1998). With the intervention of musical training, it seemed that the modified organization of tonotopy in subjects of prelingually deafened children could also be further optimized for a more delicate resolution of frequency spectrum, as is indexed by a better performance of pitch perception in the present study.

2.4.3 Effect of age and duration of cochlear implant use on pitch perception

In the present study, the performance of pitch perception is better in children with cochlear implants >6 y/o than those ≤6 y/o (Table 2). This might be due to the younger children not understanding the test itself. Actually, some of our older children appear to have longer training periods (Table 1). Our finding was in line with previous studies in which older children with cochlear implants tended to score higher on tonal-language performance (Huang et al., 2005; Lee & van Hasselt, 2005). At least partly, this could also be attributed to the aforementioned influence of auditory plasticity. In an operational context, the generally longer duration of auditory rehabilitation and thus more cognitive experiences of acoustic stimulation lead to the enhanced skills for musical perception of our older children with longer duration of cochlear implant use (Table 4c~d). Nevertheless, the effect of musical training is much more significant for children ≤6 y/o than those >6 y/o (Table 4a~b). The seemingly gender effect observed in Table 2 might actually be due to the age effect, since the mean age of boys (6.9 y/o) was larger than that of girls (6.2 y/o), though the difference was not significant ($p=0.404$, t-test). Our finding thus verified that later pitch sensations in implanted children possibly reflected higher-level and/or experience-dependent plastic changes in the auditory pathway (Reiss et al., 2007), and that musical training in the sensitive period (≤6 y/o) would be beneficial for development of pitch sensations (Baharloo et al., 2000).

2.4.4 Limits of this study

While pitch ranking was assessed, testing intervals used in this research may be too small for the evaluation of real-world music appreciation. It has been reported that postlingual cochlear implantees were generally less accurate in identification of formerly well-known music pieces than normal-hearing subjects (Gfeller et al., 2005). Further study using larger intervals/musical extracts is thus necessary to see if improvement of pitch discrimination could result in a better music perception in prelingual cochlear implantees.

Though loudness was monitored to avoid the possible effect of intensity variation in this study, it is clear that loudness matching of different tones from a piano cannot be as precise as that of computerized sounds. Since musical training could improve loudness discrimination in normal-hearing subjects (Plath, 1968), the training might also improve pitch differentiation by advancing use of available loudness differences created unintentionally by cochlear implant programming. Future research using computerized tones with a more precise matching of loudness and analyzing how the results relate to MAPs will be helpful to separate tone discrimination from loudness differences.

2.5 Conclusion

In summary, the ability to discriminate sounds was improved with musical experience in prelingually deafened children with cochlear implants. Implanted children attending music classes revealed significant differences compared with those without musical training. We suggest that structured training on music perception should begin early in life and be included in the post-operative rehabilitation program for prelingually deafened children with cochlear implants. Since auditory plasticity might play an important role in the enhancement of pitch perception, our research invites further studies on a larger group of implanted children to correlate neuroelectrical changes over time from cochlear implantation and music performance. A longitudinal study is also needed to show whether such neuroelectrical responses change with improvement of music performance in prelingually deafened children with a cochlear implant.

2.6 Acknowledgment

This study was funded by Cheng Hsin General Hospital (9522, 9631, 9739) of Taiwan. We declare that we have no conflict of interest or financial relationships with this manuscript. Special thanks to Ms Meei-Ling Kuan, Wen-Chen Chiu, Meng-Ju Lien, and Hsiu-Wen Chang for audiological assistance.

2.7 Annotations

1. Section 2.2.3: The type of ANOVA used was repeated measure ANOVA.
2. Section 2.2.3: Normal distribution of data was confirmed by using Kolmogorov-Smirnov test.
3. Section 2.3.1: The power was 0.35 for the boys/girls comparison and 0.32 for the subjects >6 yr/subjects ≤6 yr comparison.

3. Part II: Other factors related to the improvement of music perception in cochlear implantees

3.1 Effect of residual hearing preservation on music perception in cochlear implantees

There are many factors that can influence functional outcomes post-cochlear implantation including surgical techniques, variability of array placement, device coding strategies, intensity of rehabilitation and pathology of hearing loss (Wilson & Dorman, 2008a, 2008b). In addition to the variability of functional outcomes, music appreciation in cochlear implant recipients is also variable, presumably for similar reasons. While it is not possible to differentiate between all of these, technological developments of cochlear implants aim to maximize an individual's ability to reach their maximum potential. As cochlear implant candidacy is expanded with improvements in technology, individuals with increasing levels of residual low-frequency hearing (e.g those with steeply sloping severe-profound hearing loss) fall within the candidacy range (Gantz et al., 2006). In this population, where hearing is retained after surgery, combined electric and acoustic stimulation can be used which may provide access to finer spectral resolution and temporal fine structure, enhancing music perception (Gantz et al., 2005; Kong et al., 2004). Techniques aimed to preserve residual hearing include the insertion of a short electrode array (Gantz et al., 2006; Gfeller et al., 2005) or partial or full insertion of a standard electrode array combined with a soft surgery technique to minimize intracochlear trauma (Fraysse et al., 2006; Gstoettner et al., 2004).

Short electrode arrays, including the research 10mm Iowa/Nucleus Hybrid-S Cochlear Implant, have been designed to facilitate electric and acoustic stimulation in individuals with residual hearing by only entering the descending cochlear basal turn (Gantz et al., 2005). Results reported as part of the multi-centre FDA clinical trial in 47 patients with the Nucleus Hybrid implant (Gantz et al., 2006) showed hearing preservation in 45 immediately after implantation, with hearing within 10dB of pre-operative thresholds maintained in 25 and within 30dB maintained in 22 for up to 3 years in some patients. Within this study, comparisons between long-term Hybrid-S users and long-term long array users who were matched on word understanding in quiet showed a difference in speech perception in noise (using both multi-talker babble and steady-state noise), suggesting that the Hybrid-S users perform better within a more realistic listening environment. Despite these benefits, Briggs and colleagues (Briggs et al., 2006) identified the possibility that shortening of the electrode array to 10mm may cause a place-frequency mismatch because only the basal portion of the cochlea will be stimulated, causing a disproportionately higher frequency percept than with a standard array. Further, should hearing not be preserved, then concerns have been raised that speech perception outcomes will be impaired for individuals who only receive electrical stimulation in such a limited region of the cochlea (Gstoettner et al., 2009). Nonetheless, in the clinical trial of the commercially-available 16mm Hybrid-L24, Lenarz et al. (Lenarz et al., 2009) showed good post-operative hearing preservation in 24 recipients implanted with a round-window surgical approach.

A standard commercially available electrode array has also been used for hearing preservation with full or partial insertion of the array using an atraumatic surgical technique (Roland, 2005). Using a prospective multicenter study, Fraysse et al. (Fraysse et al., 2006) compared changes in hearing threshold levels after 27 patients were implanted with the Nucleus 24 Contour Advance perimodiolar electrode array. Of these, 12 were implanted with a soft surgery technique using a 17mm insertion depth. The authors demonstrated that preservation of hearing thresholds was more successful when the soft surgery technique was used with median changes in average hearing thresholds between 250-500Hz measured at 40dB for the entire group and 23dB for the soft surgery group. Success in hearing preservation has also been reported using partial insertion of other electrode arrays, including the MED-EL C40+ implant (Gstoettner et al., 2004; Skarzynski et al., 2007). However delayed loss of residual hearing has been reported in some instances even when an atraumatic surgical technique is used (Fraysse et al., 2006; Gstoettner et al., 2006).

In contrast to the standard length electrode array, Skarzynski and Podskarbi-Fayette (Skarzynski & Podskarbi-Fayette, 2010) reported on the Nucleus® Straight Research Array (Cochlear Ltd), an atraumatic electrode array. The main characteristics of this array that are different from the usual straight or Contour Advance arrays are that it is thinner and smoother which aim to reduce intracochlear trauma and kinking of the proximal end during insertion with a 20mm insertion. This study showed that of nine patients who had low-frequency residual hearing ≤50dBHL at 500Hz, the mean increase in thresholds at this frequency was 19dB. Similarly, Gstoettner and colleagues (Gstoettner et al., 2009) reported on the outcomes of 9 patients implanted with the MED-EL Flex EAS (with increased flexibility of the array) showing that 4 patients had full hearing preservation and 5 showed partial preservation. However, Baumgartner et al (Baumgartner et al., 2007) reported hearing preservation in 10 of 16 patients fitted with the MED-EL Flex*soft* at 1 month post-implantation but this declined to only 4 patients at 6 months post-implantation, suggesting variable outcomes which may or may not reflect the array *per se,* or the surgical technique or the underlying pathology or combination of the above.

To date, only limited evidence exists to support the possibility that any of these techniques result in improved music perception for implant recipients. Gfeller and colleagues (Gfeller, 2005, 2006) compared music perception in 17 normally-hearing adults, 39 with a conventional long array (from Cochlear Ltd, Advanced Bionics and Ineraid) and 4 patients with a Hybrid-S Cochlear Implant (Cochlear Ltd). The results showed that Hybrid-S recipients and NH listeners performed significantly better than those with a standard-electrode array on recognizing real-world songs with no lyrics and instrument recognition (with no significant difference observed with device or processing strategy for the standard-electrode array group). Nonetheless, it does indicate the possibility of combined electrical and acoustic stimulation for improved musical recognition in cochlear implant recipients.

3.2 Effect of bimodal hearing and/or bilateral implantation on music perception in cochlear implantees

It has long been known that bimodal hearing is better than unimodal hearing for patients with hearing impairment in terms of speech/language perception. With respect to music perception, bimodal hearing was also revealed to be superior to unimodal hearing for prelingually deafened children in one of our previous studies (Chen et al., in submission). Scores for pitch differentiation were generally higher for the condition of "simultaneous use of both hearing aid as well as cochlear implant" than that of "utilization of cochlear implant only" in the same subject, although the differences were not statistically significant enough which could possibly be ascribed to the small sample size. The performance of pitch-interval differentiation was furthermore shown to be superior in subjects with longer duration of hearing aids use and longer duration of hearing aids use prior to the cochlear implantation.

Our study was congruent with one recent research in which bimodal hearing was noted to be better than hearing with bilateral cochlear implantation regarding music perception in patients with post-lingual deafness (Cullington & Zeng, 2011). The mechanisms underlying the superior effect of bimodal hearing on music perception over unimodal hearing and hearing with bilateral cochlear implantation remained unknown. One possibility is that the low-frequency cues inherent in hearing aids can compensate for the insufficiency of low-frequency cues built-in in the contemporary systems of cochlear implant in terms of pitch discrimination (Cullington & Zeng, 2011). Another more plausible explanation is that the auditory signals transmitted by hearing aids are analog in format (Chen et al., in submission). The acoustic information enclosed is thus much more abundant than that conveyed via the "digital" devices of cochlear implant, which in turn could sound more like that a normal-hearing subject would percept.

A usable high-frequency hearing gain by using hearing aids sometimes leads to a longer duration of hearing aids use prior to the cochlear implantation (Chen et al., in submission). The implanted ear will continue to benefit the implantees with a good high-frequency hearing gain even after the cochlear implantation. Since the neuronal architects serving auditory perception are hardwired to fine-tune to subtle differences in the auditory environment (Illing & Reisch, 2006), longer duration of hearing aids use will enable our subjects to become more familiar with the presented tone pairs, which would consecutively lead to a better capability of pitch-interval differentiation.

3.3 Coding strategies

In current commercially available cochlear implant systems, four main sound coding strategies are utilized (Wilson & Dorman, 2008a, 2008b). These are: (i) SPEAK (spectral peak strategy) (ii) CIS (continuous interleaved sampling); (iii) ACE (advanced combination encoder), which extracts both spectral and temporal cues; and (iv) *n of m* (number of maxima spectral speech extractor). However, it is proposed by some researchers that two main limitations affect music perception: (1) low-frequency fine structure information is poorly represented by envelope-based strategies; and (2) insufficient numbers of independent effective channels exist to deliver fine structure due to current spread and electrode interactions (conventional arrays have been 12-22 channels). More recently, considerable attention has been focused on the development of *novel* strategies to address this. These include the development of virtual channels through current steering (Firszt et al., 2007), and fine structure processing which intends to increase access to spectral and temporal fine structure (Hochmair et al., 2006). While such strategies are continually being improved to facilitate improved music perception and appreciation, limited empirical evidence currently exists to support the role of virtual channels or fine structure coding at this stage (Berenstein et al., 2008; Firszt et al., 2007). Nonetheless, they continue to represent possibilities for the future.

3.4 Conclusion

In summary, only limited evidence exists to support the possibility that factors such as residual hearing, bimodal hearing, and coding strategies result in improved music perception for implant recipients to date. However, they continue to represent opportunities for the future. The importance of techniques aimed to preserve residual hearing thus cannot be overemphasized in cochlear implantation. Further studies are also needed to show the longitudinal effect of bimodal hearing and newly developed coding strategies to benefit music performance in cochlear implantees.

4. References

4.1 References - Part I

Baharloo, S., Service, S.K., Risch, N., Gitschier, J., & Freimer, N.B. (2000). Familial aggregation of absolute pitch. *American Journal of Human Genetics*, Vol. 67, pp. 755-758

Busby, P.A. & Plant, K.L. (2005). Dual electrode stimulation using the nucleus CI24RE cochlear implant: electrode impedance and pitch ranking studies. *Ear and Hearing*, Vol. 26, pp. 504-511

Chen, J.K., Chuang, A.Y., McMahon, C., Hsieh, J.C., Tung, T.H., & Li, L.P. (2010). Music training improves pitch perception in prelingually deafened children with cochlear implants. *Pediatrics*, Vol. 125, pp. e793-800

Donaldson, G.S., Kreft, H.A., & Litvak, L. (2005). Place-pitch discrimination of single- versus dual-electrode stimuli by cochlear implant users (L). *Journal of Acoustical Society of America*, Vol. 118, pp. 623-626

Durham, D., Park, D.L., & Girod, D.A. (2000). Central nervous system plasticity during hair cell loss and regeneration. *Hearing Research*, Vol. 147, pp. 145-159

Firszt, J.B., Koch, D.B., Downing, M., & Litvak, L. (2007). Current steering creates additional pitch percepts in adult cochlear implant recipients. *Otology Neurotology*, Vol. 28, pp. 629-636

Galvin, J.J., 3rd, Fu, Q.J., & Nogaki, G. (2007). Melodic contour identification by cochlear implant listeners. *Ear and Hearing*, Vol. 28, 302-319

Gfeller, K. & Lansing, C.R. (1991). Melodic, rhythmic, and timbral perception of adult cochlear implant users. *J Speech Hear Res*, 34, 916-920

Gfeller, K., Olszewski, C., Rychener, M., Sena, K., Knutson, J.F., Witt, S., & Macpherson, B. (2005). Recognition of "real-world" musical excerpts by cochlear implant recipients and normal-hearing adults. *Ear and Hearing*, Vol. 26, pp. 237-250

Gfeller, K., Witt, S., Adamek, M., Mehr, M., Rogers, J., Stordahl, J., & Ringgenberg, S. (2002). Effects of training on timbre recognition and appraisal by postlingually deafened cochlear implant recipients. *Journal of the American Academy of Audiology*, Vol. 13, pp. 132-145

Guiraud, J., Besle, J., Arnold, L., Boyle, P., Giard, M.H., Bertrand, O., Norena, A., Truy, E., & Collet, L. (2007). Evidence of a tonotopic organization of the auditory cortex in cochlear implant users. *Journal of Neuroscience*, Vol. 27, pp. 7838-7846

Hamzavi, J. & Arnoldner, C. (2006). Effect of deep insertion of the cochlear implant electrode array on pitch estimation and speech perception. *Acta Otolaryngolagy*, Vol. 126, pp. 1182-1187

Harrison, R.V., Ibrahim, D., & Mount, R.J. (1998). Plasticity of tonotopic maps in auditory midbrain following partial cochlear damage in the developing chinchilla. *Experimental Brain Research*, Vol. 123, pp. 449-460

Huang, C.Y., Yang, H.M., Sher, Y.J., Lin, Y.H., & Wu, J.L. (2005) Speech intelligibility of Mandarin-speaking deaf children with cochlear implants. *International Journal of Pediatric Otorhinolaryngology*, Vol. 69, pp. 505-511

Huffman, K.J. & Cramer, K.S. (2007). EphA4 misexpression alters tonotopic projections in the auditory brainstem. *Developmental Neurobiology*, Vol. 67, pp. 1655-1668

Illing, R.B. & Reisch, A. (2006). Specific plasticity responses to unilaterally decreased or increased hearing intensity in the adult cochlear nucleus and beyond. *Hearing Research*, Vol. 216-217, pp. 189-197

Koelsch, S., Wittfoth, M., Wolf, A., Muller, J., & Hahne, A. (2004). Music perception in cochlear implant users: an event-related potential study. *Clinical Neurophysiology*, Vol. 115, pp. 966-972

Lee, K.Y. & van Hasselt, C.A. (2005). Spoken word recognition in children with cochlear implants: a five-year study on speakers of a tonal language. *Ear and Hearing*, Vol. 26, pp. 30S-37S

Li, L.P, Shiao, A.S., Chen, L.F., Niddam, D.M., Chang, S.Y., Lien, C.F., Lee, S.K., & Hsieh, J.C. (2006). Healthy-side dominance of middle- and long-latency neuromagnetic fields in idiopathic sudden sensorineural hearing loss. *European Journal of Neuroscience*, Vol. 24, pp. 937-946

Li, L.P, Shiao, A.S., Lin, Y.Y., Chen, L.F., Niddam, D.M., Chang, S.Y., Lien, C.F., Chou, N.S., Ho, L.T., & Hsieh, J.C. (2003). Healthy-side dominance of cortical neuromagnetic responses in sudden hearing loss. *Annals of Neurology*, Vol. 53, pp. 810-815

McDermott, H.J. (2004). Music perception with cochlear implants: a review. *Trends in Amplification*, Vol. 8, pp. 49-82

Nardo, W.D., Cantore, I., Cianfrone, F., Melillo, P., Fetoni, A.R., & Paludetti, G. (2007). Differences between electrode-assigned frequencies and cochlear implant recipient pitch perception. *Acta Otolaryngology*, Vol. 127, pp. 370-377

Pantev, C., Dinnesen, A., Ross, B., Wollbrink, A., & Knief, A. (2006). Dynamics of auditory plasticity after cochlear implantation: a longitudinal study. *Cerebral Cortex*, Vol. 16, pp. 31-36

Pantev, C., Oostenveld, R., Engelien, A., Ross, B., Roberts, L.E., & Hoke, M. (1998). Increased auditory cortical representation in musicians. *Nature*, Vol. 392, pp. 811-814

Plath, P. (1968). [Influence of training effect on the loudness differentiation-threshold in normal hearing persons]. *Archiv fur Klinische und Experimentelle Ohren- Nasen- und Kehlkopfheilkunde*, Vol. 190, pp. 286-290

Reiss, L.A., Turner, C.W., Erenberg, S.R., & Gantz, B.J. (2007) Changes in pitch with a cochlear implant over time. *Journal of Associated Research in Otolaryngology*, Vol. 8, pp. 241-257

Singh, S., Kong, Y.Y., & Zeng, F.G. (2009). Cochlear Implant Melody Recognition as a Function of Melody Frequency Range, Harmonicity, and Number of Electrodes. *Ear and Hearing*, Vol. 30, pp. 160-168

Sucher, C.M. & McDermott, H.J. (2007). Pitch ranking of complex tones by normally hearing subjects and cochlear implant users. *Hearing Research*, Vol. 230, pp. 80-87

Yu, X., Sanes, D.H., Aristizabal, O., Wadghiri, Y.Z., & Turnbull, D.H. (2007). Large-scale reorganization of the tonotopic map in mouse auditory midbrain revealed by MRI. *Proceedings of the National Academy of Sciences USA*, Vol. 104, pp. 12193-12198

Zhang, Y., Dyck, R.H., Hamilton, S.E., Nathanson, N.M., & Yan, J. (2005). Disrupted tonotopy of the auditory cortex in mice lacking M1 muscarinic acetylcholine receptor. *Hearing Research*, Vol. 201, pp. 145-155

4.2 References - Part II

Baumgartner, W.D., Jappel, A., Morera, C., Gstottner, W., Muller, J., Kiefer, J., Van De Heyning, P., Anderson, I., & Nielsen, S.B. (2007). Outcomes in adults implanted with the FLEXsoft electrode. *Acta Otolaryngology*, Vol. 127, pp. 579-586

Berenstein, C.K., Mens, L.H., Mulder, J.J., & Vanpoucke, F.J. (2008). Current steering and current focusing in cochlear implants: comparison of monopolar, tripolar, and virtual channel electrode configurations. *Ear and Hearing*, Vol. 29, pp. 250-260

Briggs, R.J., Tykocinski, M., Xu, J., Risi, F., Svehla, M., Cowan, R., Stover, T., Erfurt, P., & Lenarz, T. (2006). Comparison of round window and cochleostomy approaches with a prototype hearing preservation electrode. *Audiology Neurootology*, Vol. 11 Suppl 1, pp. 42-48.

Chen, J.K., Chuang, A.Y., McMahon, C., Hsieh, J.C., Tung, T.H., & Li, L.P. Concomittant hearing aids use improving pitch perception in prelingually deafened children with cochlear implant. In submission.

Cullington, H.E., & Zeng, F.G. (2011). Comparison of bimodal and bilateral cochlear implant users on speech recognition with competing talker, music perception, affective prosody discrimination, and talker identification. *Ear and Hearing*, Vol. 32, pp. 16-30

Firszt, J.B., Koch, D.B., Downing, M., & Litvak, L. (2007). Current steering creates additional pitch percepts in adult cochlear implant recipients. *Otology Neurotology*, Vol. 28, 629-636

Fraysse, B., Macias, A.R., Sterkers, O., Burdo, S., Ramsden, R., Deguine, O., Klenzner, T., Lenarz, T., Rodriguez, M.M., Von Wallenberg, E., & James, C. (2006). Residual hearing conservation and electroacoustic stimulation with the nucleus 24 contour advance cochlear implant. *Otology Neurotology*, Vol. 27, pp. 624-633

Gantz, B.J., Turner, C., & Gfeller, K.E. (2006). Acoustic plus electric speech processing: preliminary results of a multicenter clinical trial of the Iowa/Nucleus Hybrid implant. *Audiology Neurootology*, Vol. 11 Suppl 1, pp. 63-68

Gantz, B.J., Turner, C., Gfeller, K.E., & Lowder, M.W. (2005). Preservation of hearing in cochlear implant surgery: advantages of combined electrical and acoustical speech processing. *Laryngoscope*, Vol. 115, pp. 796-802

Gfeller, K., Olszewski, C., Rychener, M., Sena, K., Knutson, J.F., Witt, S., & Macpherson, B. (2005). Recognition of "real-world" musical excerpts by cochlear implant recipients and normal-hearing adults. *Ear and Hearing*, Vol. 26, pp. 237-250

Gfeller, K.E., Olszewski, C., Turner, C., Gantz, B., & Oleson, J. (2006). Music perception with cochlear implants and residual hearing. *Audiology Neurootology*, Vol. 11 Suppl 1, pp. 12-15

Gstoettner, W., Helbig, S., Settevendemie, C., Baumann, U., Wagenblast, J., & Arnoldner, C. (2009). A new electrode for residual hearing preservation in cochlear implantation: first clinical results. *Acta Otolaryngology*, Vol. 129, pp. 372-379

Gstoettner, W., Kiefer, J., Baumgartner, W.D., Pok, S., Peters, S., & Adunka, O. (2004). Hearing preservation in cochlear implantation for electric acoustic stimulation. *Acta Otolaryngology*, Vol. 124, pp. 348-352

Gstoettner, W.K., Helbig, S., Maier, N., Kiefer, J., Radeloff, A. & Adunka, O.F. (2006). Ipsilateral electric acoustic stimulation of the auditory system: results of long-term hearing preservation. *Audiology Neurootology*, Vol. 11 Suppl 1, pp. 49-56

Hochmair, I., Nopp, P., Jolly, C., Schmidt, M., Schosser, H., Garnham, C., & Anderson, I. (2006). MED-EL Cochlear implants: state of the art and a glimpse into the future. *Trends in Amplification*, Vol. 10, pp. 201-219

Illing, R.B. & Reisch, A. (2006). Specific plasticity responses to unilaterally decreased or increased hearing intensity in the adult cochlear nucleus and beyond. *Hearing Research*, Vol. 216-217, pp. 189-197

Kong, Y.Y., Cruz, R., Jones, J.A., & Zeng, F.G. (2004). Music perception with temporal cues in acoustic and electric hearing. *Ear and Hearing*, Vol. 25, pp. 173-185

Lenarz, T., Stover, T., Buechner, A., Lesinski-Schiedat, A., Patrick, J., & Pesch, J. (2009). Hearing conservation surgery using the Hybrid-L electrode. Results from the first clinical trial at the Medical University of Hannover. *Audiology Neurootology*, Vol. 14 Suppl 1, pp. 22-31

Roland, J.T., Jr. (2005). A model for cochlear implant electrode insertion and force evaluation: results with a new electrode design and insertion technique. *Laryngoscope*, Vol. 115, pp. 1325-1339.

Skarzynski, H., Lorens, A., Piotrowska, A., & Anderson, I. (2007). Preservation of low frequency hearing in partial deafness cochlear implantation (PDCI) using the round window surgical approach. *Acta Otolaryngology*, Vol. 127, pp. 41-48

Skarzynski, H. & Podskarbi-Fayette, R. (2010). A new cochlear implant electrode design for preservation of residual hearing: a temporal bone study. *Acta Otolaryngology*, Vol. 130, pp. 435-442

Wilson, B.S. & Dorman, M.F. (2008a). Cochlear implants: a remarkable past and a brilliant future. *Hearing Research*, Vol. 242, pp. 3-21.

Wilson, B.S. & Dorman, M.F. (2008b) Cochlear implants: current designs and future possibilities. *Journal of Rehabilitation Research and Development*, Vol. 45, pp. 695-730

5

A Review of Stimulating Strategies for Cochlear Implants

Charles T. M. Choi[1] and Yi-Hsuan Lee[2]
[1]*National Chiao Tung University,*
[2]*National Taichung University of Education,*
Taiwan, R.O.C.

1. Introduction

Many animals use sound to communicate with each other, and hearing is particularly important for survival and reproduction. In species that use sound as a primary means of communication, their hearing is typically most acute for the range of pitches produced in calls and speech. Human is one such species and Fig. 1 shows a human ear consisting of the outer, middle and inner ear. The eardrum of an ear converts incoming acoustic pressure waves through the middle ear to the inner ear. In the inner ear the distribution of vibrations along the length of the basilar membrane is detected by hair cells. The location and intensity of these vibrations are transmitted to the brain by the auditory nerves. If the hair cells are damaged (as shown in Fig. 2(b)), the auditory system is unable to convert acoustic pressure waves to neural impulses, which results in hearing impairment. Damaged hair cells can subsequently lead to the degeneration of adjacent auditory neurons. If a large number of hair cells or auditory neurons are damaged or missing, the condition is called *profound hearing impairment* (Yost, 2000).

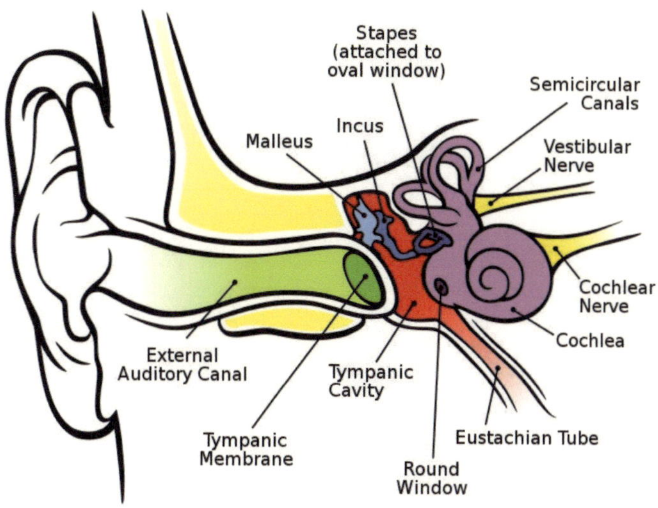

Fig. 1. A diagram of the anatomy of the human ear. (Chittka, L. & Brockmann, A. (2005))

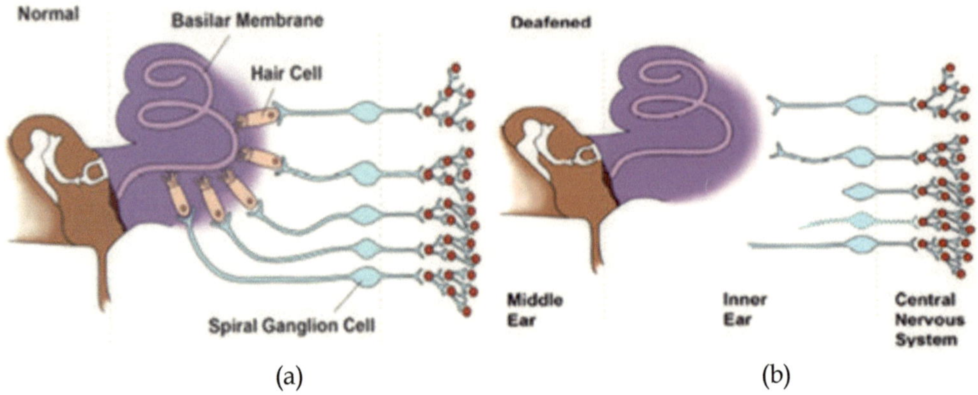

Fig. 2. (a) Normal human ear; (b) Profound hearing impairment. (Loizou, P.C. (1999))

Cochlear implants (*CI*) have been commercially available for nearly thirty years. Today cochlear implants still provide the only opportunity for people with profound hearing impairment to recover partial hearing through electrical stimulation of the auditory nerves (Loizou, 1998; Loizou, 1999; Spelman 1999; Wilson & Dorman, 2008). Fig. 3 is a diagram of a cochlear implant. The external part consists of microphones, a speech processor and a transmitter. Internally an array of up to 22 electrodes is inserted through the cochlea, and a receiver is secured to the bone beneath the skin. The microphones pick up sounds and the speech processor converts the sounds into electrical signals based on a stimulating strategy. The electrical signals, which determine the sequence in which the electrodes are activated, are then converted into electric impulses and sent to the implanted electrodes by the transmitter (Girzon, 1987; Suesserman & Spelman, 1993). The simulating strategy plays an extremely important role in maximizing a user's overall communicative potential.

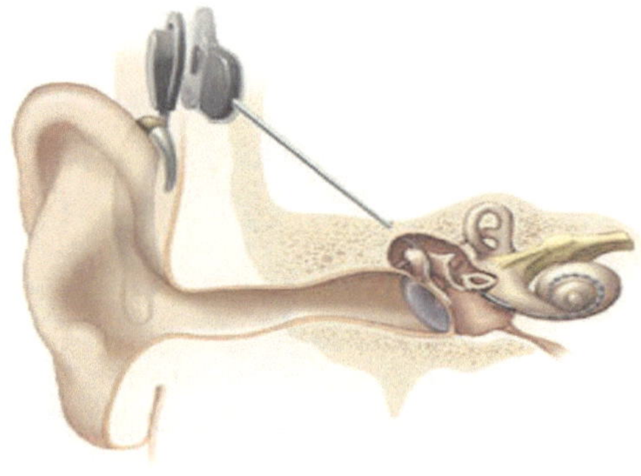

Fig. 3. A cochlear implant.

Until recently the main thrust in cochlear implant research has been to improve the hearing ability of CI users in a quiet environment (Dorman & Loizou, 1997; Loizou et al., 1999). There have been numerous improvements in the current generation of cochlear prosthesis, including the development of completely implantable cochlear implants. However, today CI users still have difficulty in listening to music and tonal languages, and in hearing in a noisy environment (Fu et al., 1998; Friesen et al., 2001; Xu et al., 2002; Kong et al., 2004; Lan et al.,

2004). One cause of these problems is that the spectral resolution perceived by CI user is not good enough. If a novel stimulating strategy is developed to increase spectral resolution, these problems can to some extent be relieved. In this literature review we first introduce basic stimulating strategies used in commercial cochlear implant systems. We then discuss a new *hybrid stimulating strategy,* and some experimental results of normal hearing tests are presented to compare the performance achieved by different stimulating strategies.

2. Stimulating strategy review

In the cochlear implant system, the stimulating strategy plays an extremely important role in generating the sounds heard by users (Wilson et al., 1991; Kiefer et al., 2001; Koch et al., 2004; Wilson & Dorman, 2008). It functions to convert sounds into a series of electric impulses which determines which electrodes should be activated in each cycle. A complete stimulating strategy should address the following:

1. The number of channels selected to reproduce the original spectrum;
2. The number of electrodes activated to generate each channel;
3. The number of consecutive clock cycles required to deliver selected channels,; and
4. The scheduling of the activating sequence of electrodes.

Many stimulating strategies have been developed over the past two decades. An ideal stimulating strategy is one that closely reproduces the original sound spectrum and allows a CI user to hear clear sounds. In the following we briefly describe and compare the *advanced combinational encoder* (*ACE*), *continuous interleaved sampling* (*CIS*), and *HiRes*120 strategies, which are frequently used in today's commercial cochlear implants.

2.1 Stimulating strategy using fixed channel

2.1.1 Advanced Combinational Encoder (ACE) (Kiefer et al., 2001)

The ACE strategy (Fig. 4), used in the Nucleus implant, is based on a so-called N of M principle. This system uses 22 implanted electrodes which can be activated to generate 22 fixed channels. The signal is processed into 22 frequency bands for each frame of recorded sound. After the envelope information for every frequency band is extracted, 8–10 (set by the audiologist) frequency bands with the largest amplitudes will be stimulated. Electrodes corresponding to the selected channels are then activated. Thus in the ACE strategy, a channel is generated by one implanted electrode, and the original spectrum is reproduced by 8–10 fixed channels.

2.1.2 Continuous Interleaved Sampling (CIS) (Wilson et al., 1991)

CIS is a strategy used in the speech processors of all major cochlear implant manufacturers. For Advanced Bionics implants, which have 16 implanted electrodes, a diagram of the strategy is shown in Fig. 5. For each frame of sound, the signal is applied through 16 band-pass filters, and the envelopes of these frequency bands are extracted by full-wave rectifying and low-pass filtering (with 200–400Hz cutoff frequency). Unlike ACE, all 16 frequency bands are then stimulated in sequence. Trains of balanced biphasic pulses modulated with extracted signal envelopes are delivered to each electrode at a constant rate in a non-overlapping sequence. The stimulation rate of each channel is relatively high, and the overlap across channels can also be eliminated. So, in the CIS strategy a channel is still generated by one implanted electrode. The original spectrum is reproduced by 16 fixed channels, and all electrodes are turned on in a predefined sequence within 16 consecutive clock cycles.

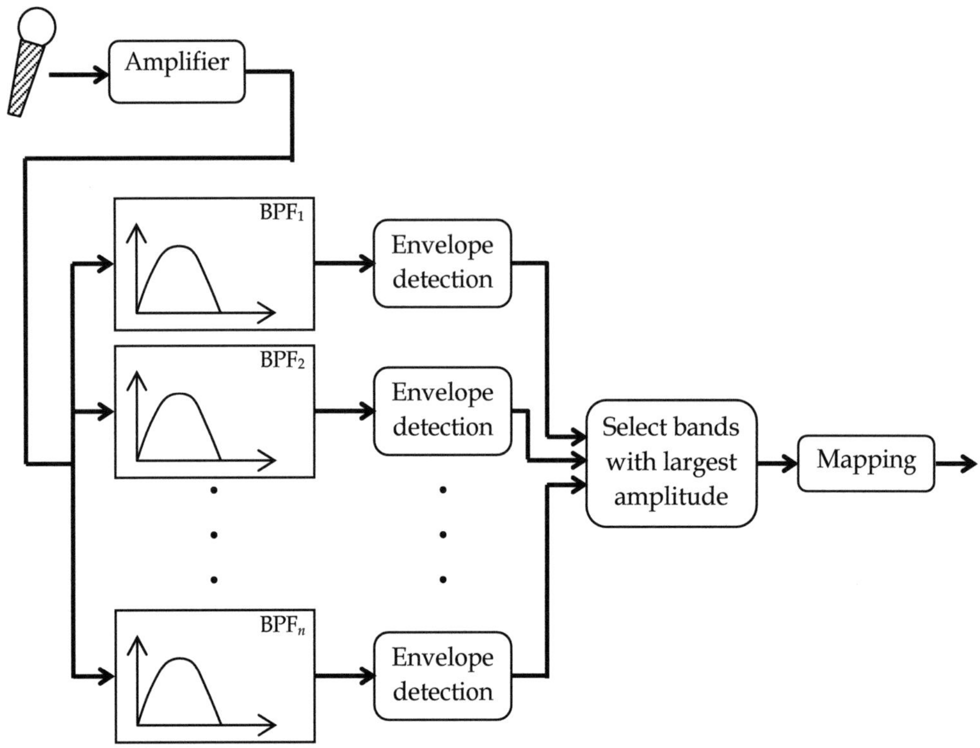

Fig. 4. A block diagram of the ACE stimulating strategy.

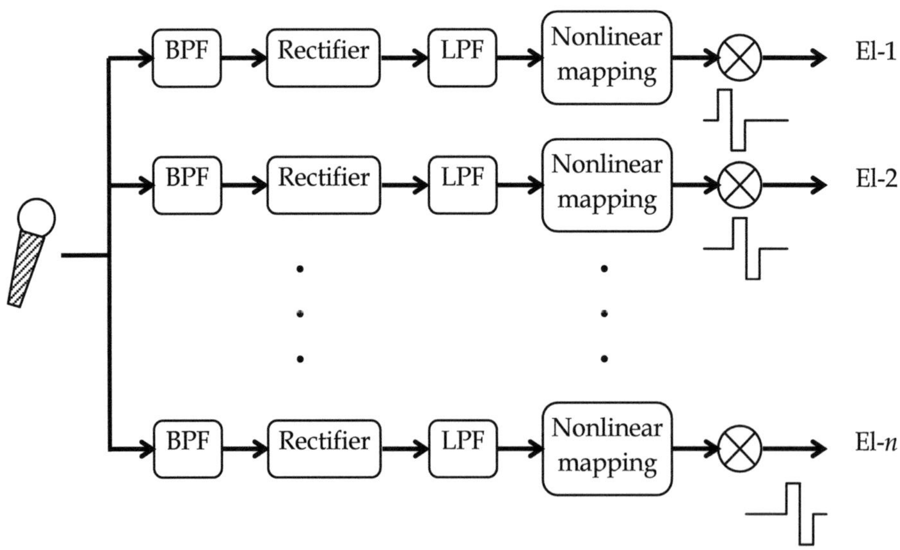

Fig. 5. A block diagram of the CIS stimulating strategy.

2.2 Stimulating strategy using virtual channel

As described above, both ACE and CIS strategies only use fixed channels to reproduce the original sound spectrum. There are, however, around 30,000 auditory nerve fibers in a human ear, but only 16–22 electrodes can currently be implanted into a CI user's ear to generate 16–22 fixed channels. Due to the limitation of the electrode design, the electrode has limited stimulation selectivity. Thus, these electrodes can only excite a small number of specific auditory nerve fibers, thus restricts the resolution and information received by a CI user is thus restricted.

2.2.1 Virtual channel technique

One possible way to achieve better spectral resolution is by increasing the number of electrodes. If, however, the number of implanted electrodes is limited and fixed, an alternative is to use the *virtual channel* technique (Donaldson et al., 2005; Koch et al., 2007). This technique uses *current steering* to control the electrical interaction. When two (or more) neighboring electrodes are stimulated in a suitable manner, intermediated channels, also known as virtual channels, are created between the electrodes. These virtual channels can enable CI users to perceive different frequencies between two fixed channels (Koch et al., 2004; Choi & Hsu, 2009). Using the virtual channel technique not only allows for more stimulating space, but also improves the reproduction of the original spectrum. This is Illustrated by the example in Fig. 6. Fig. 6(a) shows a sample original spectrum, and Figs. 6(b) and (c) show spectrums generated using fixed and virtual channel techniques, respectively. There appears to be much similarity between Fig. 6(a) and Fig. 6(c), but Fig. 6(b) is distorted from the original. Therefore, in order to better reproduce the original spectrum and increase the perceptual quality of CI users, it would be beneficial to apply the virtual channel technique to the stimulating strategies of cochlear implants.

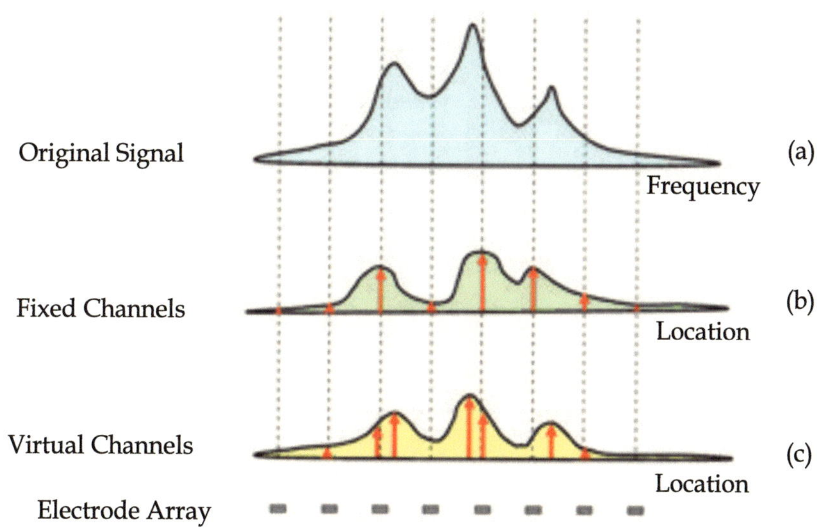

Fig. 6. A comparison of spectrums generated using different stimulating strategies. (a) A sample original spectrum; (b) A spectrum generated using fixed channels; (c) A spectrum generated using virtual channels.

2.2.2 HiRes120 (Koch et al., 2004)

To apply the virtual channel technique to a cochlear implant system, each electrode must have an independent power source to allow the current to be delivered simultaneously to more than one electrode. Theoretically, with a fine control over the current level ratio of neighboring electrodes, the locus of stimulation is steered between electrodes to create virtual channels. The HiRes120 strategy, used in the Advanced Bionics implant, is the first commercial stimulating strategy that uses the virtual channel technique. Virtual channels are created by adjusting the current level ratio of two neighboring electrodes. Since the Advanced Bionics implant has 16 implanted electrodes, there are 15 electrode pairs that can be used to steer the focus of the electrical stimulation. Fig. 7 is a diagrammatic representation of the HiRes120 strategy. For each frame of sound, the signal is divided by 15 band-pass filters and the envelope is extracted for every frequency band. In addition, 15 spectral peaks, which indicate the most important frequency within each frequency band, are also derived using the *Fast Fourier Transform* (*FFT*). These spectral peaks are then steered by corresponding electrode pairs based on the virtual channel technique. The HiRes120 strategy also delivers channels in sequence with a high stimulation rate similar to that of the CIS. Thus, in the HiRes120 strategy a channel is generated by two neighboring electrodes. The original spectrum is reproduced by 15 virtual channels, and all electrode pairs are turned on in a predefined sequence within 15 consecutive clock cycles.

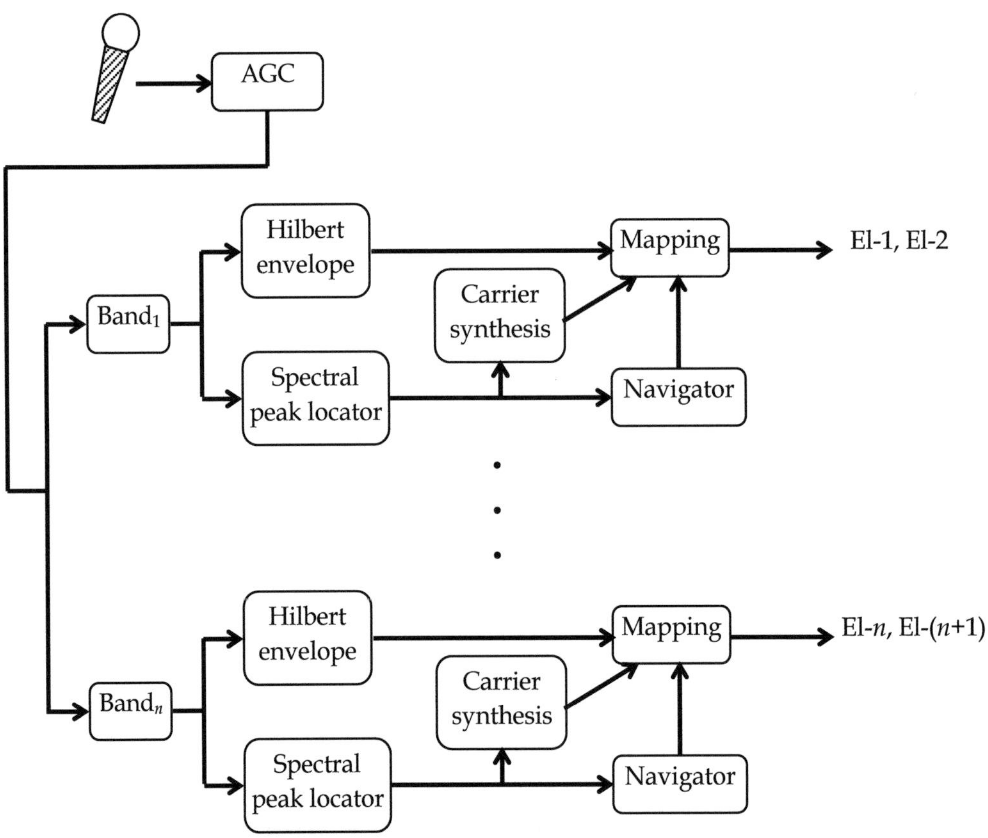

Fig. 7. A block diagram of the HiRes120 stimulating strategy.

3. Hybrid stimulating strategy

3.1 Four-Electrode Current Steering Schemes (FECSS) (Choi & Hsu, reviewing)

CI users with the HiRes120 strategy devices usually have better hearing performance compared to those with the CIS strategy devices (Koch et al., 2004; Wilson & Dorman, 2008), indicating that applying virtual channel technique does improve the perceptual quality of CI users. However, since the HiRes120 strategy only adjusts the current level ratio of two neighboring electrodes, its spectral resolution is actually not high enough due to the relatively wider stimulation region of the immediate channels. For a channel with a wider stimulation region, more auditory nerve fibers are excited. This increases the difficulty of CI users to discriminate between different channels, and limits the total number of immediate channels that can be generated. In the HiRes120 strategy only seven virtual channels are generated between two electrodes.

If more adjacent electrodes are used to steer the current, it will narrow the stimulation region to focus on firing specific auditory nerve fibers. *Four-electrode current steering schemes (FECSS)* is a current steering technique developed to control four adjacent electrodes simultaneously (Choi & Hsu, reviewing; Choi & Hsu, 2009). As shown in Fig. 8, the locus of stimulation is focused between the middle electrode pair, and the stimulation region is apparently narrower. This indicates that applying FECSS to stimulating strategies can help the CI user hear sounds with more specific frequencies, thus improving the perceptual quality and number of discriminable virtual channels.

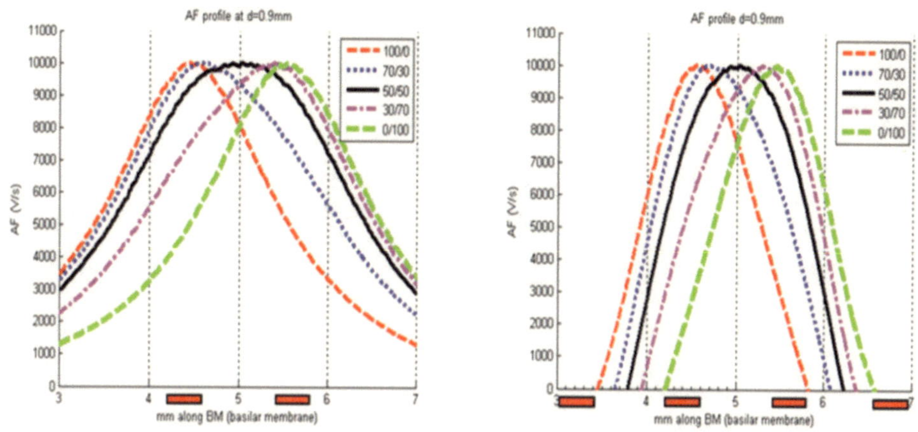

(a) (b)

Fig. 8. Current steering technique. (a) Virtual channels generated using two adjacent electrodes; (b) Virtual channels generated using four adjacent electrodes (FECSS).

3.2 Hybrid stimulating strategy (Choi et al., reviewing)

Although FECSS has the potential to achieve better hearing performance for CI users, it is primarily an algorithm to control the electrical current spread spatially and does not consider the activating sequence of the electrodes. Furthermore all current commercial stimulating strategies are highly inflexible, because the number of electrodes used to generate a channel and the number of channels delivered in every clock cycle are both fixed, which makes it difficult to closely reproduce the original sound spectrum.

In (Choi et al., reviewing) a flexible *hybrid stimulating strategy* is proposed to overcome the limitations mentioned above. This strategy utilizes a combination of the two-electrode current steering scheme (TECSS) and FECSS to reproduce the original sound spectrum. In FECSS it has been shown that it is possible to generate a sharper spectral peak by using 4-electrode stimulation (Choi & Hsu, reviewing). Hence, in the hybrid stimulating strategy algorithm, TECSS and FECSS are used to generate wider and narrower spectral peaks, respectively. The entire spectrum is delivered within eight to fifteen clock cycles, and a number of spectral peaks are delivered in each clock cycle.

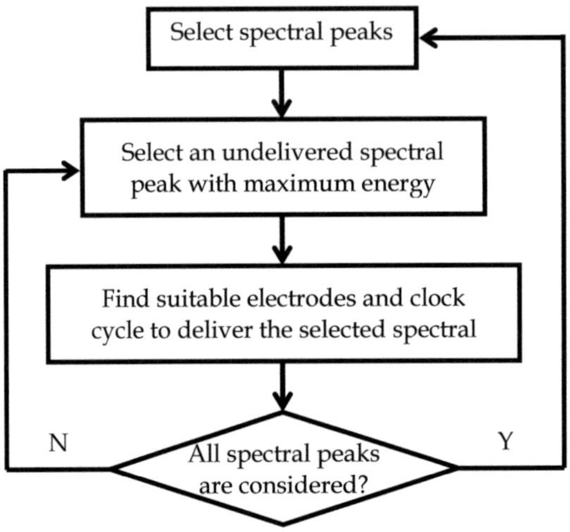

Fig. 9. A flowchart of the hybrid stimulating strategy.

		Hybrid	HiRes120	CIS	ACE
Manufacture		***	Advanced Bionics	Advanced Bionics	Cochlear
No. of implanted electrodes		*m*	16	16	22
Virtual channel technique		Yes (>300 channels)	Yes (120 channels)	No	No
To reproduce a signal frame	No. of spectral peaks	~*n* (adaptive)	15	16	8~10 (fixed) (adjustable)
	No. of electrodes to generate a channel	at most *u* (adaptive)	2	1	1
	No. of clock cycle	*k* (fixed) (adjustable)	15	16	8~10 (fixed) (adjustable)
	No. of spectral peaks per clock cycle	adaptive	1	1	1

Table 1. The characteristics of the stimulating strategy of cochlear implant system including ACE, CIS, HiRes120, and hybrid.

Fig. 9 shows a flowchart of the hybrid stimulating strategy. For each frame of sound, the signal is divided by m band-pass filters. After the envelope information for every frequency band is extracted, n ($n \geq m$) spectral peaks are derived using the FFT. A combination of TECSS and FECSS is used to duplicate these n spectral peaks within k clock cycles. Each selected spectral peak is generated by at most u adjacent electrodes (two or four electrodes) and is scheduled to be generated within 8 to 15 clock cycles, without causing temporal and spatial interactions. Notice that not all n spectral peaks will be selected at a time. Table 1 lists the characteristics of stimulating strategies including hybrid, HiRes120, CIS, and ACE.

3.3 Hybrid stimulating strategy with psychoacoustic model (Choi et al., reviewing)

Hearing is not a purely mechanical wave propagation phenomenon, but also a sensory and perceptual event. In the phenomenon called *masking*, as shown on Fig. 10, a weaker sound is masked if it is made inaudible in the presence of a louder sound (Hellman, 1972; Zwicher & Fastl, 2008).

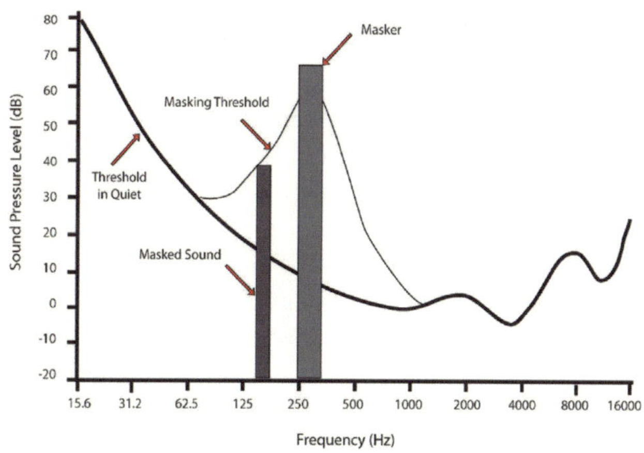

Fig. 10. An audio masking graph.

The psychoacoustic model is a computation model developed to detect the less perceptually important components of audio signals. It has been successfully used in the field of audio coding in order to reduce bandwidth requirements. Authors of the hybrid stimulating strategy also incorporate their strategy with a psycho-acoustic model (Zwicher & Fastl, 2008), and the implementation steps are shown in Fig. 11. After incorporating

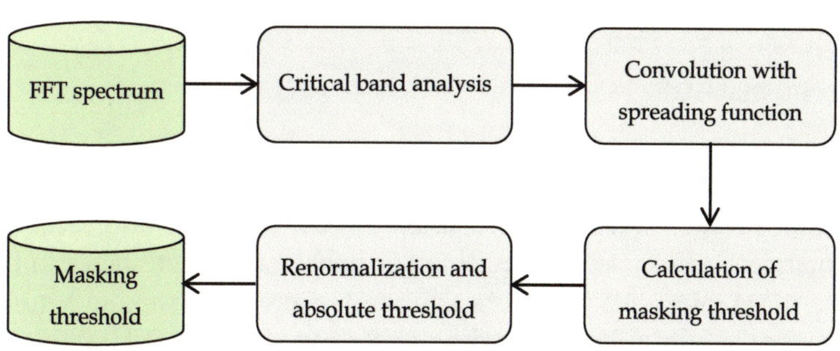

Fig. 11. A block diagram of the psychoacoustic model.

the psychoacoustic model, the number of activated electrodes is reduced compared to basic hybrid strategy, but more power is saved and the hearing performance of CI users is retained.

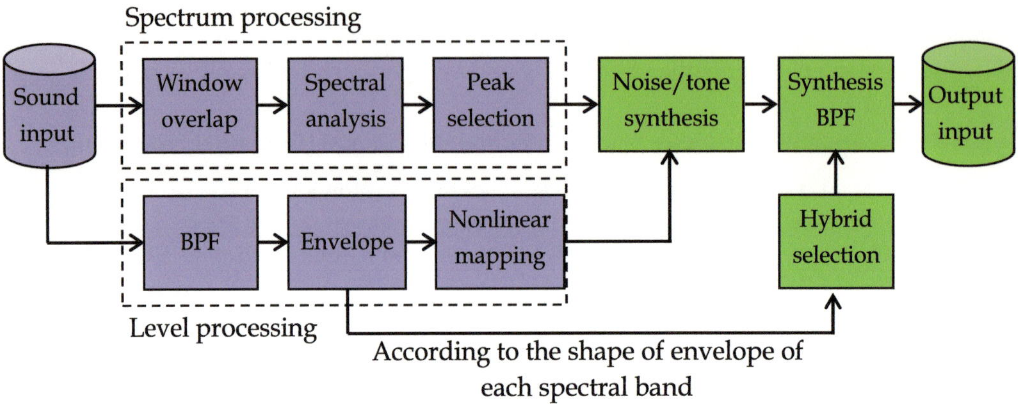

Fig. 12. A block diagram of the acoustic cochlear implant model.

4. Experimental results

4.1 Acoustic cochlear implant model

When a new stimulating strategy for cochlear implants is developed, it is impractical to apply it directly to a speech processor for testing by CI users. Researchers normally implement the strategy in an acoustic cochlear implant model (also called a vocoder), to simulate the sounds heard by CI users for conducting normal hearing tests with normal hearing subjects first.

As shown in Fig. 12, an acoustic cochlear implant model was implemented using LabVIEW (Choi et al., 2008), which contained two main paths. The *spectrum processing* path was used to derive spectral peaks using FFT, and the temporal envelope information for every frequency band was extracted in the *level processing* path. Both white noise and pure tones were used as carriers to synthesize the sounds as heard by CI users. The stimulating strategies implemented included the CIS, HiRes120, and hybrid, with and without a psychoacoustic model.

4.2 Subjects and materials

Normal hearing tests were conducted to evaluate the performance of a hybrid stimulating strategy (Choi et al., reviewing). Chinese sentences were used as test material (Tsai & Chen, 2002), and subjects were asked to listen to each sentence and recognize the final word. All sentences were mixed by multi-talker babble and white noise in 0, 5, or -5 dB SNR (signal-to-noise ratio). All normal hearing tests were conducted in a quiet room. The test subjects were 25 adults between 25 and 30 years old. SENNHEISER HD-380 PRO headphones were used.

4.3 Performance comparison of different stimulating strategies (Choi et al., reviewing)

Fig. 13 shows the results of the normal hearing tests for different stimulating strategies. The mean recognition % and standard deviation are both presented in Fig. 13, and the higher recognition % indicates more Chinese sentences can be correctly recognized. In general, the hybrid strategy showed a better performance.

The recognition % achieved in different SNRs is as follows. An SNR of -5 dB is considered a relatively noisy environment. The hybrid strategy achieved a recognition % of 50–70% at -5 dB SNR, a performance approaching that of people with normal hearing. The HiRes120 and CIS only achieved recognition % of 40–50% and < 20%, respectively. These results indicate that in a noisy environment the hybrid strategy has noticeable advantages compared to the HiRes120 and CIS. With an SNR of 0 dB, the recognition % of the hybrid strategy was 80%–85%, compared to 70%–85% for HiRes120 and <50% for CIS. With an SNR of 5 dB, a relative quiet environment, both hybrid and HiRes120 strategies had a recognition % of >85%. The CIS strategy also improved the recognition % to >50% when SNR was 5 dB.

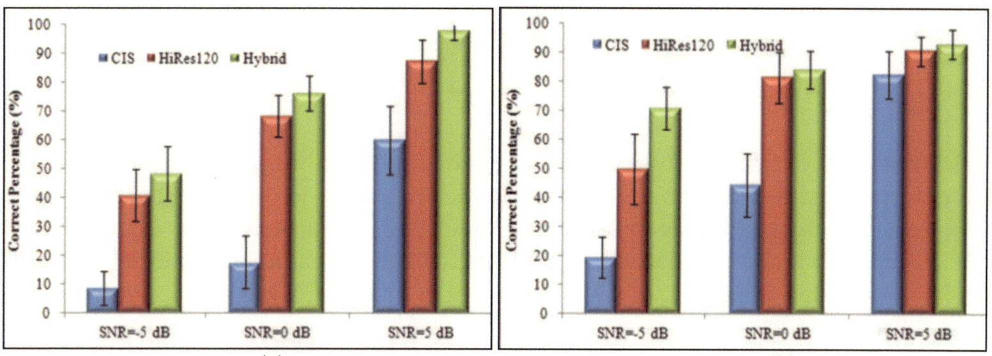

(a) (b)

Fig. 13. Results of the normal hearing tests: a comparison among stimulating strategies CIS, HiRes120, and hybrid. (a) Multi-talker babble; (b) White noise.

Two-way ANOVA and Post Hoc tests were used to further analyze the results obtained as shown in Fig. 13. ANOVA indicated a significant main effect for SNR and the strategies. The Post Hoc test indicated that there was always a statistically significant difference between the hybrid and the CIS. Between the hybrid and the HiRes120, statistically significant differences only existed at an SNR of -5 dB. When SNR was equal to 5 dB, the hybrid performed similarly to the HiRes120 and no statistically significant difference existed between them.

4.4 Performance comparison of hybrid strategy with and without psychoacoustic model (Choi et al., reviewing)

Fig. 14 shows the results of the normal hearing tests for the hybrid strategy with and without the psychoacoustic model, showing that the recognition % before and after incorporating the psychoacoustic model are almost the same. ANOVA also indicated a significant main effect for SNR, but no statistically significant difference existed between the hybrid strategy with and without the psychoacoustic model. These results indicate that incorporating the hybrid stimulating strategy with the psychoacoustic model is a feasible concept. The number of activated electrodes is reduced for power saving, and the hearing performance can be successfully retained.

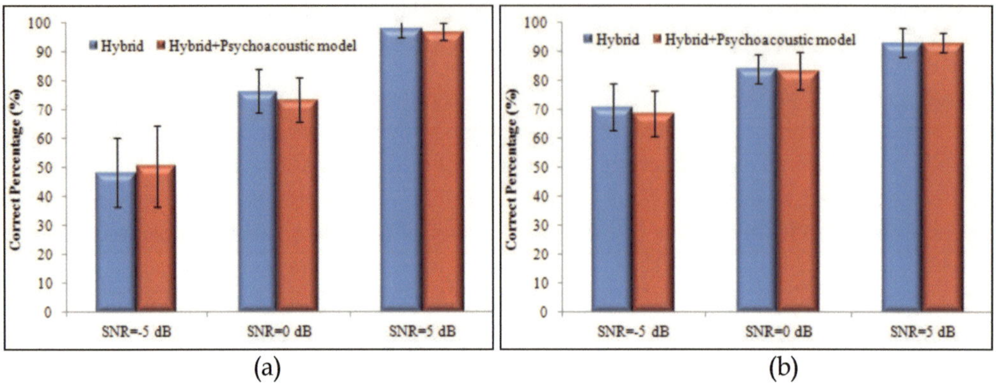

Fig. 14. Results of normal the hearing tests: the comparison between hybrid strategy with and without a psychoacoustic model. (a) Multi-talker babble; (b) White noise.

5. Conclusions

In this chapter we considered the most challenging problems currently facing CI research and demonstrated the importance of the stimulating strategy in cochlear implant systems. Some basic stimulating strategies used in commercial systems were reviewed, and a new hybrid stimulating strategy based on the virtual channel technique was introduced. The hybrid strategy can activate implanted electrodes in a more flexible way to reproduce the original sound spectrum. The results from the normal hearing experiments show the hybrid stimulating strategy achieves a better hearing performance when compared with the results from commercial stimulating strategies. The hybrid strategy can also be incorporated with a psychoacoustic model for power saving and load reduction on the stimulating cycles, without compromising the hearing performance. We therefore believe that developing a new stimulating strategy is a possible alternative to improving the hearing ability of CI users.

6. References

Chittka, L. & Brockmann, A. (2005). Perception Space - The Final Frontier, *PLoS Biology*, Vol.3, No.4, (April 2005), pp. e137 doi:10.1371/journal.pbio.0030137

Choi, C. T. M. & Hsu, C. H. (2009). Conditions for Generating Virtual Channels in Cochlear Prosthesis Systems, *Annals of Biomedical Engineering*, Vol.37, No.3, (March 2009), pp. 614-624, ISSN 0090-6964

Choi, C. T. M.; Hsu, C. H.; Tsai, W. Y. & Lee, Y. H. (2008). A Vocoder for a Novel Cochlear Implant Stimulating Strategy based on Virtual Channel Technology, *Proceedings of 13th ICBME*, ISBN 978-3-540-92840-9, Singapore, December 3-6, 2008

Choi, C. T. M. & Hsu, C. H. (reviewing). Novel Current Steering Schemes for Cochlear Prosthesis Systems, reviewing in *IEEE Transactions on Biomedical Engineering*

Choi, C. T. M.; Tsai, W. Y. & Lee, Y. H. (reviewing). A Novel Cochlear Implant Stimulating Strategy Incorporating a Hybrid Current Steering Scheme and a Psychoacoustic Model, reviewing in *Journal of Acoustic Society of America*

Donaldson, G. S.; Kreft, H. A. & Litvak, L. (2005). Place-Pitch Eiscrimination of Single-versus Dual-Electrode Stimuli by Cochlear Implant Users, *Journal of Acoustic Society of America*, Vol.118, No.22, (August 2005), pp. 623-626, ISSN 0001-4966

Dorman, M. F. & and Loizou, P. C. (1997). Speech Intelligibility as a Function of the Number of Channels of Stimulation for Normal-Hearing Listeners and Patients with Cochlear Implants, *American Journal of Otolaryngology*, Vol.18, No.6, (December 1997), ppS113-S114, ISSN 0196-0709

Friesen, L. M.; Shannon, R. V.; Baskent, D. & Wang, X. (2001). Speech Recognition in Noise as a Function of the Number of Spectral Channels: Comparison of Acoustic hearing and Cochlear Implants, *Journal of Acoustic Society of America*, Vol.110, No.2, (August 2011), pp. 1150-1163, ISSN 0001-4966

Fu, Q. J.; Shannon, R., V. & Wang, X. (1998). Effect of Noise and Number of Channels on Vowel and Consonant Recognition: Acoustic and Electric Hearing, *Journal of Acoustic Society of America*, Vol.104, No.6, (December 1998), pp. 3586-3596, ISSN 0001-4966

Girzon, G. (1987). Investigation of Current Flow in the Inner Ear during Electrical Stimulation of Intracochlear Electrodes, MS Thesis in EE&CS, MIT, Cambridge, Massachusetts

Hellman, R. P. (1972). Asymmetry of Masking between Noise and Tone, *Attention, Perception, and Psychophysics*, Vol.11, No.3, (May 1972), pp. 241-246, ISSN 1943-3921

Kiefer, J.; Hohl, S.; Sturzebecher, E.; Pfennigdorff, T. & Gstoettner, W. (2001). Comparison of Speech Recognition with Different Speech Coding Strategies (SPEAK, CIS, and ACE) and Their Relationship to Telemetric Measures of Compound Action Potentials in the Nucleus CI 24M Cochlear Implant System, *Audiology*, Vol. 40, No.1, (January/February 2001), pp. 32-42, ISSN 0020-6091

Koch, D. B.; Downing, M.; Osberger, M. J. & Litvak, L. (2007). Using Current Steering to Increase Spectral Resolution in CII and HiRes 90K Users, *Ear and Hearing*, Vol.28, No.2, (April 2007), pp. 38S-41S, ISSN 0196-0202

Koch, D. B.; Osberger, M. J.; Segal, P. & Kessler, D. (2004). HiResolution and Conventional Sound Processing in the HiResolution Bionic Ear: Using Appropriate Outcome Measures to Assess Speech Recognition Ability, *Audiology and Neurotology*, Vol.9, No.4, (July/August 2004), pp. 241-223, ISSN 1420-3030

Kong, Y. Y.; Cruz, R.; Jones, J. A. & Zeng, F. G. (2004). Music Perception with Temporal Cues in Acoustic and Electric Hearing, *Ear and Hearing*, Vol.25, No.2, (April 2004), pp. 173-185, ISSN 0196-0202

Lan, N.; Nie, K. B.; Gao, S. K. & Zeng, F. G. (2004). A Novel Speech-Processing Strategy Incorporating Tonal Information for Cochlear Implants, *IEEE Transactions on Biomedical Engineering*, Vol.51, No.5, (May 2004), pp. 752-760, ISSN 0018-9294

Loizou, P.C. (1999). Introduction to Cochlear Implant, *IEEE Engineering in Medical and Biology Magazine*, Vol.18, No.1, (January/February 1999), pp. 32-42, ISSN 0739-5175

Loizou, P. C. (1998). Mimicking the Human Ear, *IEEE Signal Processing Magazine*, Vol.15, No.5, (September 1998), pp. 101-130, ISSN 1053-5888

Loizou, P. C.; Dorman, M. and Tu, Z. (1999). On the Number of Channels Needed to Understand Speech, *Journal of Acoustic Society of America*, Vol.106, No.4, (October 1999), pp. 2097-2103, ISSN 0001-4966

Spelman, F. (1999). The Past, Present, and Future of Cochlear Prostheses, *IEEE Engineering in Medical and Biology Magazine*, Vol.18, No.3, (May/June 1999), pp.27-33, ISSN 0739-5175

Suesserman, M. F. & Spelman, F. A. (1993). Lumped-Parameter Model for in Vivo Cochlear Stimulation, *IEEE Transactions on Biomedical Engineering*, Vol.40, No.3, (March 1993), pp.237-245, ISSN 0018-9294

Tsai, C. H. & Chen, H. C. (2002). The Development of Mandarin Speech Perception in Noise Test, *Journal of Special Education*, Vol.23, (September 2002), pp. 121-140, ISSN 1026-4485 (in Traditional Chinese)

Wilson, B. S. & Dorman, M. F. (2008). Cochlear Implants: Current Designs and Future Possibilities, *Journal of Rehabilitation Research & Development*, Vol.45, No.5, (February 2008), pp.695-730, ISSN 0748-7711

Wilson, B. S.; Finley C. C.; Lawson, D. T.; Wolford, R. D.; Eddington, D. K. & Rabinowitz, W. M. (1991). Better Speech Recognition with Cochlear Implants, *Nature*, Vol.352, No.6332, (July 1991), pp. 236-238, ISSN 0028-0836

Xu, L.; Tsai, Y. J. & Pfingst, B. E. (2002). Features of Stimulation Affecting Tonal-Speech Perception: Implications for Cochlear Prostheses, *Journal of Acoustic Society of America*, Vol.112, No.1, (July 2002), pp. 247-258, ISSN 0001-4966

Yost, W. A. (2000). *Fundamentals of Hearing: An Introduction* (5th Ed.), Elsevier Academic Press, ISBN 9780123704733, San Diego

Zwicker, E. & Fastl, H. (2008). *Psychoacoustics: Facts and Models* (3rd Ed.), Springer, ISBN 978-3540650638, New York

6

A Fine Structure Stimulation Strategy and Related Concepts

Clemens Zierhofer and Reinhold Schatzer
C. Doppler Laboratory for Active Implantable Systems
University of Innsbruck
Austria

1. Introduction

The auditory system provides a natural frequency-to-place mapping which is designated as *tonotopic organisation* of the cochlea. In the normal-hearing system, the acoustic signal causes a fluid pressure wave which propagates into the cochlea. At particular positions within the cochlea, most of the energy of the wave is absorbed causing mechanical oscillations of the basilar membrane. The oscillations are transduced into electrical signals (action potentials) in neurons by the action of the inner hair cells. Waves caused by low input frequencies travel further into the cochlea than those caused by high frequencies. Thus, each position of the basilar membrane can be associated with a particular frequency of the input signal (Greenwood, 1990). This natural form of frequency-to-place mapping, together with the fact that the positioning and fixation of an intrascalar electrode array is comparatively simple, is likely one of the most important factors for the success of cochlear implants as compared to other sensory neural prostheses.

1.1 The "Continuous Interleaved Sampling" stimulation strategy

In the late 1980s, Wilson and colleagues introduced a coding strategy for cochlear implants designated as "Continuous Interleaved Sampling" (CIS) strategy (Wilson et al., 1991). Supporting significantly better speech perception in comparison to all other coding strategies at the time, CIS became and still is the de-facto standard among CI coding strategy. CIS signal processing involves splitting up of the audio frequency range into spectral bands by means of a filter bank, envelope detection of each filter output signal, and instantaneous nonlinear compression of the envelope signals (map law).

According to the tonotopic principle of the cochlea, each stimulation electrode in the scala tympani is associated with a band pass filter of the external filter bank. High-frequency bands are associated with electrodes positioned more closely to the base, and low-frequency bands to electrodes positioned more deeply in the direction of the apex. For stimulation, charge-balanced current pulses - usually biphasic symmetrical pulses - are applied. The amplitudes of the stimulation pulses are directly derived from the compressed envelope signals. These signals are sampled sequentially, and, as the characteristic CIS paradigm, the stimulation pulses are applied in a strictly non-overlapping way in time. Typically, the pulse sampling rate per channel is within the range of 0.8-1.5 kpulses/sec.

Many investigators have aimed at finding optimum CIS parameters for best speech perception, e.g., for parameters such as number of channels, stimulation rate per channel, etc. (Loizou et al., 2000). It turns out that four channels seem to be the absolute minimum number of channels for reasonable speech intelligibility, and speech perception reaches an asymptotic level of performance at about ten channels. Stimulation rates higher than about 1.5 kpulses/sec per channel also do not substantially improve speech perception.

Other approaches to improve speech recognition are based on the idea that neurons should have some activity even in the absence of an acoustic input. In a normal-hearing system such an activity is present and is generally designated as "spontaneous activity", i.e., neurons produce action potentials and cause a type of noise floor of neural activity. Following the principle of stochastic resonance (Morse & Evans, 1999), such a noise floor could provide a more natural representation of the envelope signals in the spiking patterns of neurons. In the deaf ear, there is no or very little spontaneous activity of neurons. To combine the CIS strategy with principles of stochastic resonance, it has been suggested to introduce high-frequency pulse trains with constant amplitudes - so-called "conditioner pulses" - in addition to the CIS pulses (Rubinstein et al., 1999). However, such approaches have so far not found their way into broad clinical applications, partly because no substantial improvement in speech intelligibility has been found and partly for practical reasons, because the power consumption of the implants is considerably increased.

1.2 Temporal fine structure

According to the principles of the Fourier transform, each signal can be decomposed into a sum of sinusoids of different frequencies and amplitudes. Following Hilbert (Hilbert, 1912), an alternative way of signal decomposition is to factor a signal into the product of a slowly varying *envelope* and a rapidly varying *temporal fine structure*. Hilbert's decomposition is particularly useful in the case of band pass signals as used in a CIS filter bank. Considering the response of a band pass filter to a voiced speech segment, the envelope carries mainly pitch frequency information. Temporal fine structure information is, first of all, present in the position of the zero crossings of the signal and shows the exact spectral position of the center of gravity of the signal within its band pass region, including temporal transitions of such centers of gravity. For example, the temporal transitions of formant frequencies in vowel spectra are highly important cues for the perception of subsequent plosives of other unvoiced utterances. Furthermore, a close look at the details of a band pass filter output also reveals that the pitch frequency is clearly present in the temporal structure of the zero crossings.

It is known from literature that the neurons in the peripheral auditory system are able to track analogue electrical sinusoidal signals up to about 1 kHz (Hochmair-Desoyer et al., 1983; Johnson, 1980). However, CIS is entirely based on envelope information, and temporal fine structure information is largely discarded. For example, consider the response of an ideal CIS system (filter bank composed of ideal rectangular band pass filters) to a sinusoidal input signal with constant amplitude and a frequency which is swept over the whole input frequency range. Then one channel after the other will generate an output. The CIS response reflects the approximate spectral position of the input signal (i.e., the information, *which* band filter within the filter bank is responding), but within each responding filter, there is no further spectral resolution.

Smith and colleagues (Smith et al., 2002) described an experiment with normal-hearing subjects based on a vocoder-type signal processor similar to CIS. Audio input signals were split up by means of a filter bank, and both envelope and temporal fine structure information was extracted from each channel. So-called "auditory chimaeras" were then constructed by combining, across channels, the envelopes of one sound with the temporal fine structure of a different sound. By presenting these auditory chimaeras to normal-hearing listeners, the relative perceptual importance of envelope and fine structure was investigated for speech (American English), musical melodies, and sound localization. The main outcome was that for an intermediate number of 4 to 16 channels, the envelope is dominant for speech perception, and the temporal fine structure is most important for pitch perception (melody recognition) and sound localization. When envelope information is in conflict with fine structure information, the sound of speech is heard at a location determined by the fine structure, but the words are identified according to the envelope.

In the light of these results, standard CIS is a good choice for the encoding of speech in Western languages (e.g., for American English). However, regarding music perception and perception of tone languages (e.g., Mandarin Chinese, Cantonese, Vietnamese, etc.), CIS might be suboptimal due to the lack of temporal fine structure information.

1.3 Spatial channel interaction

One basic problem in cochlear implant applications is spatial channel interaction. Spatial channel interaction means that there is considerable geometric overlap of the electrical fields at the location of the excitable neurons, if different stimulation electrodes in the scala tympani are activated. Thus, the same neurons can potentially be activated if different electrodes are stimulated. Spatial channel interaction is mainly due to the conductive fluids and tissues surrounding the stimulation electrode array.

One approach to defuse spatial channel interaction is to employ particular electrode configurations which aim at concentrating electrical fields in particular regions. Bipolar or even multipolar configurations have been investigated. These configurations have in common that active *and* return electrodes are positioned within the scala tympani of the cochlea (Miyoshi et al., 1997; van den Honert & Kelsall, 2007; van den Honert & Stypulkowski, 1987). For example, a bipolar configuration uses single sink and source electrodes which are typically separated by 1-3 mm. The main disadvantage of these approaches is that comparatively high stimulation pulse amplitudes are necessary to achieve sufficient loudness. This is because the conductivity between the active electrodes represents a low-impedance shunt conductance which causes most of the current to flow within the scala tympani and only a small portion to reach the sites of excitable neurons.

Regarding power consumption, the most effective electrode configuration is the monopolar configuration. Monopolar means that only one *active* electrode is within the scala tympani, and a remote return electrode is positioned outside. E.g., a 12-channel CIS system employing monopolar stimulation uses a 12-channel electrode array within the scala tympani and a return electrode which may by positioned under the temporal muscle and is shared by all 12 electrodes. In CIS, only one electrode of the array is active at any given time (non-overlapping pulses).

Remarkably, although spatial channel interaction in bipolar or multipolar configurations is substantially less than in monopolar configurations, this advantage in general cannot be converted to better speech perception, as has been shown in a number of studies (Loizou et al., 2003; Stickney et al., 2006; Xu et al., 2005). Thus, monopolar configurations are widely used in clinical applications.

The channel separation in systems using monopolar electrode configurations may be improved by a closer positioning of the active electrodes to the excitable structures. Such special electrode arrays are designated as "modiolus-hugging" or "perimodiolar" arrays, and a variety of designs have been developed (Lenarz et al., 2000; Wackym et al., 2004). However, one basic requirement of modiolus-hugging electrode arrays is that after implantation the array should not exert any permanent mechanical pressure on the structures within the cochlea, because mechanical pressure can damage neural tissue or cause ossification if applied to bony structures. As a matter of fact, this requirement is difficult to meet in most approaches. Temporal bone studies have shown that modiolus-hugging electrodes increase the danger of basilar membrane perforations and spiral lamina fractures (Gstoettner et al., 2001; Richter et al., 2002; Roland et al., 2000). Besides, even if the array is closer to the modiolus, the surrounding conductive fluids will still cause broad potential distributions, and it is questionable whether a substantial improvement of channel separation is possible at all.

2. Supporting concepts

Fine structure stimulation strategies require a precise representation of temporal information in individual electrode channels. Maintaining the CIS paradigm of using non-overlapping pulses, the precision of representation is limited by the minimum phase duration of sequentially applied biphasic stimuli (Zierhofer, 2001). To relax such limitations and allow the implementation of fine structure stimulation with reasonable phase durations on multiple channels, two "supporting concepts" are investigated, i.e., simultaneous stimulation in combination with "Channel Interaction Compensation" (CIC) and the "Selected Groups" (SG) concept.

Both supporting concepts may generally be useful also for envelope-based stimulation without temporal fine structure. For example, the power consumption of a cochlear implant may be reduced without compromising the hearing performance.

As a first step, the supporting concepts have been evaluated with envelope-based coding strategies and compared to a standard CIS reference strategy.

2.1 Simultaneous stimulation

2.1.1 Channel interaction compensation

For the stimulation concept presented here, the *simultaneous* activation of two or more electrodes in the scala tympani against a remote return (ground) electrode is considered. As a basic requirement for simultaneous stimulation, pulses are 100% synchronous in time and have equal phase polarities. In the following, such pulses are designated as "sign-correlated".

The injection of a stimulation current into a single electrode will cause a particular voltage distribution within the scala tympani. If currents are simultaneously injected in more than one electrode, the individual voltage distributions are superimposed.

The basic idea of CIC is to replace a particular number of sequentially applied stimulation pulses (CIS paradigm) by the same number of simultaneously applied sign-correlated pulses. However, the amplitudes of the simultaneous pulses are reduced such that the electrical potentials at the position of the electrodes remain unchanged. Regarding the practical realization in a cochlear implant with limited space- and power resources, CIC based on general assumptions regarding voltage distributions is a computational challenge.

The computational cost for CIC can be reduced significantly, if a model of voltage distributions as shown in Fig. 1 is used (Zierhofer & Schatzer, 2008).

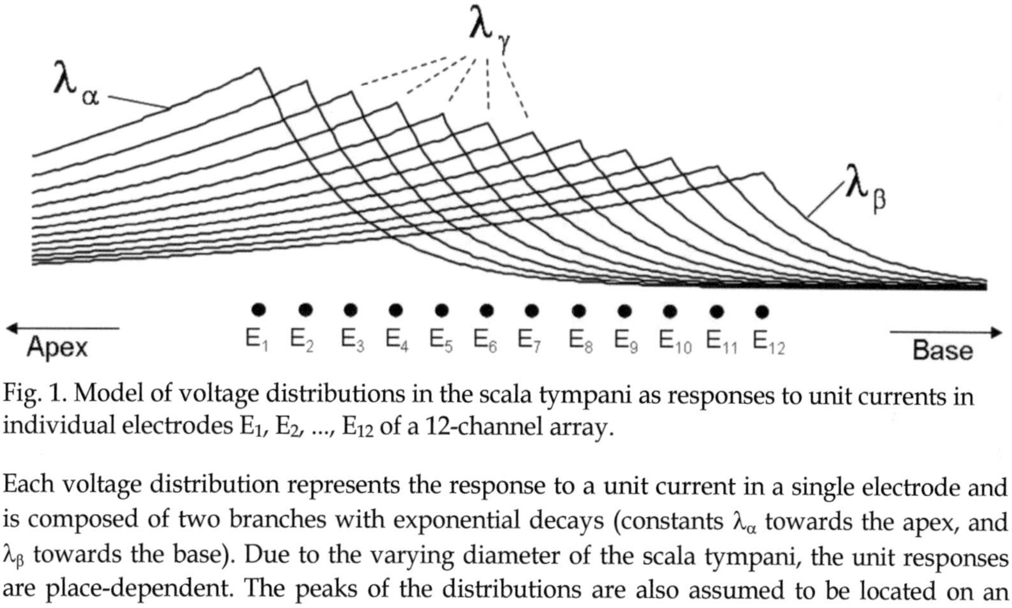

Fig. 1. Model of voltage distributions in the scala tympani as responses to unit currents in individual electrodes E_1, E_2, ..., E_{12} of a 12-channel array.

Each voltage distribution represents the response to a unit current in a single electrode and is composed of two branches with exponential decays (constants λ_α towards the apex, and λ_β towards the base). Due to the varying diameter of the scala tympani, the unit responses are place-dependent. The peaks of the distributions are also assumed to be located on an exponential characterized by constant λ_γ.

Assuming equally spaced electrodes (distance d), decay constants λ_α, λ_β, and λ_γ define CIC parameters α, β, and γ, i.e.,

$$\alpha = \exp\left(-\frac{d}{\lambda_\alpha}\right) \tag{1a}$$

$$\beta = \exp\left(-\frac{d}{\lambda_\beta}\right) \tag{1b}$$

$$\gamma = \exp\left(-\frac{d}{\lambda_\gamma}\right) \tag{1c}$$

Assuming M sequential amplitudes $I_{k,sequ}$ (k = 1, 2, ..., M) applied in M electrodes, the relation between the sequential amplitudes and the simultaneous amplitudes I_k (k = 1, 2, ..., M) is given by the set of linear equations

$$\begin{pmatrix} I_{sequ,1} \\ I_{sequ,2} \\ \cdots \\ I_{sequ,M} \end{pmatrix} = \mathbf{H} \begin{pmatrix} I_1 \\ I_2 \\ \cdots \\ I_M \end{pmatrix} \quad (2)$$

where **H** denotes the "interaction matrix"

$$\mathbf{H} = \begin{pmatrix} 1 & \gamma\alpha & (\gamma\alpha)^2 & \cdots & (\gamma\alpha)^{M-1} \\ \frac{\beta}{\gamma} & 1 & \gamma\alpha & \cdots & (\gamma\alpha)^{M-2} \\ \left(\frac{\beta}{\gamma}\right)^2 & \frac{\beta}{\gamma} & 1 & \cdots & (\gamma\alpha)^{M-3} \\ \cdots & \cdots & \cdots & \cdots & \cdots \\ \left(\frac{\beta}{\gamma}\right)^{M-1} & \left(\frac{\beta}{\gamma}\right)^{M-2} & \left(\frac{\beta}{\gamma}\right)^{M-3} & \cdots & 1 \end{pmatrix} \quad (3)$$

With (2), the simultaneous amplitudes are obtained with

$$\begin{pmatrix} I_1 \\ I_2 \\ \cdots \\ I_M \end{pmatrix} = \mathbf{H}^{-1} \begin{pmatrix} I_{sequ,1} \\ I_{sequ,2} \\ \cdots \\ I_{sequ,M} \end{pmatrix} \quad (4)$$

where $\mathbf{H}^{-1}$ represents the inverse matrix of **H**. It can be shown that, fortunately, matrix $\mathbf{H}^{-1}$ in general exists and is a tri-diagonal matrix. For a more detailed description the reader is referred to (Zierhofer & Schatzer, 2008).

2.1.2 Results

Sentence recognition in noise was assessed using the adaptive German Oldenburg sentence test (OLSA) in noise (Kollmeier & Wesselkamp, 1997). The test comprises 40 lists of 30 sentences each. The corpus is a closed set of nonsense sentences with a fixed name-verb-numeral-adjective-object word arrangement. As masker, unmodulated speech-shaped noise with the same spectral envelope as the long-term average spectrum of speech according to the standardized Comité Consultatif International Téléphonique et Télégraphique (CCITT) Rec. 227, was used (Fastl, 1993). The speech level was kept constant at comfortable loudness, while the level of the competing noise was varied adaptively. The speech reception threshold (SRT) was assessed at the 50% intelligibility point. The speech-noise mixture was fed into a MED-EL OPUS1 research processor via direct input (automatic gain control bypassed). Galvanic separation between PC sound card and speech processor was provided via an audio isolation transformer. The results of two experiments are presented here.

Experiment 1 assessed the effect of varying the number of simultaneous electrodes. Variations included 2, 3, 4, half and all electrodes stimulated simultaneously with optimum subject-specific CIC parameters α, β, and γ. In this experiment, the distances between simultaneously stimulated electrodes were maximized. For example, for configuration P2 in a ten-channel setting, the electrode addresses of simultaneously stimulated electrodes are [1, 6], [2, 7], [3, 8], [4, 9], and [5, 10].

Group results for six MED-EL CI users are shown in Fig. 2. Because the data did not meet the equal-variance criterion for the parametric analysis of variance (ANOVA) test, they were analysed with a non-parametric Friedman repeated-measures (RM) ANOVA test on ranks. This test revealed a significant effect of the number of simultaneous electrodes on speech test performance ($p < 0.05$). Post-hoc multiple comparisons using Dunn's method indicated a significantly inferior test performance with the all-simultaneous setting *Pall* in comparison to CIS.

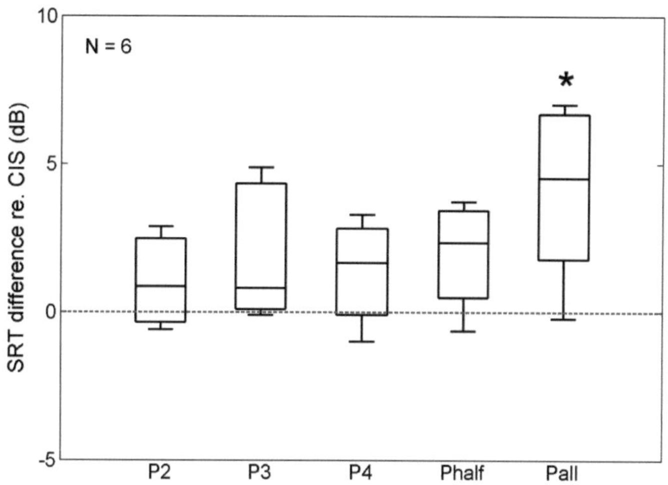

Fig. 2. SRT differences relative to CIS as a function of the number of simultaneous electrodes. Horizontal lines within the interquartile-range boxes indicate median SRT differences, whiskers encompass the ranges of SRT differences. The number of simultaneously activated electrodes was maximized. Only simultaneous stimulation of all electrodes significantly deteriorates test performance as compared to CIS (as marked by an asterisk).

Experiment 2 assessed the effect of varying the number of simultaneous channels for *adjacent* electrodes, in contrast to maximally separated electrodes as in the prior experiment. CIC parameters α, β, and γ were again individually adjusted.

Group means for five MED-EL CI users are shown in Fig. 3. A one-way RM ANOVA revealed no significant effect of electrode distances on mean SRTs ($F(2,12) = 0.016$, $p = 0.984$). Parametric test requirements for the ANOVA, i.e. normal distributions and equal variances, were verified with a Shapiro-Wilk ($p = 0.059$) and Levene test ($p = 0.963$), respectively.

However, because of the small sample size and the resulting low statistical power ($p = 0.049$) of this test, results have to be considered as preliminary.

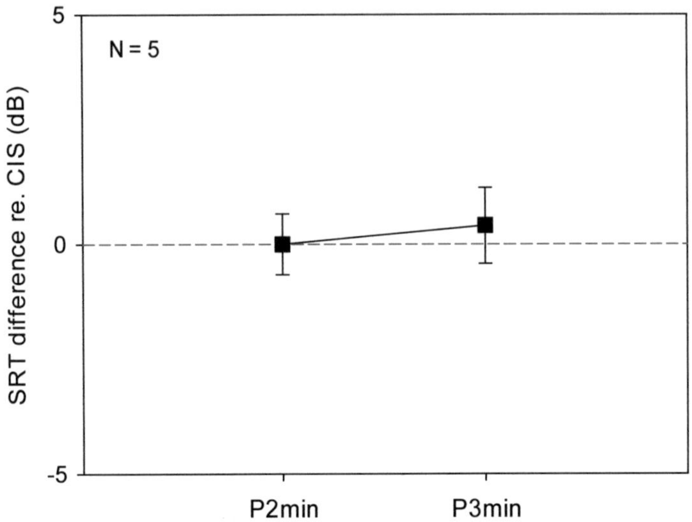

Fig. 3. SRT differences relative to CIS in a group of five subjects for two and three adjacent electrodes being stimulated simultaneously. Here, speech test performance is on a par to sequential stimulation with CIS, in contrast to the two- and three-electrodes settings P2 and P3 with maximum electrode separation in Fig. 2.

2.1.3 Discussion

Throughout all test conditions, including the CIS control condition, frame rates and phase durations were kept constant. In all configurations, the same amount of information was represented, which is why no advantage in performance of CIC as compared to CIS was expected.

Simultaneous stimulation on up to four maximally separated electrodes results in a slight, but not statistically significant, decrement in performance. When half of the electrodes are stimulated simultaneously, the decrement in performance is larger, but still not significant. The CIC configuration with all electrodes stimulated simultaneously leads to a statistically significant decrement in speech perception.

For CIC configurations with two or three neighboring electrodes the results are on a par with CIS and show no trend to a degradation of speech recognition. Thus, minimizing the distance between simultaneous electrodes is the recommended CIC configuration.

If the stimulation configuration is switched from a sequential to a simultaneous setting and the parameters are properly chosen, there should be no difference in loudness. Simultaneous stimulation *without* CIC leads to a percept that is too loud and requires an overall reduction of stimulation levels, e.g., by means of a volume control. However, this leads to an information loss in the stimulation pattern and speech perception is impaired (Zierhofer et al., 2009). On the other hand, *overcompensation* with CIC is also possible. If the spatial parameters α, β, and γ are set too high (e.g., too close to one), the perceived loudness is too low and an overall increase of stimulation levels is necessary. Also in this case, speech perception is compromised. Thus, the subjective loudness is an indication for the quality of the choice of CIC parameters α, β, and γ.

Regarding fine structure stimulation strategies, simultaneous stimulation based on CIC represents a powerful tool. The overall number of stimulation pulses per second can be increased without reducing the phase durations. For example, in a CIC configuration with two simultaneous electrodes, the overall number of stimulation pulses per second can be doubled by filling up the temporal gaps between pairs of simultaneous pulses by additional pairs of simultaneous pulses.

2.2 The "Selected Groups" approach

2.2.1 Concept

It is well known that neurons show refractory behaviour. Immediately after an action potential has been elicited, a neuron cannot fire again during the *absolute refractory period* (typically about 0.8 ms in the neurons of the auditory system). After that, the excitation threshold decreases to the normal value within the *relative refractory period* (typically 7-10 ms).

Spatial channel interaction in combination with the refractory properties of the neurons lead to pronounced masking effects. For example, in response to a first stimulation pulse, most neurons will be activated in the immediate proximity of the stimulation electrode, and the number of activated neurons will decrease with increasing distance to the electrode. These neurons cannot be retriggered during the absolute refractory period. If a second stimulation pulse in another electrode is applied in this period, its efficacy will depend on the distance between the two electrodes. If the second pulse occurs in an adjacent electrode, it will elicit additional action potentials only when the amplitude is approximately equal to or higher than the amplitude of the first pulse. If it is lower, it will be almost entirely masked by the first pulse and largely unable to elicit additional action potentials. It is intuitively clear that the neural activation pattern will not differ substantially if, as opposed to both stimulation pulses, only the pulse with the larger amplitude is applied. However, as the distance between activated electrodes is increasing, the minimum amplitude required to elicit additional neural activity gradually decreases.

The basic idea of the SG approach is to detect and avoid pulses with high masking factors (Kals et al., 2010; Zierhofer, 2007). Neighbouring stimulation channels, i.e. channels with presumably high interaction, are arranged into groups. Within each stimulation frame, a particular number of active channels with the highest amplitudes in each group are selected for stimulation. The pulses with the smaller amplitudes are omitted. With SG, a uniformly distributed stimulation activity over all cochlear regions is ensured, and a clustering of pulses at particular electrode positions is avoided.

In a formal notation, groups of channels are represented within brackets. The index after the closing bracket denotes the number of channels within a group which are selected for stimulation. For example, $[1\ 2]_1\ [3\ 4]_1\ [5\ 6]_1\ [7\ 8]_1\ [9\ 10]_1\ [11\ 12]_1$ represents a twelve-channel configuration, where two adjacent channels each form a group, resulting in six "Selected Groups". Within each one of these six groups, the channel with the larger amplitude is dynamically selected for stimulation. In short, such a configuration is denoted as SG_1/2.

Note that CIS and NofM represent special cases of the SG concept (McKay et al., 1991; Wilson et al., 1988). E.g., a twelve-channel CIS strategy would be described by $[1]_1$ $[2]_1$ $[3]_1$ $[4]_1$ $[5]_1$ $[6]_1$ $[7]_1$ $[8]_1$ $[9]_1$ $[10]_1$ $[11]_1$ $[12]_1$, corresponding to the trivial case of SG with group size one and one active channel per group (in short, this would be denoted as SG_1/1). A 6of12 strategy is described by $[1\ 2\ 3\ 4\ 5\ 6\ 7\ 8\ 9\ 10\ 11\ 12]_6$, corresponding to SG with one single group comprising all twelve channels from which six are dynamically picked (in short, this is denoted as SG_6/12).

2.2.2 Results

Speech recognition with CIS and SG was assessed by measuring SRTs for German OLSA sentences in CCITT noise. Throughout all test conditions, including the CIS control condition, frame rates were kept constant. Two experiments were conducted.

Experiment 1 assessed the effect of group size variations, using the same phase durations as for CIS. Thus, according to the SG algorithm, stimulation pulses were simply discarded, and the resulting gaps were not filled with any additional pulses.

Individual and group means of the SRTs for nine tested ears (N = 9) are shown in Fig. 4. Mean SRTs for SG_1/2, SG_1/3, and SG_1/4 increased respectively by 0.3±0.5 dB, 0.6±0.9 dB, and 1.8±1.0 dB (mean±95% confidence interval) compared to the CIS control condition. A one-way RM ANOVA (Shapiro-Wilk normality test $p = 0.326$, Levene equal variance test $p = 0.758$) revealed a significant effect of the group size on mean SRTs ($p < 0.001$, $F(3,24) = 9.275$). Post-hoc Holm-Sidak multiple comparisons against CIS indicated a significant difference for SG_1/4 only ($p = 0.004$, $\alpha = 0.017$). Conditions SG_1/2 ($p = 0.163$, $\alpha = 0.050$) and SG_1/3 ($p = 0.189$, $\alpha = 0.025$) were not significantly different from CIS.

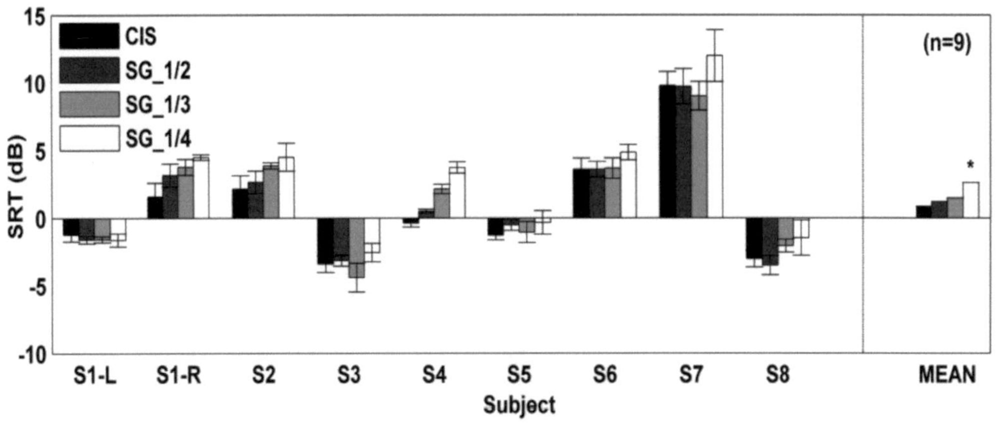

Fig. 4. SRTs for OLSA sentences in CCITT noise in eight subjects with CIS and three SG configurations including group sizes of two, three, and four. Error bars represent the standard deviations in the individual results. A significant difference among group means in comparison to CIS was found for setting SG_1/4. (From Kals et al., 2009. Used with permission of Elsevier B.V.)

Experiment 2 assessed the effect of doubling pulse phase durations with SG. Only one SG condition with a group size of two was used, and the phase durations of the stimulation pulses were doubled compared to CIS. Configurations with doubled pulse phase duration are denoted with the suffix "2DUR". For double phase duration, new MCL and THR levels were determined.

Results are summarized in Fig. 5, showing individual and group means of SRTs for six tested ears (N = 6). The mean SRT for SG_1/2-2DUR was 0.5±0.9 dB lower than the mean SRT for CIS. However, this difference was not significant ($p = 0.184$, $t(5) = 1.540$; Shapiro-Wilk normality test $p = 0.799$). Due to the small sample size and low statistical power of the test ($p = 0.155$), however, results need to be regarded as preliminary. The doubling of phase durations resulted in a significant reduction of both MCL and THR currents. MCL and THR levels were lower by 5.0±2.2 dB ($p = 0.002$) and 7.1±4.3 dB ($p = 0.008$), respectively.

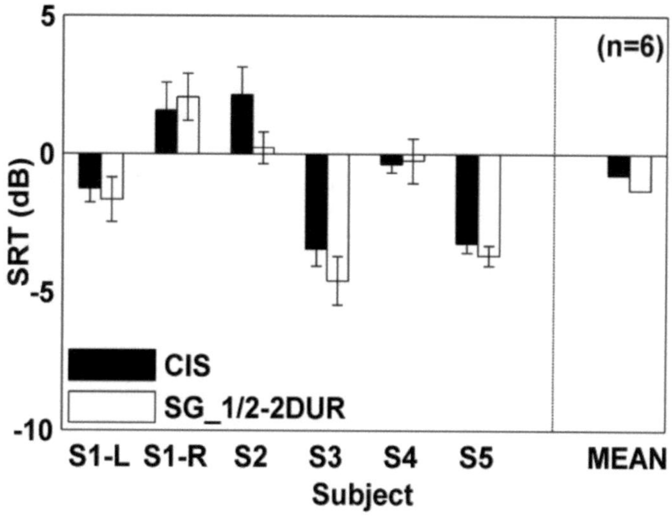

Fig. 5. SRTs for OLSA sentences in CCITT noise in five subjects with CIS and SG with doubled phase duration and a group size of two. Error bars represent the standard deviations in the individual results. No statistically significant differences between group means ($\alpha = 0.05$) were found. (From Kals et al., 2009. Used with permission of Elsevier B.V.)

2.2.3 Discussion

For group sizes two and three, SG supports the same sentence recognition in noise as CIS. This suggests that a dynamic selection of up to one third of the stimulation pulses with SG still includes all relevant pulses, at least for this particular type of test materials. SG provides a simple and robust selection algorithm for increasing the efficacy of the applied stimulation pulses and does not require any subject-specific parameters. Hence, the application in current implant designs is straightforward. With a further pulse reduction (group sizes larger than three), SG starts to suppress relevant pulses, resulting in a significant decrement in performance.

The dynamic channel-picking with SG may be utilized to increase pulse phase durations and consequently reduce pulse amplitudes, yielding to less stringent implant supply voltage requirements. In our test setup, pulse amplitude reductions of about 40% with doubled phase durations and a group size of two supported sentence recognition scores which were on a par with CIS. Such a reduction is likely to be beneficial for future designs of low-power or totally implantable cochlear implants. Additionally, longer phase durations resulted in larger electrode dynamic ranges, which may support better speech reception in CI users.

During testing, subjective sound quality was informally assessed with settings including both standard and longer phase durations. All test settings were presented multiple times in random order to the subjects, with live speech or speech test materials as input signals. Subjects did not know which setting was presented at any time. Most of them indicated SG_1/2-2DUR as their preferred setting.

3. Electric-acoustic pitch comparisons in unilateral CI subjects

In the peripheral auditory system, frequency information is thought to be encoded by a combination of two mechanisms. The first mechanism, or place principle, is based on the notion that the place of maximum excitation along the organ of Corti changes systematically as function of stimulus frequency, as previously mentioned (von Békésy, 1960; von Helmholtz, 1863). Low frequencies are "mapped" at the cochlear apex and high frequencies at the cochlear base. For humans and other mammals, cochlear frequency-place maps are well known (Greenwood, 1990, 1961). The second mechanism, or time principle, hypothesizes that stimulus frequency is encoded in the temporal structure of neural discharge patterns. Mediated by the phase locking properties of auditory nerve fibers (Johnson, 1980), neural discharges occur in synchrony to the individual harmonics of subharmonics of a stimulus waveform.

Cochlear implants implicitly assume that both place and time principles equally apply for electrical stimulation, as they do for normal acoustic stimulation. Frequency bands in implant speech processors are assigned to electrodes in tonotopic order. With CIS and related coding strategies, channel envelope modulations sampled by interleaved constant-rate pulse carriers represent a temporal code for periodic harmonic stimuli. However, due to the vastly different modality of neural excitation with electric and acoustic stimulation, the frequency-place map for electrical stimulation might differ from Greenwood's map for humans, and temporal cues to pitch mediated by phase locking may be encoded more robustly using other stimulus patterns than the CIS channel envelopes sampled at constant pulse rates. Although studies show that learning can compensate to a certain extent for a frequency-place mismatch (Svirsky et al., 2004), an optimal assignment of frequency bands based on a measured electrical frequency-place map may be beneficial in terms of CI performance and how fast asymptotic levels of performance are reached in newly implanted CI users.

In recent years, cochlear implants have become an effective treatment option for patients with single-sided deafness and intractable ipsilateral tinnitus (Van de Heyning et al., 2008). With near-normal hearing in one and a CI in the contralateral ear, direct comparisons of normal and electric hearing are possible in this unique subject population. At our laboratory, we were in the fortunate situation to study such a group of unilateral CI subjects implanted by Prof. Van de Heyning at the University Hospital Antwerp, Belgium. One aim of the study was to assess the frequency-place map for high-rate electrical stimulation, using a different methodology than similar studies in CI users with contralateral hearing (Boëx et al., 2006; Carlyon et al., 2010; Dorman et al., 2007; Vermeire et al., 2008). The second aim was to investigate the relative contributions of rate and place to pitch, in particular for low frequencies, i. e. in the apical region. Preliminary results from this study have been presented by the authors and colleagues (Schatzer et al., 2009a; Vermeire et al., 2009).

In our study group, the frequency-place maps were between Greenwood and one octave below at basal and medial electrode positions, levelling off in the apical region to on average correspond to Greenwood. This levelling-off is likely to be a consequence of the absence of any temporal code in the constant-amplitude 1.5 kpulses/sec pulse trains that could be perceived by CI users (with electrical stimulation, there seems to be a canonical pitch saturation limit of 300-500 Hz, where a further increase of pulse rate does not result in a further increase of perceived pitch, as for lower rates), but may also be due to the cochlear anatomy in the apex. Whereas in the basal cochlear turn auditory nerve fibers innervating the organ of Corti take a radial course, in the apical turn they gradually take on a more tangential course. Additionally, the spiral ganglion holding the cell bodies of the bipolar auditory neurons does not reach all the way to the apical turn, forming a cluster of cell bodies at its apical end. As electrodes sit in close proximity to the organ of Corti, current spread on apical electrodes may target more innervating fibers or spiral ganglion cells as on basal electrodes, producing a broader and less distinct pitch percept.

The most interesting finding emerging from the second experiment was that for electrical stimulation place and rate, or in other words spatial and temporal cues, may have to match to produce a robust pitch percept. For instance, most subjects could only match electrical stimuli reliably to low-frequency pure tones ranging from 100 to 200 Hz, if those electrical stimuli had a correspondingly low pulse rate and were applied on electrodes inserted more than 360 degrees from the round window into the cochlea. Thus, in order to produce low pitch percepts in the F0 range, electrodes need to be placed beyond the first cochlear turn. This finding is of particular relevance to the design of coding strategies that represent within-channel temporal fine structure information as channel-specific rate codes on apical electrodes, as discussed in in the following section.

This observation is consistent with findings in normal-hearing listeners. Oxenham and colleagues (Oxenham et al., 2004) demonstrated that pitch discrimination thresholds for "transposed" acoustic stimuli, where the temporal information of low-frequency sinusoids is presented to locations in the cochlea tuned to high frequencies, are significantly deteriorated compared to discrimination thresholds for pure tones. Also, using harmonic transposed stimuli, they found that subjects were largely unable to extract the fundamental frequency from multiple low-frequency harmonics presented to high-frequency cochlear regions. These results also indicate the importance of a match between temporal and tonotopic cues for a robust pitch perception.

4. Temporal fine structure with Channel Specific Sampling Sequences

4.1 Concept

The basic idea of a stimulation strategy based on "Channel Specific Sampling Sequences" (CSSS) is to add fine time information to the envelope information already present in a speech processor, at least in the low-frequency filter bands (Zierhofer, 2003). For this, a particular stimulation pulse sequence composed of high-rate biphasic pulses (typically 5 kpulses/sec per channel) is associated to the filter channel. Such a sequence is designated as "Channel Specific Sampling Sequence" and has a programmable length (number of pulses) and a programmable amplitude distribution. The length of a CSSS sequence can be anywhere from a single-pulse to a sequence of 16 pulses.

For stimulation, the sequences are triggered by the zero-crossings (e.g., negative-to-positive) of the band pass filter output signal. The individual sequences are weighted by the instantaneous envelopes of the output signal. Note that such a stimulation sequence contains both envelope- and temporal fine structure information. An example is shown in Fig. 6, where the sampling sequence is a pair of pulses. The sampling sequences are started at every other zero crossing of the band pass filter output (upper panel). The weights of the sequences are derived from the envelope of the band pass output signal.

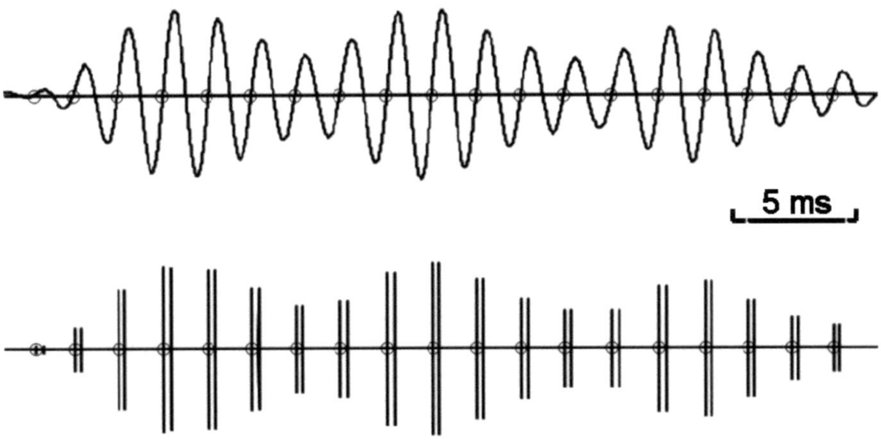

Fig. 6. Example for stimulation according to the CSSS concept. Upper panel: Output of a band pass filter from 450 to 603 Hz. Lower panel: CSSS stimulation sequence. Each vertical line represents a biphasic stimulation pulse. Here, the sampling sequences are double pulses, separated by 0.25 ms. The sequences are started at every other zero crossing of the band pass output.

Given the phase-locking limit of primary auditory neurons (Johnson, 1980) and the finding that in CI subjects the so-called "rate pitch" shows an upper boundary at about 300-500 pulses/sec in most subjects (Wilson et al., 1997; Zeng, 2002), but can also extend up to about 1 kpulses/sec (Hochmair-Desoyer et al., 1983; Kong & Carlyon, 2010), a stimulation based on CSSS seems appropriate only for stimulation channels below about 1 kHz. For higher-frequency channels, CIS stimulation based on envelope information only is applied. Thus, in practical implementations, a mixture between low-frequency CSSS channels and high-frequency CIS channels will be reasonable. For convenience, such a mixture between CSSS and CIS channels is designated as CSSS concept in the following.

4.2 Results

Effects of CSSS fine structure stimulation on speech recognition in competing-voice backgrounds and for the recognition of tonal languages have been investigated in recent studies, conducted at our laboratories and at Queen Mary Hospital in Hong Kong, China (Schatzer et al., 2010).

4.2.1 CSSS study in our laboratories

Subjects and strategy settings

In eight MED-EL implant subjects, SRTs were measured for OLSA sentences using a female-talker sentence as masker. Strategies were fitted and tested acutely with no listening experience for the subjects.

The overall frequency range for both CIS and CSSS settings was 80 to 8500 Hz. For CSSS, 4 CSSS channels from 80 to 800 Hz were arranged in two selected groups $[1\ 2]_1$ and $[3\ 4]_1$. Maximum pulse rates were 4545 and 1515 pulses/sec on CSSS and CIS channels, respectively. Sequences were double pulses on CSSS channels 1 and 2 and single pulses on CSSS channels 3 and 4.

Results and discussion

Individual and group results for the eight subjects are shown in Fig. 7. A paired *t*-test revealed a statistically significant difference among group means of 1.0 dB ($p = 0.008$, $t(12) = 3.192$, Shapiro-Wilk normality test $p = 0.675$), with better performance for the CSSS condition.

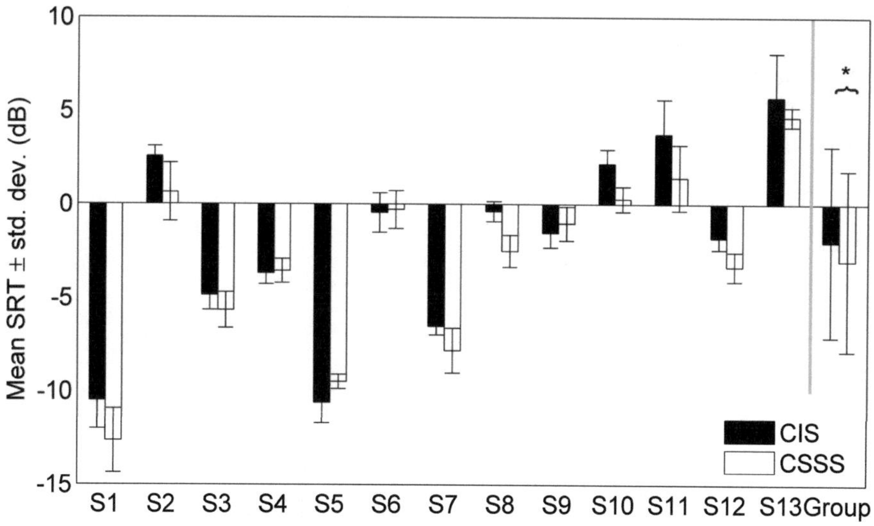

Fig. 7. Individual and group results for OLSA sentences presented with a competing female-talker masking sentence.

In this study a significant improvement in speech perception was found in acute tests. Results reported in literature often do not find an initial benefit for CSSS (Schatzer et al., 2009b), but an improvement over time (Lorens et al., 2010; Riss et al., 2011).

4.2.2 CSSS study in Hong Kong

Subjects and test materials

Twelve adult and experienced implant users participated in this study. All subjects are native speakers of Cantonese and implanted with MED-EL C40+ or $PULSAR_{CI}{}^{100}$ devices with full electrode insertions. At the time of testing, all participants were users of the MED-EL TEMPO+ speech processor and had no prior exposure to temporal fine structure stimulation.

Test materials included the Cantonese lexical tone identification test and the Cantonese Hearing in Noise (CHINT) sentence test. The tone identification test was presented at a subject-specific constant SNR, i.e. CCITT noise was added on a per-subject basis to avoid ceiling effects, if necessary. Acutely compared test settings comprised CIS and CSSS.

The overall frequency range for both CIS and CSSS settings was 100 to 8500 Hz. For CSSS, 4 CSSS channels from 100 to 800 Hz were arranged in two selected groups $[1\ 2]_1$ and $[3\ 4]_1$. Maximum pulse rates were 4545 and 1515 pulses/sec on CSSS and CIS channels, respectively. Sequences on CSSS channels were quarter-sine shaped. For further details, the reader is referred to (Schatzer et al., 2010).

Results and discussion

Group results of CIS and CSSS performance for Cantonese tones and sentences are illustrated in Fig. 8. Mean identification scores of Cantonese lexical tones in 12 subjects were 59.2±15.2 % (mean±standard deviation) with CIS and 59.2±15.3 % with CSSS, indicating identical intelligibility with CIS and fine structure stimulation (paired t-test on percent-correct scores, $p = 0.972$, $t(11) = 0.036$; Shapiro-Wilk normality test $p = 0.873$). Mean identification scores for CHINT sentences were 54.2±27.7 % with CIS and 55.9±22.8 % with CSSS, indicating no significant difference (paired t-test, $p = 0.676$, $t(7) = 0.436$; Shapiro-Wilk normality test $p = 0.539$).

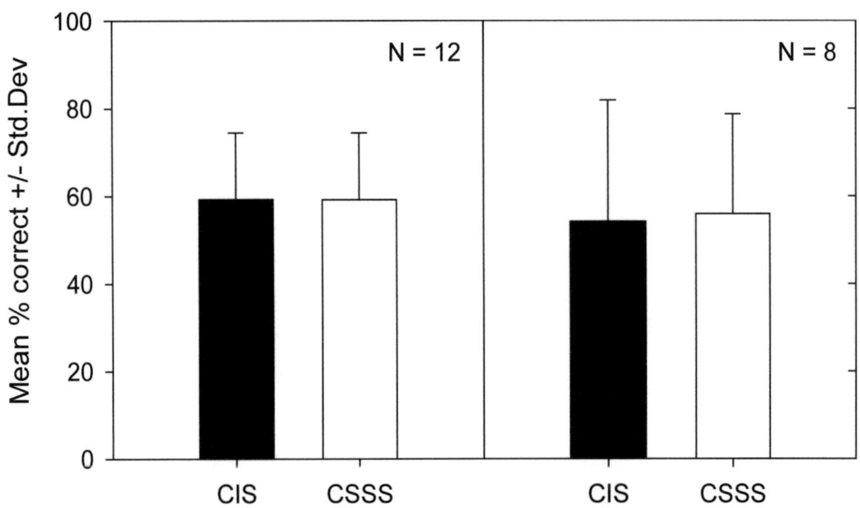

Fig. 8. Group results for Cantonese tone identification (left panel, 12 subjects) and CHINT sentences (right panel, 8 subjects) with CIS and CSSS, respectively.

These findings are consistent with results from studies in which experienced CI users were switched from CIS to fine structure stimulation, showing equal performance for the two coding strategies at baseline, and a statistically significant benefit with fine structure stimulation only after weeks or even months of fine structure use (Arnoldner et al., 2007).

4.2.3 Expanded pitch range with CSSS

When being switched from CIS to fine structure stimulation with CSSS, many CI recipients report an overall pitch shift towards lower frequencies. This effect was explored and quantified.

Subjects and methods

Seven experienced cochlear implant subjects participated in the study. The stimuli were 500 ms harmonic tone complexes with a spectral roll-off of 9 dB per octave, presented via the direct input of an OPUS1 research speech processor. All stimuli were carefully balanced for equal loudness before running the actual experiment. Additionally, in order to prevent the participants from basing their decisions on residual loudness differences, amplitudes were roved by 2 dB during the main experiment.

For pitch comparisons, a method of constant stimuli was utilized. Subjects were asked to compare the pitch of the harmonic tone complexes presented in two 500-ms intervals separated by 300 ms. In the first interval a harmonic tone was presented with the first strategy (either CSSS or CIS), in the second interval another harmonic tone was presented with the second strategy. Based on psychometric functions fitted to the data, points of subjective equivalence were derived. These indicated which pair of F0s elicited the same pitch when one of them was processed with the CSSS strategy and the other one was processed with the CIS strategy. For a more detailed description of the study the reader is referred to (Krenmayr et al., 2011).

Results and discussion

A summary of the results is illustrated in Fig. 9. For each one of the four reference frequencies, the frequency difference between CSSS and CIS required for identical pitch is plotted.

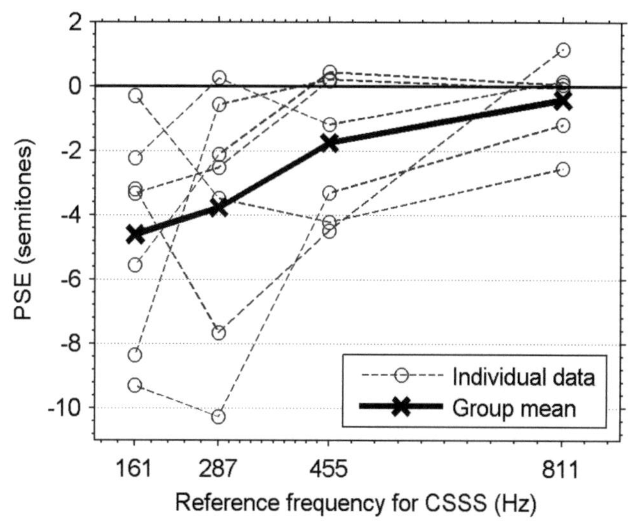

Fig. 9. Pitch differences between CSSS and CIS, expressed in semitones, as a function of F0. Dotted lines represent the individual data, the solid black line indicates the group mean. The pitch difference is most pronounced at low frequencies and vanishes towards higher frequencies, where the stimulation patterns of CSSS and CIS become more and more alike. (From Krenmayr et al., 2011. Used with permission of Maney Publishing.)

The results indicate that the pitch of a given harmonic tone complex decreases when presenting it with CSSS compared to when presenting it with CIS. On average, this pitch shift was 5 semitones or one perfect fourth at the lowest tested F0 (161 Hz). As expected, this pitch shift decreased at higher F0s. At 287 Hz it was 4 semitones or one major third, while at 455 Hz it was already reduced to 2 semitones or one major second. At the "blank trial" frequency of 811 Hz, the group mean was 0.5 semitones. Since these data were collected with one strategy as reference stimulus only, they can still contain possible subjective response bias. However, this response bias is expected to average out when calculating the group mean. Therefore the blank trial gives an estimate for the accuracy of the method.

The study quantitatively shows that explicitly stimulating the fine structure component of the lowest partials decreases the pitch of harmonic tone complexes with fundamental frequencies below 811 Hz. Since the pitches produced by both coding strategies converge at 811 Hz, it can be concluded that fine structure stimulation expands the range of perceivable pitches as compared to CIS.

As the present results are only based on a small number of subjects, further studies are needed to support the findings. However, the robustness of F0 representation with CSSS has also been demonstrated in another, more recent study (Bader et al., 2011). There, two pulse trains of *equal rates* have been applied in two neighbouring apical electrodes. In a ranking experiment, pitch percepts have been compared for dual-electrode pulse trains which were almost in phase (they were not completely in phase because of sequential stimulation) and dual-electrode pulse trains which were out of phase (phase shift π). Remarkably, the pitch percept in the latter case did not correspond to that of a stimulus with twice the rate of the individual pulse trains as could be expected in the case of spatial channel interaction, but just shifted slightly towards higher frequencies. Interestingly, Macherey and Carlyon found similar results of very low temporal channel interaction at low rates for phase-shifted pulse trains on electrode pairs which are not positioned in the apical, but the middle range of the cochlea (Macherey & Carlyon, 2010).

5. Conclusion

The introduction of the CIS strategy certainly represented a breakthrough in the field of cochlear implants. In its standard version, CIS provides an optimized level of speech perception for Western languages. CIS is first of all based on the tonotopic principle of hearing. The temporal information is limited to envelope signals.

Fine structure stimulation aims at representing temporal cues beyond envelopes and thus is based on the periodicity principle of hearing. Experiences with early cochlear implants (i.e., with single channel devices) and also more recent studies show that such temporal cues indeed can be used in a frequency range up to about 1 kHz. This essentially covers the ranges of the fundamental frequency F0 and the first formant frequency F1.

The need for a precise representation of both envelope and fine structure information lead to the development of two supporting concepts, i.e., simultaneous stimulation based on CIC and SG. Both concepts have been evaluated with envelope-based stimulation strategies without temporal fine structure. Among CIC settings, configurations with neighbouring simultaneous channels resulted in speech test performance on a par with CIS. So far, only two and three neighbouring channels have been investigated, and studies with even more simultaneous channels are currently conducted. SG settings yielded no statistically significant difference to CIS for group sizes of two and three. However, also for these group sizes, a tendency to a reduction of speech perception scores was observed.

Implant subjects with unilateral deafness and contralateral normal hearing provide the possibility to directly compare electrical and acoustic hearing. An important finding from pitch matching studies in unilaterally deaf subjects was that the perception of low frequencies in the F0 range requires electrode insertion depths greater than 360 degrees, in combination with adequate low-frequency temporal cues. Thus, a sufficient insertion depth of the electrodes represents a *necessary condition*. If electrodes are not inserted deeply enough, low rate temporal cues alone do not produce low pitch percepts.

A strategy based on CSSS combines fine structure and envelope information. High-rate pulse packages are triggered at every other zero crossing of the band pass output signals, and the weights of the sequences are derived from the band pass envelopes. Practical configurations are mixtures of CSSS channels in the low frequency region (e.g., 100-800 Hz covering the F0 and F1 regions) and CIS channels for the higher frequencies (e.g., 800-8500 Hz). When being switched from a CIS to a CSSS stimulation setting, most patients perceive an immediate downward pitch shift. This effect has been quantified. On average, pitch shifts of five semitones at the low frequency end were measured. This is a clear indication that the additional temporal information represented in the low frequency CSSS channels can indeed be perceived despite the presence of spatial channel interaction. Besides, many patients are reporting an improvement in sound quality with fine structure stimulation. Typically, they report the sound being fuller and more natural as compared to their CIS settings. In acute tests, speech perception with CSSS is often on a par with CIS. However, there is increasing evidence that with fine structure stimulation, speech performance does improve over time, even in CI users with long-term implant experience.

6. Acknowledgements

The authors would like to acknowledge the contributions of Mathias Kals, Andreas Krenmayr, and Daniel Visser in conducting many of the experiments and evaluating the results. In addition, we would like to thank all of the subjects participating in our studies for their time and dedication.

7. References

Arnoldner, C.; Riss, D.; Brunner, M.; Durisin, M.; Baumgartner, W. D. & Hamzavi, J. S. (2007). Speech and music perception with the new fine structure speech coding strategy: preliminary results. *Acta Otolaryngol*, Vol. 127, No. 12, (Dec), pp. 1298-303, ISSN 0001-6489 (Print)

Bader, P.; Schatzer, R.; Vermeire, K.; Van de Heyning, P.; Visser, D.; Krenmayr, A.; Kals, M. & Zierhofer, C. (2011). Pitch of dual-electrode stimuli as a function of rate and electrode separation, *Conference on Implantable Auditory Prostheses,* Pacific Grove, CA, July 24-29, 2011

Boëx, C.; Baud, L.; Cosendai, G.; Sigrist, A. & Kós, M.-I. (2006). Acoustic to electric pitch comparisons in cochlear implant subjects with residual hearing. *J Assoc Res Otolaryngol,* Vol. 7, No. 2, (Jun), pp. 110-124, ISSN 1525-3961 (Print)

Carlyon, R. P.; Macherey, O.; Frijns, J. H.; Axon, P. R.; Kalkman, R. K.; Boyle, P.; Baguley, D. M.; Briggs, J.; Deeks, J. M.; Briaire, J. J.; Barreau, X. & Dauman, R. (2010). Pitch comparisons between electrical stimulation of a cochlear implant and acoustic stimuli presented to a normal-hearing contralateral ear. *J Assoc Res Otolaryngol,* Vol. 11, No. 4, (Dec), pp. 625-640, ISSN 1525-3961 (Print)

Dorman, M. F.; Spahr, T.; Gifford, R.; Loiselle, L.; McKarns, S.; Holden, T.; Skinner, M. & Finley, C. (2007). An electric frequency-to-place map for a cochlear implant patient with hearing in the nonimplanted ear. *J Assoc Res Otolaryngol,* Vol. 8, No. 2, (Jun), pp. 234-240, ISSN 1525-3961 (Print)

Fastl, H. (1993). A masking noise for speech intelligibility tests, *Proceedings of TC Hearing,* H-93–70, Acoust. Society of Japan

Greenwood, D. D. (1990). A cochlear frequency-position function for several species--29 years later. *J Acoust Soc Am,* Vol. 87, No. 6, (Jun), pp. 2592-2605, ISSN 0001-4966 (Print)

Greenwood, D. D. (1961). Critical bandwidth and the frequency coordinates of the basilar membrane. *J Acoust Soc Am,* Vol. 33, No. 10, pp. 1344-1356, ISSN 0001-4966 (Print)

Gstoettner, W. K.; Adunka, O.; Franz, P.; Hamzavi, J., Jr.; Plenk, H., Jr.; Susani, M.; Baumgartner, W. & Kiefer, J. (2001). Perimodiolar electrodes in cochlear implant surgery. *Acta Otolaryngol,* Vol. 121, No. 2, (Jan), pp. 216-219

Hilbert, D. (1912). *Grundzüge einer allgemeinen Theorie der linearen Integralgleichungen,* B. G. Teubner, Leipzig, Berlin

Hochmair-Desoyer, I. J.; Hochmair, E. S.; Burian, K. & Stiglbrunner, H. K. (1983). Percepts from the Vienna cochlear prosthesis. *Ann N Y Acad Sci,* Vol. 405, pp. 295-306, ISSN 0077-8923 (Print)

Johnson, D. H. (1980). The relationship between spike rate and synchrony in responses of auditory-nerve fibers to single tones. *J Acoust Soc Am,* Vol. 68, No. 4, pp. 1115-1122, ISSN 0001-4966 (Print)

Kals, M.; Schatzer, R.; Krenmayr, A.; Vermeire, K.; Visser, D.; Bader, P.; Neustetter, C.; Zangerl, M. & Zierhofer, C. (2010). Results with a cochlear implant channel-picking strategy based on "Selected Groups". *Hear Res,* Vol. 260, No. 1-2, (Feb), pp. 63-69, ISSN 1878-5891 (Electronic)

Kollmeier, B. & Wesselkamp, M. (1997). Development and evaluation of a German sentence test for objective and subjective speech intelligibility assessment. *J Acoust Soc Am,* Vol. 102, No. 4, pp. 2412-2421

Kong, Y. Y. & Carlyon, R. P. (2010). Temporal pitch perception at high rates in cochlear implants. *J Acoust Soc Am,* Vol. 127, No. 5, (May), pp. 3114-23, ISSN 1520-8524 (Electronic)

Krenmayr, A.; Visser, D.; Schatzer, R. & Zierhofer, C. (2011). The effects of fine structure stimulation on pitch perception with cochlear implants. *Cochlear Implants International,* Vol. 12, No. Suppl. 1, pp. S70-72, ISSN 1467-0100 (Print). Available online at www.maney.co.uk/journals/cim and www.ingentaconnect.com/content/maney/cii

Lenarz, T.; Battmer, R. D.; Goldring, J. E.; Neuburger, J.; Kuzma, J. & Reuter, G. (2000). New electrode concepts (modiolus-hugging electrodes), in *Updates in Cochlear Implantation.* vol. 57, C. S. Kim & S. O. Chang, Eds., ed Basel: Karger, 2000, pp. 347-353

Loizou, P. C.; Poroy, O. & Dorman, M. (2000). The effect of parametric variations of cochlear implant processors on speech understanding. *J Acoust Soc Am,* Vol. 108, No. 2, pp. 790-802

Loizou, P. C.; Stickney, G.; Mishra, L. & Assmann, P. (2003). Comparison of speech processing strategies used in the Clarion implant processor. *Ear Hear,* Vol. 24, No. 1, (Feb), pp. 12-19

Lorens, A.; Zgoda, M.; Obrycka, A. & Skarzynski, H. (2010). Fine Structure Processing improves speech perception as well as objective and subjective benefits in pediatric MED-EL COMBI 40+ users. *Int J Pediatr Otorhinolaryngol,* Vol. 74, No. 12, (Dec), pp. 1372-8, ISSN 1872-8464 (Electronic)

Macherey, O. & Carlyon, R. P. (2010). Temporal pitch percepts elicited by dual-channel stimulation of a cochlear implant. *J Acoust Soc Am,* Vol. 127, No. 1, (Jan), pp. 339-49, ISSN 1520-8524 (Electronic)

McKay, C.; McDermott, H.; Vandali, A. & Clark, G. (1991). Preliminary Results with a Six Spectral Maxima Sound Processor for the University of Melbourne/Nucleus Multiple-Electrode Cochlear Implant. *J Otolaryng Soc Austral,* Vol. 6, No. 5, pp. 254-359, ISSN 0030-6614

Miyoshi, S.; Sakajiri, M.; Ifukube, T. & Matsushima, J. (1997). Evaluation of the tripolar electrode stimulation method by numerical analysis and animal experiments for cochlear implants. *Acta Otolaryngol Suppl,* Vol. 532, pp. 123-125, ISSN 0365-5237 (Print)

Morse, R. P. & Evans, E. F. (1999). Additive noise can enhance temporal coding in a computational model of analogue cochlear implant stimulation. *Hear Res,* Vol. 133, No. 1-2, (Jul), pp. 107-119, ISSN 0378-5955 (Print)

Oxenham, A. J.; Bernstein, J. G. & Penagos, H. (2004). Correct tonotopic representation is necessary for complex pitch perception. *Proc Natl Acad Sci U S A,* Vol. 101, No. 5, (Feb 3), pp. 1421-1425, ISSN 0027-8424 (Print)

Richter, B.; Aschendorff, A.; Lohnstein, P.; Husstedt, H.; Nagursky, H. & Laszig, R. (2002). Clarion 1.2 standard electrode array with partial space-filling positioner: radiological and histological evaluation in human temporal bones. *J Laryngol Otol,* Vol. 116, No. 7, (Jul), pp. 507-513, ISSN 0022-2151 (Print)

Riss, D.; Hamzavi, J. S.; Katzinger, M.; Baumgartner, W. D.; Kaider, A.; Gstoettner, W. & Arnoldner, C. (2011). Effects of fine structure and extended low frequencies in pediatric cochlear implant recipients. *Int J Pediatr Otorhinolaryngol,* Vol. 75, No. 4, (Apr), pp. 573-8, ISSN 1872-8464 (Electronic)

Roland, J. T., Jr.; Fishman, A. J.; Alexiades, G. & Cohen, N. L. (2000). Electrode to modiolus proximity: a fluoroscopic and histologic analysis. *Am J Otol,* Vol. 21, No. 2, (Mar), pp. 218-225, ISSN 0192-9763 (Print)

Rubinstein, J. T.; Wilson, B. S.; Finley, C. C. & Abbas, P. J. (1999). Pseudospontaneous activity: stochastic independence of auditory nerve fibers with electrical stimulation. *Hear Res,* Vol. 127, No. 1-2, pp. 108-118

Schatzer, R.; Krenmayr, A.; Au, D. K.; Kals, M. & Zierhofer, C. (2010). Temporal fine structure in cochlear implants: preliminary speech perception results in Cantonese-speaking implant users. *Acta Otolaryngol,* Vol. 130, No. 9, (Feb 9), pp. 1031-9, ISSN 0001-6489 (Print)

Schatzer, R.; Vermeire, K.; Van de Heyning, P.; Voormolen, M.; Visser, D.; Krenmayr, A.; Kals, M. & Zierhofer, C. (2009a). A tonotopic map of the electrically stimulated cochlea from CI users with contralateral normal hearing, *Conference on Implantable Auditory Prostheses*, Lake Tahoe, CA, July 12-17, 2009

Schatzer, R.; Visser, D.; Krenmayr, A.; Kals, M.; Vermeire, K.; Neustetter, C.; Zangerl, M.; Bader, P. & Zierhofer, C. (2009b). Recognition of speech with a competing talker using fine structure in cochlear implants, *Conference on Implantable Auditory Prostheses*, Lake Tahoe, CA, July 12-17, 2009

Smith, Z. M.; Delgutte, B. & Oxenham, A. J. (2002). Chimaeric sounds reveal dichotomies in auditory perception. *Nature,* Vol. 416, No. 6876, (Mar 7), pp. 87-90, ISSN 0028-0836 (Print)

Stickney, G. S.; Loizou, P. C.; Mishra, L. N.; Assmann, P. F.; Shannon, R. V. & Opie, J. M. (2006). Effects of electrode design and configuration on channel interactions. *Hear Res,* Vol. 211, No. 1-2, (Jan), pp. 33-45, ISSN 0378-5955 (Print)

Svirsky, M. A.; Silveira, A.; Neuburger, H.; Teoh, S. W. & Suarez, H. (2004). Long-term auditory adaptation to a modified peripheral frequency map. *Acta Otolaryngol,* Vol. 124, No. 4, (May), pp. 381-386, ISSN 0001-6489 (Print)

Van de Heyning, P.; Vermeire, K.; Diebl, M.; Nopp, P.; Anderson, I. & De Ridder, D. (2008). Incapacitating unilateral tinnitus in single-sided deafness treated by cochlear implantation. *Ann Otol Rhinol Laryngol,* Vol. 117, No. 9, (Sep), pp. 645-652, ISSN 0003-4894 (Print)

van den Honert, C. & Kelsall, D. C. (2007). Focused intracochlear electric stimulation with phased array channels. *J Acoust Soc Am,* Vol. 121, No. 6, (Jun), pp. 3703-3716, ISSN 1520-8524 (Electronic)

van den Honert, C. & Stypulkowski, P. H. (1987). Single fiber mapping of spatial excitation patterns in the electrically stimulated auditory nerve. *Hear Res,* Vol. 29, pp. 195-206, ISSN 0378-5955 (Print)

Vermeire, K.; Nobbe, A.; Schleich, P.; Nopp, P.; Voormolen, M. H. & Van de Heyning, P. H. (2008). Neural tonotopy in cochlear implants: an evaluation in unilateral cochlear implant patients with unilateral deafness and tinnitus. *Hear Res,* Vol. 245, No. 1-2, (Nov), pp. 98-106, ISSN 0378-5955 (Print)

Vermeire, K.; Schatzer, R.; Visser, D.; Krenmayr, A.; Kals, M.; Neustetter, C.; Bader, P.; Zangerl, M.; Van de Heyning, P. & Zierhofer, C. (2009). Contributions of temporal and place cues to pitch in the apical region, *Conference on Implantable Auditory Prostheses,* Lake Tahoe, CA, July 12-17, 2009

von Békésy, G. (1960). *Experiments in Hearing,* McGraw-Hill Book Company, Inc., ISBN 978-0070043244, New York

von Helmholtz, H. (1863). *Die Lehre von den Tonempfindungen als physiologische Grundlage für die Theorie der Musik,* Friedrich Vieweg und Sohn, Braunschweig, Germany,

Wackym, P. A.; Firszt, J. B.; Gaggl, W.; Runge-Samuelson, C. L.; Reeder, R. M. & Raulie, J. C. (2004). Electrophysiologic effects of placing cochlear implant electrodes in a perimodiolar position in young children. *Laryngoscope,* Vol. 114, No. 1, (Jan), pp. 71-76, ISSN 0023-852X (Print)

Wilson, B. S.; Finley, C. C.; Farmer, J. C., Jr.; Lawson, D. T.; Weber, B. A.; Wolford, R. D.; Kenan, P. D.; White, M. W.; Merzenich, M. M. & Schindler, R. A. (1988). Comparative studies of speech processing strategies for cochlear implants. *Laryngoscope,* Vol. 98, No. 10, (Oct), pp. 1069-1077, ISSN 0023-852X (Print)

Wilson, B. S.; Finley, C. C.; Lawson, D. T.; Wolford, R. D.; Eddington, D. K. & Rabinowitz, W. M. (1991). Better speech recognition with cochlear implants. *Nature,* Vol. 352, No. 6332, (Jul 18), pp. 236-238, ISSN 0028-0836 (Print)

Wilson, B. S.; Zerbi, M.; Finley, C. C.; Lawson, D. T. & van den Honert, C. (1997). *Speech processors for auditory prostheses: Relationships between temporal patterns of nerve activity and pitch judgments for cochlear implant patients,* Eighth Quarterly Progress Report, NIH project N01-DC-5-2103, Neural Prosthesis Program, National Institutes of Health, Bethesda, MD

Xu, L.; Zwolan, T. A.; Thompson, C. S. & Pfingst, B. E. (2005). Efficacy of a cochlear implant simultaneous analog stimulation strategy coupled with a monopolar electrode configuration. *Ann Otol Rhinol Laryngol,* Vol. 114, No. 11, (Nov), pp. 886-893, ISSN 0003-4894 (Print)

Zeng, F. G. (2002). Temporal pitch in electric hearing. *Hear Res,* Vol. 174, No. 1-2, (Dec), pp. 101-6, ISSN 0378-5955 (Print)

Zierhofer, C. (2001). Analysis of a Linear Model for Electrical Stimulation of Axons - Critical Remarks on the "Activating Function Concept". *IEEE Trans Biomed Eng,* Vol. 48, No. 2, pp. 173-184, ISSN 0018-9294 (Print)

Zierhofer, C.; Kals, M.; Krenmayr, A.; Vermeire, K.; Zangerl, M.; Visser, D.; Bader, P.; Neustetter, C. & Schatzer, R. (2009). Simultaneous Pulsatile Stimulation with "Channel Interaction Compensation", *9th European Symposium on Paediatric Cochlear Implantation,* Warsaw, Poland, May 14-17, 2009

Zierhofer, C. M. (2003). Electrical nerve stimulation based on channel specific sampling sequences, U.S. Patent 6,594,525

Zierhofer, C. M. (2007). Electrical stimulation of the acoustic nerve based on selected groups, U.S. Patent 7,283,876

Zierhofer, C. M. & Schatzer, R. (2008). Simultaneous intracochlear stimulation based on channel interaction compensation: analysis and first results. *IEEE Trans Biomed Eng*, Vol. 55, No. 7, (Jul), pp. 1907-16, ISSN 1558-2531 (Electronic)

Section 3

Other Research Updates

7

Acoustic Simulations of Cochlear Implants in Human and Machine Hearing Research

Cong-Thanh Do
Idiap Research Institute, Centre du Parc, Martigny
Switzerland

1. Introduction

Cochlear implant is an instrument which can be implanted in the inner ear and can restore partial hearing to profoundly deaf people (Loizou, 1999a) (see Fig. 1). Acoustic simulations of cochlear implants are widely used in cochlear implant research. Basically, they are acoustic signals which simulate what the profoundly deaf people could hear when they wear cochlear implants. Useful conclusions can be deduced from the results of experiments performed with acoustic simulations of cochlear implants. There are two typical applications in cochlear implant research which use acoustic simulations of cochlear implants. In the first one, acoustic simulations of cochlear implants are used to define how many independent channels are needed in order to achieve high levels of speech understanding (Loizou et al., 1999). The second application of acoustic simulations in cochlear implants research is for determining the effect of electrode insertion depth on speech understanding (Baskent & Shannon, 2003; Dorman et al., 1997b). In this chapter, we review briefly these conventional applications of acoustic simulations in cochlear implants research and, on the other hand, introduce novel applications of acoustic simulations of cochlear implants, both in cochlear implants research and in other domains, such as automatic speech recognition (ASR) research. To this end, we present quantitative analyses on the fundamental frequency (F0) of the cochlear implant-like spectrally reduced speech (SRS) which are, essentially, acoustic simulations of cochlear implants (Loizou, 1999a). These analyses support the report of (Zeng et al., 2005), which was based on subjective tests, about the difficulty of cochlear implant users in identifying speakers. Following the results of our analyses, the F0 distortion in state-of-the-art cochlear implants is large when the SRS, which is acoustic simulation of cochlear implant, is synthesized only from subband temporal envelopes (Do, Pastor & Goalic, 2010a). The analyses revealed also a significant reduction of F0 distortion when the frequency modulation is integrated in cochlear implant, as proposed by (Nie et al., 2005). Consequently, the results of such quantitative analyses, performed on relevant acoustic traits, could be exploited to conduct subjective studies in cochlear implant research. On the other hand, we investigate the automatic recognition of the cochlear implant-like SRS. Actually, state-of-the-art ASR systems rely on relevant spectral information, extracted from original speech signals, to recognize input speech in a statistical pattern recognition framework. We show that from certain SRS spectral resolution, it is possible to achieve (automatic) recognition performance as good as that attained with the original clean speech even though the cochlear implant-like SRS is synthesized only from subband temporal envelopes of the original clean speech (Do, Pastor & Goalic, 2010b; Do, Pastor, Le Lan & Goalic, 2010). Basing on this result, a novel framework for noise robust ASR, using cochlear implant-like SRS, has been proposed in (Do et al., 2012). In this novel framework, cochlear implant-like SRS is used in both the training and testing conditions. Experiments show that the (automatic) recognition results are significantly improved, compared to the baseline system which does not employ the SRS (Do et al., 2012).

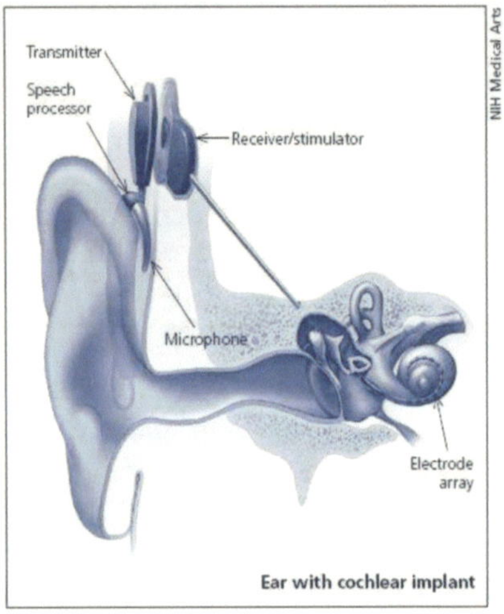

Fig. 1. Cochlear implant is an instrument which can be implanted in the inner ear and can restore partial hearing to profoundly deaf people (Loizou, 1999a) (image source: NIH Medical Arts, USA).

2. Conventional applications of acoustic simulations of cochlear implants

2.1 Researching the number of independent channels needed to achieve high levels of speech understanding

It has been known that the speech understanding does not require highly detailed spectral information of speech signal since much of the information in the speech spectrum is redundant (Dudley, 1939). On the other hand, the fine spectral cues, presented in naturally produced utterances, are not required for speech recognition (Zeng et al., 2005). In general, the signal processing in cochlear implant divides the speech spectrum into several spectral subbands, from 4 to 12 depending on the device, and then transmits the energy in all the subbands. However, knowing how many independent channels are needed in order to achieve high levels of speech understanding is an important issue. In fact, it is difficult to answer this question basing on the results of subjective tests performed by cochlear implant users, since their performance might be affected by many cofounding factors (e.g. number of surviving ganglion cells). For example, if a cochlear implant user obtains poor auditory performance using 4 channels of stimulation, the rationale might be that 4 stimulating channels are not enough but it could probably be blamed for the lack of surviving ganglion cells near the stimulating electrodes (Loizou et al., 1999). Using acoustic simulations can help in separating the rationale coming from the lack of surviving ganglion cells.

In (Shannon et al., 1995), the authors showed that high levels of speech understanding (e.g. 90% correct for sentences) could be achieved using a few as four spectral subbands. The subband temporal envelopes of speech signal were extracted from a small number (1-4) of frequency subbands, and used to modulate noise of the same bandwidth. In their signal processing strategy, the temporal cues within each subband are preserved but the fine spectral cues within each subband are eliminated. In another study, (Dorman et al., 1997a) used subband temporal envelopes to modulate sine waves rather than noise bands, and then, summed these subband modulated signals. As in (Shannon et al., 1995), sentence recognition using four channels was found to be 90% correct.

Typically, in the subjective tests for determining the necessary number of frequency subbands needed for understanding speech, normal hearing listeners listened to stimulus consisting of consonants, vowels, and simple sentences in each of the signal conditions (Faulkner et al., 1997; Loizou et al., 1999; Shannon et al., 2004; 1995). In these tests, consonants and vowels were presented in a random order to each listener. The listeners were instructed to identify the presented stimulus by selecting it from the complete set of vowels or consonants (Shannon et al., 1995). In the sentence recognition tests, sentences were presented once and the listeners were asked to repeat as many words in the sentence as they could. Training (i.e. practice) is a factor that needs to be taken into account when interpreting the speech recognition results mentioned previously, since the normal hearing listeners cannot recognize immediately the speech signals with spectro-temporal distortion. For example, in (Shannon et al., 1995), the listeners were trained on sample conditions to familiarize them with the testing environment; after about two or three sessions, for a total of 8 to 10 hours, when the listeners' performance stabilized, the training can be stopped. No feedback was provided in any of the test conditions.

On the other hand, (Zeng et al., 2005) showed that although subband temporal envelopes (or amplitude modulations - AMs) from a limited number of spectral subbands may be sufficient for speech recognition in quiet, frequency modulations (FMs) significantly enhances speech recognition in noise, as well as speaker and tone recognition. The result of (Zeng et al., 2005) suggested that FM components provide complementary information which supports robust speech recognition under realistic listening situations. A novel signal processing strategy, named FAME (frequency amplitude modulation encoding), was proposed which integrates not only AMs but also FMs into the cochlear implants (Nie et al., 2005; Zeng et al., 2005). More details about the FAME strategy will be presented in section 3.1.

2.2 Simulating the effect of electrodes insertion depth on speech identification accuracy

The second application of acoustic simulations in cochlear implants research is for determining the effect of electrode insertion depth on speech understanding. In cochlear implantation, electrode arrays are inserted only partially to the cochlea, typically 22-30 mm, depending on the state of the cochlea. Acoustic simulations of cochlear implants could be used to simulate the effect of depth of electrode insertion on identification accuracy. In this respect, normal hearing listeners performed identification tasks with an acoustic simulation of cochlear implant whose electrodes are separated by 4 mm (Dorman et al., 1997b). Insertion depth was simulated by outputting sine waves from each channel of the processor at a frequency determined by the cochlear place of electrode inserted 22-25 mm into the cochlea, through the Greenwood's frequency-to-place equation (Greenwood, 1990). The results indicated that simulated insertion depth had a significant effect on speech identification performance (Dorman et al., 1997b).

The mapping of acoustic frequency information onto the appropriate cochlear place is a natural biological function in normal acoustic hearing. However, in cochlear implant, this mapping is controlled by the speech processor. Indeed, the length and insertion depth of the electrode arrays are important factors which determine the cochlear tonotopic range (Baskent & Shannon, 2003). A 25 mm insertion depth of the electrode arrays is usually used in the design of conventional cochlear implant. This design would place the electrodes in a cochlear region corresponding to an acoustic frequency range of 500-6000 Hz. While this mapping preserves the entire range of acoustic frequency information, it also results in a compression of the tonotopic pattern of speech information delivered to the brain. The effects of such a compression of frequency-to-place mapping on speech recognition are studied in (Baskent & Shannon, 2003) using acoustic simulations of cochlear implants.

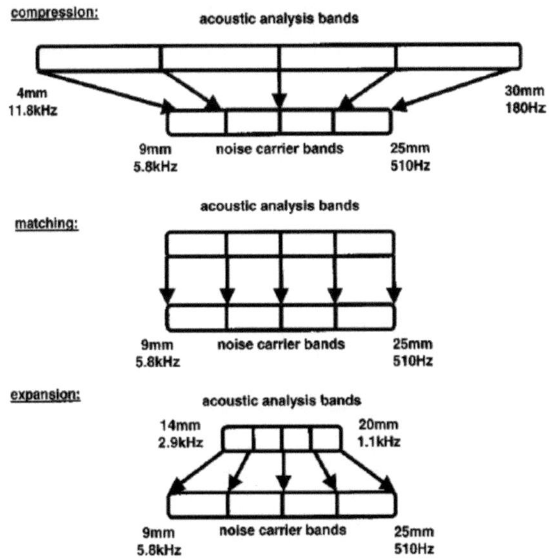

Fig. 2. Frequency-place mapping conditions for 4-channel processor at the simulated 25-mm electrode insertion depth (Baskent & Shannon, 2003). In this condition, the noise carrier bands are fixed (9-25 mm: 510-5800 Hz). The speech envelope was extracted from the analysis subbands and used to modulate the noise carrier subbands. The three panels, in top-down order, show the three mapping conditions, compression, matched and expansion, respectively. In the top panel where there is a compression of +5 mm, the analysis subbands are mapped onto narrower carrier subbands. The middle panel shows the 0 mm condition, in which the analysis and carrier bands are matched. The lower panel shows the -5 mm expansion condition, in which analysis subbands are mapped onto wider carrier subbands.

In (Baskent & Shannon, 2003), speech recognition was measured as a function of linear frequency-place compression and expansion using phoneme and sentence stimulus. Cochlear implant with different number of electrode channels and different electrode insertion depths were simulated by noise-subband acoustic simulations and presented to normal hearing listeners. Indeed, it was found that in the matched condition where a considerable amount of acoustic information was eliminated, speech recognition was generally better than any condition of frequency-place expansion and compression. This result demonstrates the dependency of speech recognition on the mapping of acoustic frequency information onto the appropriate cochlear place (Baskent & Shannon, 2003).

3. Novel applications of acoustic simulations of cochlear implants

In this section, we introduce novel applications of acoustic simulations of cochlear implants, henceforth abbreviated cochlear implant-like spectrally reduced speech (or simply SRS), both in cochlear implant research and other domains, such as automatic speech recognition (ASR). In this respect, section 3.1 presents our SRS synthesis algorithm, based on the frequency amplitude modulation encoding (FAME) algorithm (Nie et al., 2005), that is use through out the rest of this chapter. Section 3.2 introduces an analysis of the speech fundamental frequency (F0) in the SRS and its application in cochlear implant research. In addition, another application of the acoustic simulations of cochlear implants, in ASR, is introduced in section 3.3. Finally, section 4 concludes the chapter.

3.1 Cochlear implant-like SRS synthesis algorithm

A speech signal, $s(t)$, is first decomposed into N subband signals $s_i(t), i = 1, \ldots, N$, by using an analysis filterbank consisting of N bandpass filters with N taking values in $\{4, 8, 16, 24, 32\}$. The analysis filterbank is aimed at simulating the motion of the basilar membrane (Kubin & Kleijn, 1999). In this respect, the filterbank consists of nonuniform bandwidth bandpass filters that are linearly spaced on the Bark scale. In the literature, gammatone filters (Patterson et al., 1992) or elliptic filters (Nie et al., 2005; Shannon et al., 1995) have been used to design such a filterbank. In this chapter, each bandpass filter in the filterbank is a second-order elliptic bandpass filter having a minimum stop-band attenuation of 50-dB and a 2-dB peak-to-peak ripple in the pass-band. The lower, upper and central frequencies of the bandpass filters are calculated as in (Gunawan & Ambikairajah, 2004). An example of the analysis filterbank is given in Fig. 3.

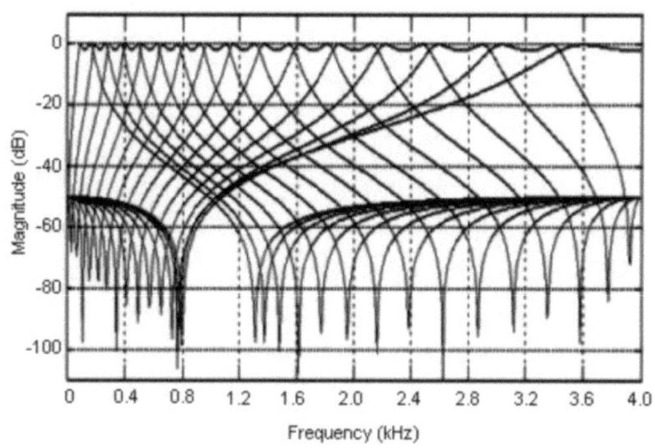

Fig. 3. Frequency response of an analysis filterbank consisting of 16 second-order elliptic bandpass filters used for speech signal decomposition. The speech signal is sampled at 8 kHz.

The subband signals, $s_i(t), i = 1, \ldots, N$, are supposed to follow a model that contains both amplitude and frequency modulations

$$s_i(t) = m_i(t)cos\left(2\pi f_{ci}t + 2\pi \int_0^t g_i(\tau)d\tau + \theta_i\right) \tag{1}$$

where $m_i(t)$ and $g_i(t)$ are the amplitude and frequency modulation components of the i-th subband whereas f_{ci} and θ_i are the i-th subband central frequency and initial phase,

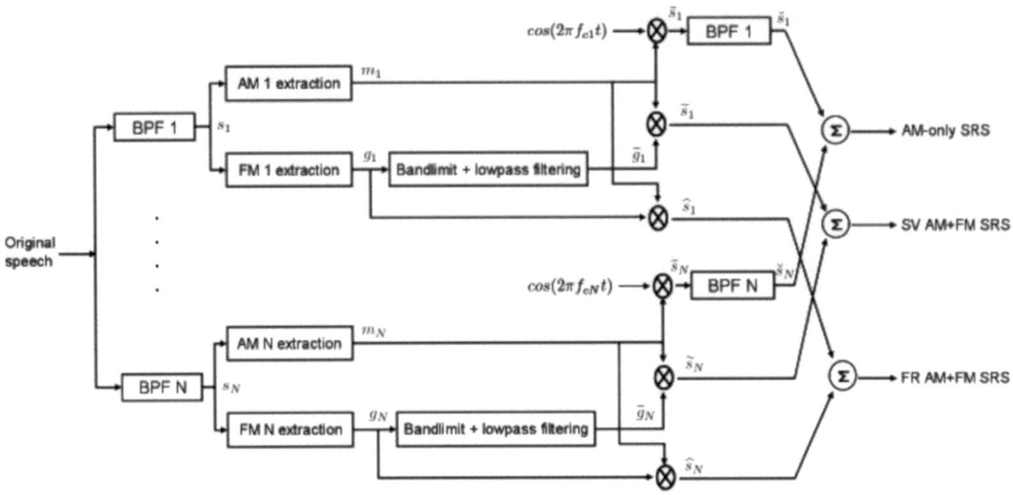

Fig. 4. The SRS synthesis algorithm derived from the Frequency Amplitude Modulation Encoding (FAME) strategy proposed in (Nie et al., 2005). The speech signal is decomposed by a filterbank consisting of N bandpass filters. AM and FM components are extracted from each subband signal. The AM components are used to modulate a fixed sinusoid, or a carrier with or without rapidly varying FM components, then summed up to synthesize the AM-only SRS, the FR AM+FM SRS, or the SV AM+FM SRS, respectively. The $f_{c1}, f_{c2}, \ldots, f_{cN}$ are the central frequencies of the bandpass filters in the analysis filterbank. The FR AM+FM SRS synthesis is our proposition.

respectively. Each AM component m_i of the subband signal s_i is extracted by full-wave rectification and subsequently, lowpass filtering of the subband signal s_i with a 50- or 500-Hz cutoff frequency. In the other way, the subband FM components, g_i, is extracted by first removing the central frequency, f_{ci}, from the subband signal s_i, thanks to a quadrature oscillator consisting of a pair of orthogonal sinusoidal signals whose frequencies equal the central frequency of the i-th subband (Nie et al., 2005). At the outputs of the quadrature oscillator, two lowpass filters are subsequently used to limit the frequency modulation range. The cutoff frequencies of these two lowpass filters equal 500 Hz or the bandwidth of the bandpass filter used in the analysis stage, whenever the latter is less than 500 Hz. The full rate (FR) FM signal, g_i, is then band-limited and filtered by using a 400-Hz cutoff frequency lowpass filter to derive the slowly varying (SV) band-limited FM signal, $\widetilde{g}_i$, as in (Nie et al., 2005). In the synthesis stage, the subband AM signal, m_i, is used to modulate a carrier containing the subband FR FM signal, g_i, or the subband SV FM signal, $\widetilde{g}_i$, to obtain the subband modulated signals, $\widehat{s}_i$, or $\widetilde{s}_i$, respectively. The sum of the subband modulated signals, $\widehat{s}_i, i = 1, \ldots, N$, gives the SRS with FR FM components, called FR AM+FM SRS. Similarly, SV AM+FM SRS is the SRS achieved when summing the subband modulated signals, $\widetilde{s}_i, i = 1, \ldots, N$, which are obtained by modulating the subband SV FMs with the subband AMs. All the lowpass filters used in the AM and FM extractions are fourth-order elliptic lowpass filters having a minimum stop-band attenuation of 50-dB and a 2-dB peak-to-peak ripple in the pass-band.

In the synthesis of the AM-based SRS, the subband modulated signal, $\bar{s}_i$, is obtained by using the subband AM signal, m_i, to modulate a sinusoid whose frequency equals the central frequency, f_{ci}, of the corresponding analysis bandpass filter of the i-th subband. The subband modulated signal, $\bar{s}_i$, is then spectrally limited by the same bandpass filter used for the original analysis subband to derive the spectrally limited subband modulated signal, $\breve{s}_i$ (Shannon et al., 1995). The AM-based SRS is the sum of all the spectrally limited subband modulated signals, $\breve{s}_i, i = 1, \ldots, N$. This type of SRS is called the AM-only SRS to indicate that the SRS is synthesized by using only AM cues. This description is summarized by the schema of Fig. 4.

3.2 Normalized mean squared error (NMSE) analysis of F0 in the acoustic simulations of cochlear implants

3.2.1 Motivation for the analysis

It is known that cochlear implant listeners do not have sufficient information about the voice fundamental frequency (F0) for their speech recognition task. Meanwhile, F0 information is useful for speaker discrimination and provides critical cues for the processing of prosodic information. Most present-day cochlear implants extract the speech temporal envelope and are not designed to specifically deliver speech F0 information to the listener. Cochlear implant listeners have therefore difficulties to perform the tasks needing F0 information, such as speaker recognition, gender recognition, tone recognition, or intonation recognition, etc (Chatterjee & Peng, 2008; Nie et al., 2005).

The modulation in speech, especially the frequency modulation, is expected to carry speaker-specific information. In (Nie et al., 2005), the authors proposed a speech processing strategy, FAME (for Frequency Amplitude Modulation Encoding), which encodes the speech temporal fine structure by extracting slowly varying band-limited frequency modulations (FMs) and incorporates these components in the cochlear implant. The acoustic simulations of cochlear implant, called spectrally reduced speech (SRS), can be synthesized either by using the FAME strategy or by using conventional AM-based SRS synthesis algorithm (Nie et al., 2005). In (Zeng et al., 2005), the authors performed speaker recognition tests by using these types of SRS. Experimentally, normal hearing listeners achieved significant better speaker recognition scores when listening to the FAME-based SRS, compared to when listening to the SRS synthesized from only AM components. Meanwhile, cochlear implant users could only achieve an average recognition score of 23% when they performed the same speaker recognition tests but listening to the original clean speech (Zeng et al., 2005). These results showed that current cochlear implant users have difficulties in identifying speakers (Zeng et al., 2005).

We thus want to quantitatively clarify the report of (Zeng et al., 2005) on the speaker recognition tasks of cochlear implant users, by performing a comparative study on the speech F0, extracted from the AM-based and FAME-based SRSs. The AM-based and the FAME-based SRSs were synthesized from a set of original clean speech utterances selected from the TI-digits, which is a multi-speaker speech database (Leonard, 1984). The selected speech utterances contain a large number of speakers to take into account the intra-speaker F0 variation. Next, the Normalized Mean Square Errors (NMSEs) between the F0 extracted from the original clean speech and from the SRS were calculated and analyzed.

3.2.2 Data for analysis

A set of 250 utterances was selected from the TI-digits clean speech database. TI-digits is a large speech database of more than 25 thousand connected digits sequences, spoken by over 300 men, women, and children (Leonard, 1984). The data were collected in a quiet environment and digitized at 20 kHz. In this study, the data are downsampled to 8 kHz. These 250 utterances were selected so that they had been spoken by both adults (men, women) and children (boy, girls) speakers. The lengths of the utterances in the set vary from the minimum length (isolated digit sequence) to the maximum length (seven-digit sequence) of the sequences in the TI-digits. The AM-only SRS, the FR AM+FM SRS, and the SV AM+FM SRS were synthesized from these 250 utterances by using the algorithm described in section 3.1. We thus have 250 AM-only SRS, 250 FR AM+FM SRS, and 250 SV AM+FM SRS utterances.

3.2.3 F0 NMSE analysis

The F0 values are extracted from the voiced speech frames of the original clean speech and the SRS utterances by using the Praat software. Praat is a computer program to analyse, manipulate speech signal and compute acoustic features, developed by Boersma and Weenink (Boersma & Weenink, 2009). The Praat F0 extraction algorithm, based on the autocorrelation method, is standard and accurate. A detailed description of the Praat F0 extraction algorithm can be found in (Boersma, 2004). Let $\mathbf{X} = [\mathbf{t}_X \; \mathbf{f}_X]$ and $\mathbf{Y} = [\mathbf{t}_Y \; \mathbf{f}_Y]$ be the vectors extracted from the voiced speech frames (of length 10 ms) of a clean speech utterance and the corresponding SRS utterance, respectively. The vectors $\mathbf{t}_X = [t_X(1), \ldots, t_X(L)]^T$ and $\mathbf{f}_X = [f_X(1), \ldots, f_X(L)]^T$ contain the time instants and the extracted F0 values, respectively, of the voiced speech frames in the original clean speech utterance. Similarly, $\mathbf{t}_Y = [t_Y(1), \ldots, t_Y(M)]^T$ and $\mathbf{f}_Y = [f_Y(1), \ldots, f_Y(M)]^T$ contain the time instants and the extracted F0 values, respectively, of the voiced speech frames in the corresponding SRS utterance. The Praat script for extracting the vectors $\mathbf{X}$ and $\mathbf{Y}$ can be found at `http://www.icp.inpg.fr/~loeven/ScriptsPraat.html`. The superscript ^{T} denotes the transpose whereas L and M are the lengths of the vectors $\mathbf{X}$ and $\mathbf{Y}$, respectively. In general, $\mathbf{X}$ and $\mathbf{Y}$ do not have the same lengths ($L \neq M$) even though the SRS utterance is synthesized from the same original clean speech utterance. The time instant values in $\mathbf{t}_X$ and $\mathbf{t}_Y$ are not identical, either. Without losing the generality, we suppose that $L < M$. In order to correctly calculate the NMSE between the F0 vectors of an original clean speech and a SRS utterance, we calculate the vector $\widehat{\mathbf{Y}} = \left[\widehat{\mathbf{t}}_Y \; \widehat{\mathbf{f}}_Y\right]$ as follows

Algorithm 1 Calculating $\widehat{\mathbf{Y}} = \left[\widehat{\mathbf{t}}_Y \; \widehat{\mathbf{f}}_Y\right]$ from $\mathbf{t}_X, \mathbf{t}_Y$ and $\mathbf{f}_Y$

FOR $i = 1 \rightarrow L$

1: $\widetilde{j} = \underset{j=1..M}{\arg\min} |t_Y(j) - t_X(i)|$

2: $\widehat{t}_Y(i) = t_Y(\widetilde{j})$

3: $\widehat{f}_Y(i) = f_Y(\widetilde{j})$

END

where $\widehat{\mathbf{t}}_Y = [\widehat{t}_Y(1), \ldots, \widehat{t}_Y(L)]^T$ and $\widehat{\mathbf{f}}_Y = \left[\widehat{f}_Y(1), \ldots, \widehat{f}_Y(L)\right]^T$ are the new time instants and F0 values vectors of the SRS utterance. The purpose of algorithm 1 is to calculate $\widehat{\mathbf{Y}} = \left[\widehat{\mathbf{t}}_Y \; \widehat{\mathbf{f}}_Y\right]$ from $\mathbf{t}_X, \mathbf{t}_Y$ and $\mathbf{f}_Y$ so that the temporal lags between the identical index elements of $\mathbf{t}_X$ and $\widehat{\mathbf{t}}_Y$ are minimal. The NMSE is then calculated between the two vectors of F0 values, $\mathbf{f}_X$ and $\widehat{\mathbf{f}}_Y$, now having the same length L.

$$\text{NMSE} = 20\log_{10}\left(\frac{1}{L}\sum_{i=1}^{L}\left|\frac{f_X(i) - \widehat{f}_Y(i)}{f_X(i)}\right|^2\right) \qquad (2)$$

The temporal lag minimization performed by algorithm 1 makes it possible to achieve an accurate NMSE calculation, following formula (2). The averages of the NMSEs on the selected 250 utterances were calculated and represented as a function of the SRS number of frequency subbands in Fig. 5 and Fig. 6.

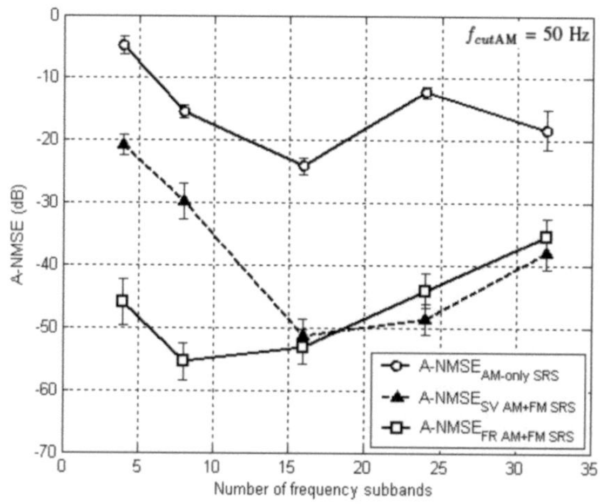

Fig. 5. Averages of the NMSEs (A-NMSEs) between the F0 vectors, extracted from the clean speech utterances and those extracted from the AM-only SRS (A-NMSE$_{\text{AM-ONLY SRS}}$), SV AM+FM SRS (A-NMSE$_{\text{SV AM+FM SRS}}$), and FR AM+FM SRS (A-NMSE$_{\text{FR AM+FM SRS}}$), calculated on 250 utterances (section III.A). The AM used for the SRS synthesis were extracted by using a 50-Hz cutoff frequency lowpass filter. Error bars indicate 95% of the confidence interval (Cumming et al., 2007) around each A-NMSE.

The curves in Fig. 5 represent the averages of the NMSEs (A-NMSEs) calculated between the original clean speech F0 vectors and those of the synthesized SRSs, which used 50-Hz cutoff frequency for the AM extraction lowpass filter ($f_{cut\text{AM}}$ = 50 Hz). Similarly, the A-NMSEs calculated between the synthesized SRS, having $f_{cut\text{AM}}$ = 500 Hz, and the original clean speech, are represented by the curves in Fig. 6. Henceforth, we use the terms A-NMSE$_{\text{AM-ONLY SRS}}$, A-NMSE$_{\text{SV AM+FM SRS}}$, and A-NMSE$_{\text{FR AM+FM SRS}}$ to designate the A-NMSEs calculated between the F0 vectors of the original clean speech and those of the AM-only SRS, SV AM+FM SRS, and FR AM+FM SRS, respectively. An one-way ANOVA reveals that the overall difference between the A-NMSEs is significant $[F(2,12) = 14.5, p < 0.001]$ for $f_{cut\text{AM}}$ = 50 Hz. Similarly, when $f_{cut\text{AM}}$ = 500 Hz, the A-NMSEs overall difference is also significant $[F(2,12) = 9.8, p < 0.005]$. Further, the A-NMSE$_{\text{AM-ONLY SRS}}$ is significantly greater than the A-NMSE$_{\text{SV AM+FM SRS}}$ $[F(1,8) = 12.1, p < 0.01]$, and the A-NMSE$_{\text{FR AM+FM SRS}}$ $[F(1,8) = 43.9, p < 0.0005]$, for $f_{cut\text{AM}}$ = 50 Hz. For $f_{cut\text{AM}}$ = 500 Hz, the same conclusion can be reported: the A-NMSE$_{\text{AM-ONLY SRS}}$ is significantly greater than the A-NMSE$_{\text{SV AM+FM SRS}}$ $[F(1,8) = 17.6, p < 0.005]$, and the A-NMSE$_{\text{FR AM+FM SRS}}$ $[F(1,8) = 17.9, p < 0.005]$. However, no significant difference is revealed between the

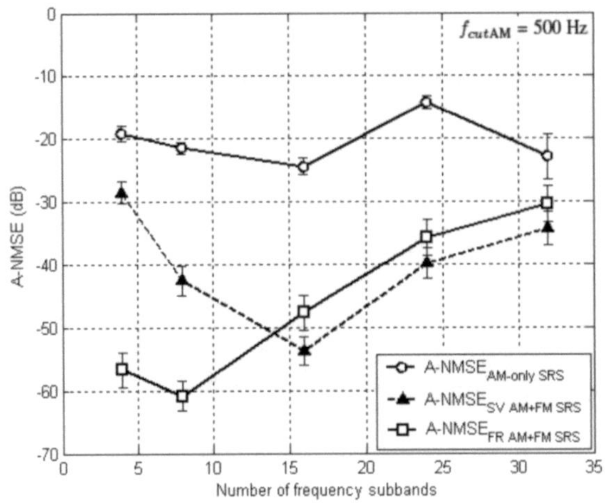

Fig. 6. The A-NMSE$_{\text{AM-ONLY SRS}}$ (solid-line + circle), A-NMSE$_{\text{SV AM+FM SRS}}$ (dashed-line + triangular), and A-NMSE$_{\text{FR AM+FM SRS}}$ (solid-line + square), calculated on 250 utterances (section III.A). The AM extraction lowpass filter cutoff frequency, $f_{cut\text{AM}}$, equals 500 Hz. As in Fig. 5, the error bars indicate 95% of the confidence interval around each A-NMSE.

A-NMSE$_{\text{SV AM+FM SRS}}$ and the A-NMSE$_{\text{FR AM+FM SRS}}$, both with $f_{cut\text{AM}}$ = 50 Hz $[F(1,8) = 1.8, p > 0.2]$, and $f_{cut\text{AM}}$ = 500 Hz $[F(1,8) = 0.8, p > 0.35]$.

In addition, for every number of SRS frequency subbands, we can remark that A-NMSE$_{\text{AM-ONLY SRS}}$ is always the greatest amongst the three A-NMSEs. This gap reflects that the distortion of F0 information in the state-of-the-art cochlear implant acoustic simulation (AM-only SRS), is greater than the FAME-based SRS (SV AM+FM SRS and FR AM+FM SRS). This is a quantitative evidence which supports the report of (Zeng et al., 2005), about the low speaker recognition score (23%) of the cochlear implant users. This evidence supports also the fact that the normal hearing listeners, listening to the FAME-based SV AM+FM SRS, achieved significant better recognition scores, compared to when listening to the AM-only SRS, in the same speaker recognition task (Zeng et al., 2005). Further, we can remark that at low spectral resolution (4 and 8 subbands), the A-NMSE$_{\text{SV AM+FM SRS}}$ (dashed-line + triangular) is significantly greater than the A-NMSE$_{\text{FR AM+FM SRS}}$ (solid line + square), both for $f_{cut\text{AM}}$ = 50 Hz $[F(1,2) = 15.2, p = 0.06]$ and for $f_{cut\text{AM}}$ = 500 Hz $[F(1,2) = 10.01, p = 0.087]$. Even though the p-values in these two cases are slightly greater than 0.05, we can still state the latter conclusion since the error bars, which indicate 95% of the confidence interval around each A-NMSE, do not overlap (Cumming et al., 2007). This phenomenon suggests that the presence of rapidly varying FM components (above 400 Hz) in the FR AM+FM SRS, help in reducing the speech F0 distortion at low spectral resolution. However, at high SRS spectral resolution (16 subbands and above), the difference between the A-NMSE$_{\text{SV AM+FM SRS}}$ and the A-NMSE$_{\text{FR AM+FM SRS}}$ is not significant ($[F(1,4) = 0.08, p > 0.75]$, $f_{cut\text{AM}}$ = 50 Hz, and $[F(1,4) = 0.37, p > 0.55]$, $f_{cut\text{AM}}$ = 500 Hz). The presence of rapidly varying FM components in the SRS is therefore not significant to reduce the F0 distortion.

3.2.4 Examples

Fig. 7 and Fig. 8 show the spectrograms of a continuous speech utterance, original clean speech and the corresponding SRSs ($f_{cut\text{AM}}$ = 50 Hz), spoken by a female speaker, selected from the set of 250 utterances as mentioned in section III.A. The blue curves in the spectrograms, estimated by using the Praat software (Boersma & Weenink, 2009), represent the speech F0 vectors, $\mathbf{f}_X, \mathbf{f}_Y$, extracted from the original clean speech and the synthesized SRS utterances. The range of the F0 is labeled on the right-hand side vertical axis of each spectrogram. Using the extracted F0 curve of the original clean speech as the reference, we can qualitatively remark that the F0 values are not correctly estimated from the AM-only SRS, whether we use 4 subbands [NMSE = -17.4 dB] or 16 subbands [NMSE = -13.1 dB]. Another concern is related to the extracted F0 values in the AM+FM SRS. The F0 information is less well estimated in the 4-subband SV AM+FM SRS (5(c)) [NMSE = -20 dB] than in the 4-subband FR AM+FM SRS (5(d)) [NMSE = -35.3 dB]. This remark is consistent with the fact that the rapidly varying FM components help in reducing the F0 distortion at low spectral resolution, as mentioned previously. This phenomenon does not happen with the 16-subband SV AM+FM SRS (6(c)) [NMSE = -72.6 dB] and the 16-subband FR AM+FM SRS (6(d)) [NMSE = -73.2

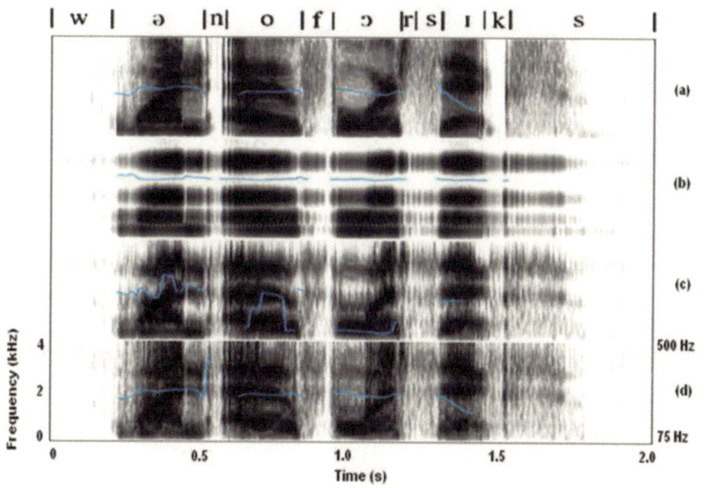

Fig. 7. Spectrograms of the original clean speech and the SRSs of the speech utterance "one oh four six", selected from the set of 250 utterances mentioned in section III.A, spoken by a female speaker; (a) original clean speech, (b) 4-subband AM-only SRS, (c) 4-subband SV AM+FM SRS, (d) 4-subband FR AM+FM SRS. The blue curves, estimated by Praat (Boersma & Weenink, 2009), represent the speech F0 vectors. The $f_{cut\mathrm{AM}}$ = 50 Hz and the F0 frequency range is [75 Hz - 500 Hz] (see the right-hand side vertical axis).

dB] where the F0 estimation is sufficiently good. Again, the fact that the rapidly varying FM components are not significant for reducing the F0 distortion at high SRS spectral resolution, compared to the slowly varying FM components, is typically verified in this example.

3.2.5 Concluding remarks

We have quantitatively analyzed the speech fundamental frequency, F0, in the cochlear implant-like spectrally reduced speech. The NMSE is calculated between the F0 values extracted from the original clean speech and those of the SRSs using algorithm 1, proposed in section III.B. NMSE analysis showed that amongst the three types of SRS studied in this chapter, the AM-only SRS is the SRS in which the speech F0 distortion is the greatest. The great distortion of F0 information in the state-of-the-art cochlear implant-like SRS, supports

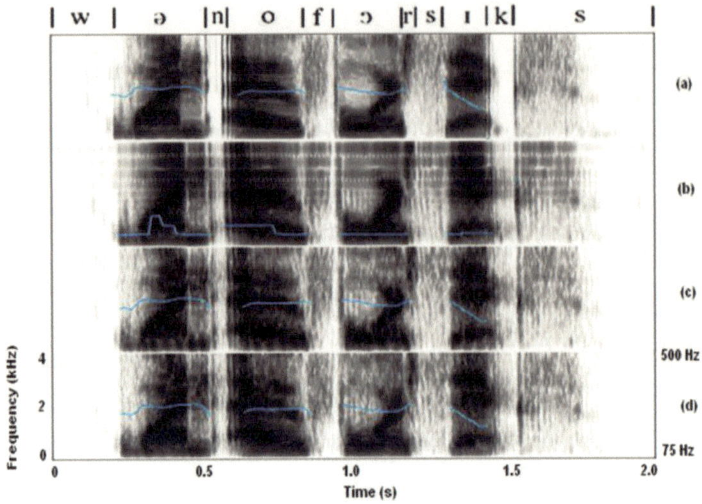

Fig. 8. Spectrograms of the original clean speech and the SRSs of the same utterance as in Fig. 8; (a) original clean speech, (b) 16-subband AM-only SRS, (c) 16-subband SV AM+FM SRS, (d) 16-subband FR AM+FM SRS. The $f_{cut\text{AM}}$ = 50 Hz and the F0 frequency range is [75 Hz - 500 Hz].

the report of (Zeng et al., 2005): " [...] *current cochlear implant users can largely recognize what is said, but they cannot identify who say it."* The FAME strategy (Nie et al., 2005), which proposes to extract the slowly varying FM components and integrates them in the cochlear implant, help in reducing the F0 distortion in the SV AM+FM SRS, compared to the AM-only SRS. However, at low spectral resolution (4 and 8 subbands), the rapidly varying FM components are beneficial to reduce the F0 distortion in the FR AM+FM SRS. At high SRS spectral resolution (16 subbands and above), there is no significant difference between the SV AM+FM SRS and the FR AM+FM SRS in terms of F0 distortion. The results obtained in this chapter might help improve the FAME strategy (Nie et al., 2005) for better performance in a speaker recognition task, by keeping the rapidly varying FM components when the SRS spectral resolution is low. Even though rapidly varying FM components cannot be perceived by cochlear implant listeners, their presence could improve speaker recognition performance of cochlear implant listeners. Obviously, further subjective studies are needed to confirm this suggestion. A similar remark can be found in a study of Chang, Bai and Zeng in which the authors, by a subjective study, have shown that the low-frequency sound component below 300 Hz, *"although unintelligible when presented alone, could improve the functional signal-to-noise ratio by 10-15 dB for speech recognition in noise when presented in combination with a cochlear implant simulation"* (Chang et al., 2006).

The speech F0 NMSE analysis performed on the cochlear implant-like SRS is a quantitative evidence supporting the speaker recognition subjective tests, performed in (Zeng et al., 2005). On the other hand, quantitative studies on other speech acoustic features could also be performed, in advance, on the acoustic simulation of cochlear implant (SRS) to orient subjective tests. The results of such quantitative analysis could be exploited to conduct subjective studies in cochlear implant research.

3.3 Automatic recognition of acoustic simulations of cochlear implants

3.3.1 Relevant speech spectral information for ASR

It is important to reduce speech signal variability, due to speech production (accent and dialect, speaking style, etc.) or environment (additive noise, microphone frequency response, etc.), in order to guarantee stable ASR performance. Therefore, in an ASR system, the speech analysis module is aimed at reducing the speech signal variability and extracting the ASR relevant spectral information into speech acoustic features. However, despite the speech variability reduction achieved by such standard speech signal analyses, ASR performance is still adversely affected by noise and other sources of acoustic variability (Raj & Stern, 2005). Since most standard speech processing analyses for ASR are performed in the spectral domain, it is natural to seek the relevant spectral information that is sufficient for ASR, in the speech signal.

In ASR based on Hidden Markov Models (HMMs) (Rabiner, 1989), one way to estimate the ASR relevant speech spectral information is to evaluate the ASR performance on spectrally reduced speech (SRS) signals when the acoustic models (the HMMs) are trained on a clean speech (full spectrum) database. As usual, the tested signals must not belong to the training database. Such an approach was first investigated by Barker and Cooke in (Barker & Cooke, 1997) where the authors *"consider how acoustic models trained on original clean speech can be adapted to cope with a particular form of spectral distortion, namely reduction of clean speech to sin-wave replicas"*. The ASR results were, however, not satisfactory in train-test unmatched conditions. The cepstral coding techniques are, following the authors, *"inappropriate for dealing with drastic alterations to the shape of the spectral profile caused by spectral reduction"* (Barker & Cooke, 1997).

The acoustic simulation of cochlear implant is a spectrally reduced transform of original speech (Shannon et al., 1995). This type of SRS should be appropriate to evaluate the relevant spectral information needed by an HMM-based ASR whose acoustic models are trained on a given clean speech database and which uses the Mel frequency cepstral coefficients (MFCCs) (Davis & Mermelstein, 1980) or the perceptual linear prediction (PLP) coefficients (Hermansky, 1990) as acoustic features. The rationale is twofold. On the one hand, cochlear implant-like SRS can be recognized by normal hearing listeners. The recognition scores then depend on the spectral resolution (or the number of frequency subbands) of the SRS (Shannon et al., 1995). Furthermore, human cochlear implant listeners relying on primarily temporal cues can achieve a high level of speech recognition in quiet environment (Zeng et al., 2005). The foregoing facts suggest that the cochlear implant-like SRS could contain sufficient information for human speech recognition, even though such an SRS is synthesized from the speech temporal envelopes only. On the other hand, in ASR, certain speech analyses, such as the Bark or Mel-scale warping of the frequency axis or the spectral amplitude compression, performed on the conventional speech acoustic features (MFCCs or PLP coefficients), derive from the model of the human auditory system. Such auditory-like analyses, which mimic the speech processing performed by the human auditory system, are basically aimed at reducing speech signal variability and emphasizing the most relevant spectral information for ASR (Morgan et al., 2004). As a result, the cochlear implant-like SRS should contain sufficient spectral information for ASR based on conventional acoustic features, such as the MFCCs or the PLP coefficients.

3.3.2 Experimental data

In this section, the SRSs are synthesized from 250 original utterances (see 3.2.2) by using the AM-only SRS synthesis algorithm described in section 3.1. With 5 values (4, 8, 16, 24 and 32) of the number of frequency subbands and 4 values (16, 50, 160 and 500 Hz) for the bandwidth of the subband temporal envelope (AM), we have thus 20 sets of synthesized AM-only SRS signals, each set contains 250 utterances. These sets will be used for the spectral distortion analyses and the ASR tests in the next sections.

3.3.3 Spectral distortion analysis

Given an original clean speech utterance x_i and the corresponding SRS utterance $\widehat{x}_i$ which is synthesized from x_i, assume that f_j and $\widehat{f}_j$ are the spectra of two speech frames of x_i and $\widehat{x}_i$, respectively. The spectral distortion between these two speech frames can be measured on their spectra $\mathrm{d}_{x_i,\widehat{x}_i}(f_j, \widehat{f}_j)$. A good spectral distortion measure should have the following properties (Nocerino et al., 1985):

1. $\mathrm{d}_{x_i,\widehat{x}_i}(f_j, \widehat{f}_j) \geq 0$, with equality when $f_j = \widehat{f}_j$;
2. $\mathrm{d}_{x_i,\widehat{x}_i}(f_j, \widehat{f}_j)$ should have a reasonable perceptual interpretation;
3. $\mathrm{d}_{x_i,\widehat{x}_i}(f_j, \widehat{f}_j)$ should be numerically tractable and easy to compute.

Amongst the available spectral distortion measures (Nocerino et al., 1985), the weighted slope metric (WSM) distortion measure (Klatt, 1982), which is a perceptually based distortion measure, satisfies well these three properties. This spectral distortion measure reflects the spectral slope difference near spectral peaks in a critical-band spectral representation (Nocerino et al., 1985). It is also shown that the WSM distortion measure correlates well with the perceptual data (Klatt, 1982). Further, the WSM distortion measure is one of the spectral distortion measures that gave the highest recognition score with a standard dynamic time warping (DTW) based, isolated word, speech recognizer (Nocerino et al., 1985). In this respect, we use the WSM distortion measure to assess the spectral distortion between two speech frames extracted from an original clean speech utterance and a synthesized SRS utterance, respectively. The mathematical formula of the WSM distortion measure has the form (Klatt, 1982; Nocerino et al., 1985)

$$\mathrm{d}_{x_i,\widehat{x}_i}(f_j, \widehat{f}_j) = k_E \left| E_{f_j} - E_{\widehat{f}_j} \right| + \sum_{q=1}^{Q} k_s(q) \left(s_{f_j}(q) - s_{\widehat{f}_j}(q) \right)^2 \tag{3}$$

where Q is the number of frequency subbands, k_E is a weighting coefficient on the absolute energy difference, $\left| E_{f_j} - E_{\widehat{f}_j} \right|$, between f_j and $\widehat{f}_j$, $k_s(q)$ is a weighting coefficient for the difference, $s_{f_j}(q) - s_{\widehat{f}_j}(q)$, between the two critical band spectral slopes of f_j and $\widehat{f}_j$ (Nocerino et al., 1985).

Henceforth, $\mathrm{d}_{x_i,\widehat{x}_i}(f_j, \widehat{f}_j)$ designates the WSM distortion measure. The length of the speech frames for the WSM distortion measure is 10 ms and the number of frequency subband $Q =$ 24. The Matlab programs for calculating the WSM spectral distortion can be found at (Loizou, 1999b). The spectral distortion $\eta_{x_i,\widehat{x}_i}$ between two speech utterances x_i and $\widehat{x}_i$ can be defined as the mean of the WSM spectral distortion measures between the speech frames $\mathrm{d}_{x_i,\widehat{x}_i}(f_j, \widehat{f}_j)$:

$$\eta_{x_i,\widehat{x}_i} = \frac{1}{M}\sum_{j=1}^{M} \mathrm{d}_{x_i,\widehat{x}_i}(f_j, \widehat{f}_j) \tag{4}$$

where M is the number of speech frames in the speech utterances x_i and $\widehat{x}_i$. We define the overall spectral distortion $\bar{\eta}$ as the average of the $\eta_{x_i,\widehat{x}_i}$ calculated for all the $N = 250$ utterances in each set of SRS signals:

$$\bar{\eta} = \frac{1}{N}\sum_{i=1}^{N} \eta_{x_i,\widehat{x}_i} = \frac{1}{N}\frac{1}{M}\sum_{i=1}^{N}\sum_{j=1}^{M} \mathrm{d}_{x_i,\widehat{x}_i}(f_j, \widehat{f}_j) \tag{5}$$

We then calculate the overall spectral distortion $\bar{\eta}$ for all 20 sets of SRS utterances (see section 3.3.2). The values of $\bar{\eta}$ are illustrated in Fig. 9. The error bars in Fig. 9 represent the standard deviations of $\eta_{x_i,\widehat{x}_i}$. An ANOVA revealed no significant difference between the overall spectral distortion $\bar{\eta}$ when the bandwidth of the subband temporal envelopes are changed from 16 Hz to 500 Hz [$F(3,16) = 0.64$, $p > 0.5$]. Generally, the overall spectral distortion $\bar{\eta}$ decreases when the number of frequency subbands of the SRS increases. Since the WSM distortion measure is perceptually based and is correlated with the perceptual data (Klatt, 1982), we can deduce that the value of $\bar{\eta}$ reflects more or less the level of perceptual distortion that the listeners have to deal with when listening to the SRS signals. In addition, we can remark that $\eta_{x_i,\widehat{x}_i}$ varies intensively when the number of frequency subbands of the SRS is small (4- and 8-subband SRS), since the standard deviations of $\eta_{x_i,\widehat{x}_i}$ are large at low spectral resolutions of the SRS (4 and 8 subbands).

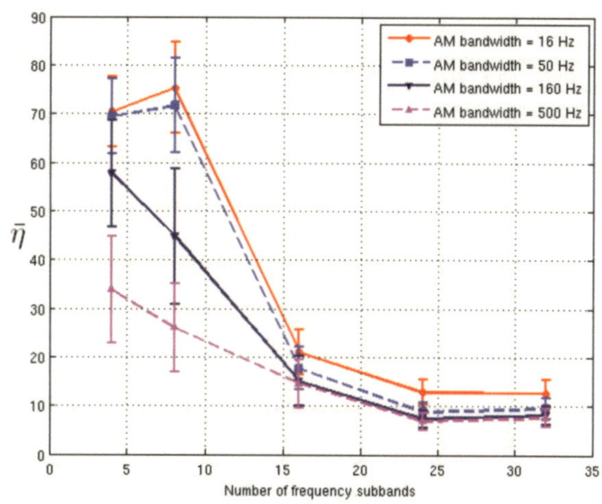

Fig. 9. Overall spectral distortion $\bar{\eta}$, which is defined as the average of the spectral distortion $\eta_{x_i,\widehat{x}_i}$, are calculated on all the 250 utterances of each set of SRS signals. There would be no overall spectral distortion if $\bar{\eta} = 0$. Error bars indicate standard deviations.

3.3.4 Automatic speech recognition results

We used the HTK speech recognition toolkit (Young et al., 2006) to train a speaker-independent HMM-based ASR system on the TI-digits speech database (Leonard, 1984). TI-digits is a large speech database of more than 25 thousand connected digits sequences spoken by over 300 men, women, and children. This speech database is widely used in the literature to assess ASR algorithms on small-vocabulary tasks (Barker et al., 2005; Cooke et al., 2001; Smit & Barnard, 2009). The data were collected in a quiet environment and digitized at 20 kHz. In this study, the data were downsampled to 8 kHz. The ASR system used a bigram language model and the acoustic models were the context-dependent three-state left-to-right triphone HMMs. These models were trained by using both MFCCs and PLP coefficients. The output observation distributions were modelled by Gaussian mixture models (GMMs) (Rabiner, 1989). In each state, the number of mixture components was 16. The feature vectors consist of 13 MFCCs or 13 PLP coefficients. For the MFCCs and the PLP coefficients calculation, the standard filterbank consisting of 26 filters was used (Young et al., 2006). The MFCCs and the PLPs coefficients were calculated from every Hamming windowed speech frame of 25 ms length and with an overlap of 15 ms between two adjacent frames. The first (delta) and second (acceleration) difference coefficients were appended to the static MFCCs and PLP coefficients to provide 39-dimensional feature vectors. This configuration for the feature vectors was used in both training and testing conditions. Next, the ASR tests were taken on the 20 sets of synthesized SRS signals. The recognition results with the MFCCs and PLP coefficients are shown in Table 1 and Table 2, respectively.

	Number of frequency subbands				
AM bandwidth	4	8	16	24	32
16 Hz	35.44	68.33	96.22	96.22	96.29
50 Hz	35.57	84.23	99.82	99.70	99.57
160 Hz	37.76	95.86	99.63	99.70	99.63
500 Hz	39.34	97.56	99.57	99.70	99.63

Table 1. ASR word accuracies (in %) computed on the 250 SRSs synthesized from 5 values for the number of frequency subbands and 4 values for the bandwidth of the subband temporal envelopes (AM). The ASR system was trained on the TI-digits clean speech training database. The speech feature vectors were MFCC-based. The ASR word accuracy computed on the 250 original clean speech utterances is 99.76%.

	Number of frequency subbands				
AM bandwidth	4	8	16	24	32
16 Hz	35.32	87.27	97.99	98.66	98.48
50 Hz	35.57	98.36	99.57	99.57	99.57
160 Hz	35.69	98.96	99.57	99.63	99.70
500 Hz	41.17	99.15	99.57	99.63	99.57

Table 2. ASR word accuracies (in %) computed on the 250 SRSs synthesized from 5 values for the number of frequency subbands and 4 values for the bandwidth of the subband temporal envelopes (AM). The ASR system was trained on the TI-digits clean speech training database. The speech feature vectors were PLP-based. The ASR word accuracy computed on the 250 original clean speech utterances is 99.70%.

For the ASR results with MFCC-based speech feature vectors, an ANOVA performed on the lines of Table I revealed that changing the bandwidth of the subband temporal envelopes had no significant effect in terms of ASR word accuracy [$F(3,16) = 0.11$, $p > 0.95$]. However, another ANOVA performed on the columns of Table I indicated that changing the number of frequency subbands had a significant effect across all tests [$F(4,15) = 73.9$, $p < 0.001$]. Protected t-tests (or Least Significant Difference (LSD) tests) (Keren & Lewis, 1993) were thus performed and showed that the 8-subband SRS yielded significant better ASR word accuracies compared to the 4-subband SRS [$t_{obs(4,8)} = 11.23 > t_{crit(15)} = 4.07, \alpha = 0.001$], where $t_{obs(4,8)}$ is the protected t-test value calculated between the 4-subband SRS and the 8-subband SRS word accuracies, $t_{crit(15)}$ is the critical value at the desired α level for 15 degrees of freedom. In contrast, no significant difference was revealed amongst the 16, 24, and 32-subband SRSs in terms of ASR word accuracy [$t_{obs(16,24)} \approx t_{obs(24,32)} \approx t_{obs(16,32)} \approx 0 < t_{crit(15)} = 2.13, \alpha = 0.05$]. The ASR word accuracies of each SRS in this group are significant better than those of the 8-subband SRS [$t_{obs(8,16)} = 2.79, t_{obs(8,24)} = 2.80, t_{obs(8,32)} = 2.78, t_{crit(15)} = 2.13, \alpha = 0.05$].

For the ASR results with PLP-based speech feature vectors, the same statistical analyses had been performed on the ASR word accuracies in Table 2 and the same conclusions would be revealed. In summary, increasing the number of the SRS frequency subbands from 4 to 16 made significant improvement in terms of ASR word accuracy. Interestingly, the 16, 24, and 32-subband SRSs could achieve an ASR word accuracy comparable to that attained with the original clean speech signals (the ASR word accuracies computed on the 250 original clean speech utterances with MFCC-based and PLP-based speech feature vectors were 99.76% and 99.70%, respectively).

3.3.5 Conclusions and perspectives

We have investigated the automatic recognition of cochlear implant-like SRS, which is synthesized from subband temporal envelopes of the original clean speech. The MFCCs and the PLP coefficients were used as speech features and the ASR system, which is speaker-independent and HMM-based, was trained on the original clean speech training database of TI-digits. It was shown that changing the bandwidth of the subband temporal envelopes had no significant effect on the ASR system word accuracy. In addition, increasing the number of frequency subbands of the SRS from 4 to 16 improved significantly the performance of the ASR system. However, there was no significant difference amongst the 16, 24, and 32-subband SRS in terms of ASR word accuracy. It was possible to achieve an ASR word accuracy as good as that attained with the original clean speech by using SRS with 16, 24, or 32 frequency subbands and by using both MFCC-based and PLP-based speech features.

The MFCCs or the PLP coefficients, along with the delta and acceleration coefficients, were concatenated together in the acoustic feature vector and were used in both the training and the testing conditions. The results presented in this chapter suggest that SRS with 16, 24, and 32 subbands contain sufficient spectral information for speech recognition with HMM-based ASR system using the MFCCs or the PLP coefficients along with the delta and acceleration coefficients. The SRS and original clean speech are quite different in the signal domain since the SRS is synthesized from original clean speech temporal envelopes, only. The spectral distortion analysis, based on the WSM distortion measure, showed that there are significant spectral distortions in the synthesized SRS compared to the original clean speech signal. Despite of these spectral distortions which are induced by the SRS synthesis, and although the ASR acoustic models are trained on the clean speech training database (TI-digits), the ASR word accuracy, computed on original clean speech signals of a testing set of TI-digits, is still maintained with the synthesized SRS of 16, 24, and 32 subbands.

Therefore, the 16-, 24-, and 32-subband SRS models might lead to the design of new acoustic features and suggest new speech models, for ASR, that could be robust to noise and other sources of acoustic variability. In this respect, performing ASR with HMMs trained on SRS could assess the relevance of SRS as a model for speech recognition. In addition, the fact that cochlear implant-like SRS is synthesized from speech temporal envelopes, only, might help in reducing ASR irrelevant spectral information due to environment. In (Do et al., 2012), we perform the ASR experiments with the noise contaminated speech signal. The SRS are used in both training and testing conditions. That is, the ASR system is trained on the SRS which was synthesized from the training original clean speech. This system is be used to recognize the SRS which is synthesized from noisy contaminated speech signals. Experimental results show that the use of SRS helps in improving significantly the ASR performance in the recognition of noisy speech (Do et al., 2012).

4. General conclusions and discussions

In this chapter, we have introduced the applications of acoustic simulations of cochlear implants in human and machine hearing research. We have reviewed the conventional applications of the acoustic simulations of cochlear implants in (1) determining the number of independent channels needed to achieve high levels of speech understanding, and in (2) simulating the effect of electrodes insertion depth on speech identification accuracy. In addition, we have introduced novel applications of acoustic simulations of cochlear implants, abbreviated as SRS, both in cochlear implant research and machine hearing research (or automatic speech recognition). Conventional as well as recently proposed synthesis algorithms have been used to synthesize the SRS signals (Nie et al., 2005; Shannon et al., 1995). These novel applications show that the acoustic simulation of cochlear implant is an important tool, not only for cochlear implant research but also for other hearing-related applications, namely noise robust ASR (Do et al., 2012).

However, for any studies performed on acoustic simulations of cochlear implants, the results should be interpreted with cautions when applied on human subjects who are cochlear implant users. In fact, the results could be slightly different due to the changes that occur in their auditory system following the severe and profound deafness. In this respect, results of the studies performed with acoustic simulations should be used as general indicators to conduct useful subjective studies. Authentic conclusions could be afterward interpreted from the results of studies performed on human subjects. On the other hand, in section 3.3, it was shown that changing the bandwidth of the subband temporal envelopes has no significant effect on the ASR word accuracies. In addition, changing the number of subband from 8 to 16 increases significantly the ASR word accuracies. Physically, these facts suggest that ASR word accuracies are more affected by the change of spectral information distributing on the whole spectral band rather than the change of local spectral information in each subband.

5. Acknowledgements

Some parts of the work in this chapter have been performed when the author was with Télécom Bretagne, Brest, France, in collaboration with Dominique Pastor and André Goalic.

6. References

Barker, J. & Cooke, M. (1997). Modelling the recognition of spectrally reduced speech, *Proc. ISCA Eurospeech 1997, September 22 - 25, Rhodes, Greece*, pp. 2127–2130.

Barker, J., Cooke, M. & Ellis, D. (2005). Decoding speech in the presence of other sources, *Speech Communication* 45(1): 5–25.

Baskent, D. & Shannon, R. V. (2003). Speech recognition under conditions of frequency-place compression and expansion, *J. Acoust. Soc. Am.* Vol. 113(4): 2064–2076.

Boersma, P. (2004). Accurate Short-term Analysis of the Fundamental Frequency and the Harmonics-to-noise Ratio of a Sampled Sound, *Proc. of Institut of Phonetic Sciences, University of Amsterdam*, Vol. 17, pp. 97–110.

Boersma, P. & Weenink, D. (2009). Praat, Doing Phonetic by Computer (Version 5.1.12)[computer program], *http://www.praat.org* .

Chang, J. E., Bai, J. Y. & Zeng, F.-G. (2006). Unintelligible Low-frequency Sound Enhances Simulated Cochlear-implant Speech Recognition in Noise, *IEEE Trans. Biomed. Eng.* 53(12): 2598–2601.

Chatterjee, M. & Peng, S.-C. (2008). Processing F0 with Cochlear Implant: Modulation Frequency Discrimination and Speech Intonation Recognition, *Hearing Research* 235(1-2): 143–156.

Cooke, M., Green, P., Josifovski, L. & Vizinho, A. (2001). Robust automatic speech recognition with missing and unreliable acoustic data, *Speech Communication* 34(3): 267–285.

Cumming, G., Fidler, F. & Vaux, D. L. (2007). Error Bars in Experimental Biology, *The Journal of Cell Biology* 177(1): 7–11.

Davis, S. B. & Mermelstein, P. (1980). Comparison of parametric representations for monosyllabic word recognition in continuous spoken sentences, *IEEE Trans. Acoustics, Speech, Signal Processing* 28(4): 357–366.

Do, C.-T., Pastor, D. & Goalic, A. (2010a). On normalized MSE analysis of speech fundamental frequency in the cochlear implant-like spectrally reduced speech, *IEEE Trans. on Biomedical Engineering* Vol. 57(No. 3): 572–577.

Do, C.-T., Pastor, D. & Goalic, A. (2010b). On the recognition of cochlear implant-like spectrally reduced speech with MFCC and HMM-based ASR, *IEEE Trans. on Audio, Speech and Language Processing* Vol. 18(No. 5): 2993–2996.

Do, C.-T., Pastor, D. & Goalic, A. (2012). A novel framework for noise robust ASR using cochlear implant-like spectrally reduced speech, *Speech Communication* 54(1): 119–133.

Do, C.-T., Pastor, D., Le Lan, G. & Goalic, A. (2010). Recognizing cochlear implant-like spectrally reduced speech with HMM-based ASR: experiments with MFCCs and PLP coefficients, *Proc. Interspeech 2010, September 26 - 30, Makuhari, Japan.*

Dorman, M. F., Loizou, P. C. & Rainey, D. (1997a). Speech intelligibility as a function of the number of channels of stimulation for signal processors using sine-wave and noise-band outputs, *J. Acoust. Soc. Am.* 102(4): 2403–2411.

Dorman, M., Loizou, P. C. & Rainey, D. (1997b). Simulating the effect of cochlear-implant electrode insertion depth on speech understanding, *J. Acoust. Soc. Am.* Vol. 102(No. 5): 2993–2996.

Dudley, H. (1939). Remarking speech, *J. Acoust. Soc. Am.* (11): 169–177.

Faulkner, A., Rosen, S. & Wilkinson, L. (1997). Effects of the number of channels and speech-to-noise ratio on rate of connected discourse tracking through a simulated cochlear implant speech processor, *Ear & Hearing* pp. 431–438.

Greenwood, D. D. (1990). A cochlear frequency-position function for several species - 29 years later, *J. Acoust. Soc. Am.* Vol. 87(No. 6): 2592–2605.

Gunawan, T. S. & Ambikairajah, E. (2004). Speech Enhancement using Temporal Masking and Fractional Bark Gammatone Filters, *Proc. 10th Australian International Conference on Speech Science & Technology, December 8 - 10, Sydney, Australia*, pp. 420–425.

Hermansky, H. (1990). Perceptual linear predictive (plp) analysis of speech, *J. Acoust. Soc. Am.* 87(4): 1738–1752.

Keren, G. & Lewis, C. (1993). *A handbook for data analysis in the behavioral sciences: statistical issues*, Lawrence Erlbaum Associates, Publishers, Hillsdale, New Jersey Hove & London.

Klatt, D. H. (1982). Prediction of perceived phonetic distance from critical band spectra: A fisrt step, *Proc. IEEE ICASSP 1982, May 03 - 05, Paris, France*, Vol. 2, pp. 1278–1281.

Kubin, G. & Kleijn, W. B. (1999). On Speech Coding in a Perceptual Domain, *Proc. IEEE ICASSP, March 15 - 19, Phoenix, AZ, USA*, Vol. 1, pp. 205–208.

Leonard, R. (1984). A Database for Speaker-independent Digit Recognition, *Proc. IEEE ICASSP, March 19 - 21, San Diego, USA*, Vol. 9, pp. 328–331.

Loizou, P. C. (1999a). Introduction to cochlear implants, *IEEE Engineering in Medicine and Biology Magazine* 18(1): 32–42.

Loizou, P. C. (1999b). COLEA: A Matlab software tool for speech analysis [Computer program] [Online]. Available: http://www.utdallas.edu/ loizou/speech/colea.htm.

Loizou, P. C., Dorman, M. & Tu, Z. (1999). On the number of channels needed to understand speech, *J. Acoust. Soc. Am.* Vol. 106(No. 4): 2097–2103.

Morgan, N., Bourlard, H. & Hermansky, H. (2004). Automatic speech recognition: an auditory perspective, *Speech processing in the auditory system (S. Greenberg, W. A. Ainsworth, A. N. Popper, and R. R. Fay, Eds.)* SPRINGER pp. 309–338.

Nie, K., Stickney, G. & Zeng, F.-G. (2005). Encoding frequency modulation to improve cochlear implant performance in noise, *IEEE Trans. on Biomedical Engineering* Vol. 52(No. 1): 64–73.

Nocerino, N., Soong, F. K., Rabiner, L. R. & Klatt, D. H. (1985). Comparative study of several distortion measures for speech recognition, *Speech Communication* 4(4): 317–331.

Patterson, R. D., Robinson, K., Holdsworth, J., Zhang, C. & Allerhand, M. H. (1992). Complex sounds and auditory images, *Auditory physiology and perception (Y. Cazals, L. Demany, and K. Horner, eds.)* OXFORD, PERGAMON pp. 429–446.

Rabiner, L. R. (1989). A tutorial on hidden Markov models and selected applications in speech recognition, *Proc. IEEE* 77(2): 257–286.

Raj, B. & Stern, R. M. (2005). Missing-feature approaches in speech recognition, *IEEE Signal Processing Magazine* 22(5): 101–116.

Shannon, R. V., Fu, Q.-J. & Ganvil, J. (2004). The number of spectral channels required for speech recognition depends on the difficulty of the listening situation, *Acta Otolaryngol. Suppl.* (552): 50–54.

Shannon, R. V., Zeng, F.-G., Kamath, V., Wygonski, J. & Ekelid, M. (1995). Speech recognition with primarily temporal cues, *Science* Vol. 270(No. 5234): 303–304.

Smit, W. & Barnard, E. (2009). Continuous speech recognition with sparse coding, *Computer Speech and Language* 23(2): 200–219.

Young, S., Evermann, G., Gales, M., Hain, T., Kershaw, D., Liu, X., Moore, G., Odell, J., Ollason, D., Povey, D., Valtchev, V. & Woodland, P. (2006). *The HTK book (for HTK version 3.4)*, Cambridge University Engineering Department, Cambridge, UK.

Zeng, F.-G., Nie, K., Stickney, G., Kong, Y.-Y., Vongphoe, M., Bhargave, A., Wei, C. & Cao, K. (2005). Speech recognition with amplitude and frequency modulations, *PNAS* Vol. 102(No. 7): 2293–2298.

8

The Cochlear Implant in Action: Molecular Changes Induced in the Rat Central Auditory System

Robert-Benjamin Illing and Nicole Rosskothen-Kuhl
Neurobiological Research Laboratory,
Department of Otorhinolaryngology,
University of Freiburg
Germany

1. Introduction

1.1 Hearing and learning

Learning is the essence of life. Throughout evolution, all species learn to adapt to a particular environment. As a consequence, organs are formed and reformed, and cellular function extends to respond to a broadening spectrum of types of energy and chemical compounds and focuses on particular stimulus configurations to respond to them in ever subtler ways. In ontogeny, chemical and spatial orientation is essential for the cells of an embryo so that it can grow all parts at the right time and at the right location. Postnatally, the radius from which an organism needs to learn expands from itself to the world surrounding it. For mammals, there appear to be two distinctly different phases of learning from the environment: early in life, or approximately before sexual maturity, and later in life, or post puberty. It has been a remarkable neuroscientific discovery that the molecular machinery employed by organism during their development is subtly but effectively modified to provide neuroplasticity later in life.

We learn to hear in ontogeny beginning at prenatal times (Peña et al., 2003), and patients receiving a cochlear implant (CI) need to learn or to re-learn hearing, depending on whether they never heard or they originally had a normal hearing experience. Both challenges require specific forms of learning. Learning implies appropriate adjustments of nervous networks to reflect differences and changes in patterns of sensory activity. Neuroscience looks for molecular, structural, and functional consequences of learning in the nervous system and refers to these changes as indicators of neuronal plasticity. To study sensory-evoked learning and plasticity we need to look at the molecular profile and cellular dynamic of neurons to identify its lasting traces in the brain.

One molecular marker associated to the initiation of sensory-evoked neuronal remodeling is the early response gene product c-Fos. Among the markers reflecting a growth-response of nerve cells and their synapses is the growth-associated protein GAP-43.

1.2 Auditory brainstem plasticity

Although earlier reports already suggested the possibility of structural plasticity in the adult mammalian brainstem (Wall & Egger, 1971; Pollin & Albe-Fessard, 1979), this mode of learning remained largely unacceptable into the 1980s. However, evidence slowly began to accumulate that structural plasticity is a general phenomenon of the adult mammalian brain, including all ages and all levels of the cerebral hierarchy. Equally important was the discovery that adult plasticity reuses many molecular mechanisms and regulatory circuits on which embryogenesis relies. However, important differences exist between juvenile and adult brain plasticity with respect to speed, breadth, and type of changes inducible by internal or external stimuli (e.g. Harris et al., 2005; 2008). At all developmental stages, neuroplasticity has many facets and includes the mutability on virtually all levels of neuronal organization, including volume growth, modifications of topographical maps, axon rerouting, dendritic outgrowth or retraction, cell death, mitosis, synaptogenesis, and molecular changes of various sorts. We finally appreciate the brain as an instrument of change.

1.3 c-Fos

1.3.1 c-Fos and learning

Immediate early genes are essential actors mediating learning-associated cellular processes and neuroplasticity. Although the immediate early gene product c-Fos has, together with phosphorylated extracellular signal-related kinase (p-ERK), been used as a marker for central sensitization, particularly in studies using nociception (Gao & Ji, 2009), its expression signifies not just electrophysiological activity but also cellular activity on different levels. Expression of c-Fos, like other early response genes, links fleeting changes of neuronal activity to lasting modifications of structure and function in the mammalian nervous system. Zuschratter et al. (1995) compared the spatial distribution of c-Fos immunoreactive neurons with the density of 2-desoxy-D-glucose (2DG) autoradiography after 1h of acoustic stimulation. While the pattern of the highest density of c-Fos labeled cells in the auditory cortex matched the peak labeling of autoradiographs, a spreading of c-Fos expression in neurons across the tonotopic maps was observed in primary auditory cortex and in the rostral and caudal fields of the auditory cortex. Corresponding to its role beyond indicating electrophysiological activity, c-Fos has been reported to be involved in the learning correlate of long term potentiation (Racaniello et al., 2010). Watanabe et al. (1996) found that homozygous mice carrying a null mutation of *c-fos* fail to show much of functional and structural plasticity seen in normal mice.

Auditory cortical neurons were shown to turn c-Fos positive following behaviorally significant sounds (Fichtel & Ehret, 1999; Wan et al., 2001; Geissler & Ehret, 2004). Sound recognition was compared with perception of exactly the same sound in mice. They showed that sound recognition, relying on memory, entails less but well focused Fos-positive cells in a primary auditory cortical field and significantly more labeling in higher order fields.

1.3.2 Regulation of c-Fos

The immediate early gene *c-fos* has, as part of its promoter, a transcription factor binding site called the cAMP response element (CRE; Ginty et al., 1994; Gispen et al., 1991). Thus, glutamate binding on NMDA receptors may activate the *c-fos* gene in neurons through the calcium-dependent phosphorylation of the CRE binding protein CREB by ERK and/or CaMKIV kinase pathways. CREB phosphorylation is modulated in cochlear nucleus and superior olivary complex as a consequence of electrical stimulation in the cochlea (Illing & Michler, 2001). Apart from CRE, the *c-fos* promoter contains a sis inducible element (SIE), a serum response element (SRE), and an activator protein-1 (AP-1)-like sequence (FAP) (Herdegen & Leah, 1998.). Besides its acting on the *c-fos* promoter, p-CREB may also affect expression of other genes containing a CRE site. Among them are the genes coding for the brain derived neurotrophic factor BDNF (Tao et al., 1998; Xu et al., 2000) and the early growth response protein-1 (Egr-1) (Sakamoto et al., 1991; Schwachtgen et al., 2000), another immediate-early gene product which is also known as Krox-24, Zif268, Zenk, NGFI-A, and Tis8. Apart from its CRE site, the promoter of the Egr-1 gene contains a SRE site and an AP-1 site (Schwachtgen et al., 2000; Weber & Skene, 1998). Competing with the activating transcription factor-2 (ATF-2; van Dam & Castellazzi, 2001), the protein c-Fos may dimerize with still another immediate-early gene product, c-Jun, to constitute a powerful transcription factor complex, called AP-1. The AP-1 factor, in turn, differentially triggers the expression of a large number of genes in a variety of functional aspects (Wisdom, 1999), with ATF-2:Jun and Fos:Jun complexes having differential binding preferences for heptameric or octameric AP-1 binding sites (van Dam and Castellazzi, 2001). Among the genes controlled by AP-1 are genes coding for the basic fibroblast growth factor bFGF (Shibata et al., 1991) and the growth and plasticity associated protein GAP-43 (Nedivi et al., 1992; Weber & Skene, 1998). Deficiency in ATF-2, in turn, leads to neurodegeneration of subsets of somatic and visceral motorneurons of the brainstem (Ackermann et al., 2011). There are conditions under which c-Fos may appear in glial cells (Edling et al., 2007).

Looking further upstream of c-Fos expression, cellular growth factors come into focus (Sharpe et al., 1993; Ginty et al., 1994). Interestingly, p-CREB is involved in regulating BDNF transcription (Tao et al., 1998), which in turn binds to TrkB receptors, modulating synaptic long-term potentiation (Xu et al., 2000) and driving the expression of c-Fos and other early response genes.

Illustrating the richness of molecular changes due to manipulating sensory input, the expression of immediate early genes, among them *egr-1* and *c-fos*, and neuronal plasticity-related genes such as those encoding for Arc, Syngr-1, and BDNF, was decreased by 2 weeks but increased again by 4 weeks in rat auditory cortex following bilateral cochlear ablation (Oh et al., 2007). ATF-2 is involved in the molecular underpinning of neuronal stability, cell death, and cellular growth (Yuan et al., 2009). Its expression goes down in retinal ganglion cells after their axotomy. Those cells capable of regrowing their axon show a return to high ATF-2 expression, indicating their return to normal conditions (Robinson GA, 1996). Members of the family of mitogen-activated protein kinases (MAPK) are ERK and p38 MAPK. ERK expression and phosphorylation reflects cellular changes associated to learning in an fear conditioning paradigm (Ota et al., 2010) and is co-regulated with c-Fos in several systems (Yang et al., 2008; Brami-Cherrier et al., 2009). Signals induced as a consequence of unilateral cochlear ablation are transduced mainly through the neuronal ERK pathway (Suneja & Potashner, 2003).

According to data available in the literature, the half- life of *c-fos* mRNA is 10-15 min (Müller et al., 1984; Sheng and Greenberg, 1990), whereas the c-Fos protein has a half-life of around 2 h (Curran et al., 1984; Müller et al., 1984).

1.3.3 Sensory stimulation of the auditory pathway

Sound-induced c-Fos expression has been employed to investigate the functional anatomy of the central auditory system of the mammalian brain. Expression of c-Fos has been seen in central auditory neurons after acoustical or electrical stimulation of the ear. Using pure-tone stimulation of mice or rats, the locations of neurons that turn positive for c-Fos or its mRNA were found to match the electrophysiologically established tonotopic maps in the ventral and dorsal cochlear nucleus (Rouiller et al., 1992; Brown & Liu, 1995; Miko et al., 2007), the superior olive (Adams, 1995), the dorsal nucleus of the lateral lemniscus (Saint Marie et al., 1999A), the inferior colliculus (Ehret & Fischer, 1991; Friauf, 1995; Pierson & Snyder-Keller, 1994; Saint Marie et al., 1999B), and the auditory cortex (Zuschratter et al., 1995). It was also induced in the vestibular nuclei (Sato et al., 1993). On exposing rats to specific behavioral tasks dependent on auditory stimuli, expression of c-Fos was also found in auditory centers of the diencephalon and telencephalon (Campeau & Watson, 1997; Carretta et al., 1999; Scheich & Zuschratter, 1995).

The amount of c-Fos mRNA also reflects habituation following stressful auditory stimulation (Campeau et al., 2002). Expression of c-Fos has also been used to estimate the driving force of axonal projections inside the central auditory system (Sun et al., 2009; Clarkson et al., 2010) and to localize the target site of audiogenic seizure (Kai & Niki, 2002) or the origin of tinnitus-related over-activity (Wu et al., 2003). The neuronal response reflected by c-Fos expression is related to the selective response of different subpopulations of neurons to sounds of time-varying properties (Lu et al., 2009) and may be induced by disinhibition following nerve lesions (Luo et al., 1999). The precision of a tonotopic c-Fos response to pure tone stimulation appears to be under the control of EphA4 and ephrin-B2 (Miko et al., 2007).

1.3.4 Electrical stimulation of the auditory pathway

Electrical intracochlear stimulation (EIS) as done with CIs in humans was shown to be similarly effective as acoustical stimulation in driving cells to express c-Fos (Roullier et al., 1992; Illing & Michler, 2001; Nakamura et al., 2003). Subsequent studies showed a marked variability in the pattern of stimulation-dependent c-Fos expression in the auditory brainstem. Some studies reported massive induction of c-Fos in dorsal cochlear nucleus (DCN), with little expression in ventral cochlear nucleus (VCN), and a substantial increase of c-Fos immunoreactivity in the external nuclei of the inferior colliculus (IC), with little staining in its central nucleus CIC (Vischer et al., 1994; 1995; Zhang et al., 1996). Others reported distinctly different patterns of c-Fos expression upon EIS (Illing & Michler, 2001; Saint Marie et al., 1999A, 1999B; Saito et al., 1999; Zhang et al., 1998). In several studies involving electrical stimulation, tonotopic patterns of c-Fos expression were found (Saito et al., 1999; Nagase et al., 2000; Saito et al., 2000; Illing & Michler, 2001), but others did not report it (Nakamura et al., 2005). c-Fos has also been induced after neonatal auditory deprivation (Keilmann & Herdegen, 1995; 1997) and in kanamycin-deafened rats (Fujii et al., 1997; Nagase et al., 2003). Like EIS, directly stimulating the dorsal cochlear nucleus is effective in driving tonotopic c-Fos expression (Takagi et al., 2004) and produces hearing in rats (Zhang & Zhang, 2010).

1.4 GAP-43

In pre- and early postnatal development of the mammalian brain, expression of the membrane phosphoprotein GAP-43, also known as B-50, F1, pp46, P-57, or neuromodulin, is high in neuronal somata, axons, and growth cones (Gispen et al., 1991; Kinney et al., 1993). Brain areas known for their adult potential for plasticity are characterized by high levels of GAP-43 (Benowitz et al., 1988; Benowitz and Routtenberg, 1997). This protein is a neuron-specific calmodulin-binding phosphoprotein and substrate for protein kinase C (Gispen et al., 1991; Schaechter & Benowitz, 1993). There are several lines of evidence relating this protein to axonal growth as well as to plasticity. It is produced at high levels in every nerve cell during neurite outgrowth and early stages of synaptogenesis (Skene and Willard, 1981; Mahalik et al., 1992) and represents a major constituent of the isolated growth cone (De Graan et al., 1985; Meiri et al., 1998). With maturation, its expression is down-regulated by most neurons (Skene, 1989; Benowitz & Perrone-Bizzozero, 1991). When a sense construct of GAP-43 mRNA was transiently expressed in non-neuronal cultured cells, these cells grow filopodial-like processes (Yankner et al., 1990; Verhaagen et al., 1994). If cells were transfected with a mutated construct of GAP-43 which prevented attachment of GAP-43 into the cell membrane, GAP-43 did not accumulate in pseudopods and no changes in cell morphology were induced (Widmer & Caroni, 1993). The attenuation of endogenous GAP-43 by an antibody that was raised against this protein and injected intracellularly has been found to reduce the degree of neurite outgrowth in a dose-dependent manner (Shea et al., 1992). The over-expression of GAP-43 in transgenic mice results in the formation of additional and aberrant neuronal connections (Aigner et al., 1995). Conversely, a knock out of the GAP-43 gene is survived by only 5-10% beyond weaning (Strittmatter et al., 1995). Whereas GAP-43 (-/-) mice show significant impairments in muscle strength, limb coordination and balance, and exhibit hyperactivity and reduced anxiety, GAP-43 (+/-) mice are only moderately impaired as compared with wild-type animals (Metz & Schwab, 2004). However, significant memory deficits were reported of heterozygous GAP-43 knockout mice with GAP-43 levels reduced by one-half, providing further evidence that GAP-43 exerts a crucial role in the bidirectional regulation of mnemonic processing (Rekart et al., 2005).

Expression of GAP-43 runs, at least partially, over activation of an AP-1 binding site. This identifies GAP-43 as a potential gene influenced by c-Fos. Further upstream, cooperation between p75(NTR) and TrkA results in an increased NGF-mediated TrkA autophosphorylation (Diolaiti et al., 2007). This cooperation also leads to a sustained activation of ERK-1/2 by phosphorylation and accelerates neurite outgrowth concomitant with a selective enhancement of the AP-1 activity and the transcriptional activation of genes such as GAP-43.

We discovered that unilateral deafness inflicted by a total sensory deafferentation of the cochlear nucleus in the mature rat invokes expression of GAP-43 (Illing & Horváth, 1995; Illing et al., 1997; see also Gil-Loyzaga et al., 2010). Since then, we found that this GAP-43 resides in presynaptic endings (Hildebrandt et al., 2011), is expressed by cholinergic neurons (Meidinger et al., 2006) residing in the ventral nucleus of the trapezoid body (Kraus & Illing, 2004), and innervate only specific subtypes of neurons in the cochlear nucleus (Illing et al., 2005). Altogether, these results clearly indicate that sensory deafferentation is followed by a specific reorganization of the neuronal network in the cochlear nucleus. Realizing that there is an impressive potential of neuroplasticity in the adult mammalian brainstem we wondered if other modifications of the pattern of sensory-evoked neuronal activity might be answered by a comparable response of the auditory brainstem in terms of synaptic reorganization and, as a consequence, signal representation and analysis. We therefore turned to EIS.

1.5 Linking c-Fos with GAP-43

Much is known about molecular networks regulating cellular growth and differentiation processes in general, but we still know little about the organization of the switch stands of activity-dependent molecular regulation in vivo. Regulatory molecules preceding c-Fos expression include p-CREB, p-ERK-1/2, p38 MAPK, and p-ATF-2. Molecules whose expression may be influenced by c-Fos include GAP-43, neuroskeletal elements, and cell adhesion molecules (Illing, 2001).

Williams et al. (1991) already suggested that an early response to sciatic nerve injury consisting of c-Fos expression in the spinal cord is transformed into a GAP-43 response emerging in the same spinal region of Rexed's lamina II, if not the same cells. It remained open if axonal sprouting mediated by GAP-43 is beneficial to the lesioned systems or accounts for sensory disorders following nerve injury (Woolf et al., 1990).

Demonstrating a succession of c-Fos and GAP-43 in functional states of neurons related to activity-dependent modifications of brain structure more directly, Kleim et al. (1996) showed that the number of synapses per neuron and the percentage of Fos-positive cells within motor cortex was elevated in rats raised in conditions requiring acrobatic motor activity as compared to rats raised without such requirement. Their data suggest that Fos may be involved in the biochemical processes underlying skill acquisition and that motor learning, as opposed to motor activity, leads to increases in synapse number in the motor cortex. Correspondingly, Black et al. (1990) see a relation between c-Fos expression and synaptogenesis, and synaptogenesis, in turn, relies on the presence and action of GAP-43 (Benowitz & Routenberg, 1997). Diets improving spatial cognition of rats concomitantly raise the number of c-Fos positive neurons in hippocampus, resulting in a statistically significant negative correlation between the number of c-Fos positive neurons and the frequency of reference memory errors (Tanabe et al., 2004).

Watanabe et al. (1996) used a kindling model of epilepsy in which changes of neuronal activity in the form of brief focal seizures lead to lifelong structural and functional reorganization of the mammalian brain (McNamara et al., 1993). Brains thus affected by patterns of activity deviating from the normal develop axonal sprouting in hippocampal granule cells. However, when c-Fos was made unavailable for these brains due to a null-mutation, axonal sprouting is strongly reduced. Their data are consistent with the hypothesis that the lack of c-Fos reduces functional plasticity as well as a structural plasticity. This study again supports the hypothesis that the absence of c-Fos leads to a substantial attenuation of axonal plasticity due to a failure to activate growth-related genes such as GAP-43.

As a consequence of BDNF binding on the TrkB receptor, the expression of both c-Fos and GAP-43 is modulated (Edsjö et al., 2001; Koponen et al., 2004). Another feature shared by c-Fos mRNA and GAP-43 mRNA is to be stabilized by the same protein HuD (Chung et al., 1996; Mobarak et al., 2000; Smith et al., 2004). Binding of HuD apparently leads to increased levels of the respective protein under constant transcriptional conditions. This opens the possibility that c-Fos and GAP-43 share part of the regulation controlling their presence and availability, a feature that deserves attention in future research.

2. Methods

2.1 Animals

The region of the brain in which we looked for stimulation-dependent changes on the molecular and cellular level is the rat auditory brainstem. Wistar rats of either sex aged 6 to 12 weeks were used. Care and use of the animals as reported here were approved by the appropriate agency (Regierungspräsidium Freiburg, permission number 37/9185.81/G-10/83). Rats were anesthetized with a mixture of ketamin (i.p., 50 mg/kg body weight; Bela-Pharm GmbH & Co. KG, Vechta, Germany) and xylazine (i.p., 5 mg/kg body weight; Rompun, Bayer-Leverkusen, Germany) before auditory brainstem response (ABR) measurements were done. For experiments involving acute EIS, anesthesia was induced by urethane (i.p., 1.5 g/kg body weight; Fluka AG, Buchs, Schwitzerland).

2.2 Deafness model

Between postnatal day (P) 10 and P20 (inclusive), neonatal Wistar rats received daily injections of kanamycin (i.p., 400 mg/kg body weight; Sigma, Taufkirchen, Germany) (Fig. 1). Due to hair cell destruction caused by this antibiotic (Matsuda et al., 1999; Osaka et al., 1979), a rise of hearing threshold was seen against normal hearing rats when rats have grown to adulthood (Fig. 2 A, B).

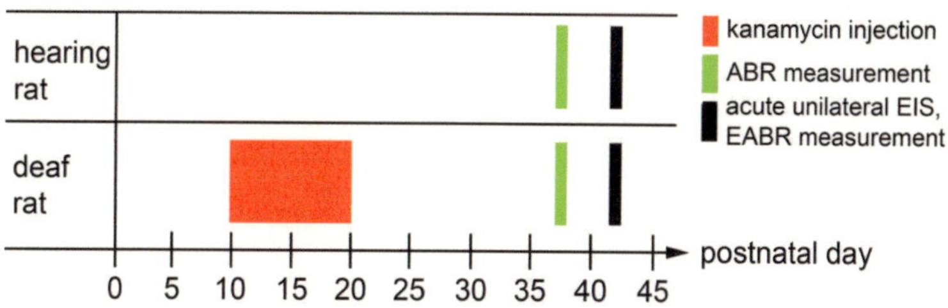

Fig. 1. Protocol to establish hearing and deaf experimental groups. Neonatal deafness was induced by daily kanamycin treatment between postnatal days 10 to 20. Measurement of acoustically or electrically evoked brainstem responses (ABR/EABR) were made around P33 and P42, respectively.

2.3 Electrical Intracochlear Stimulation (EIS)

Brains of hearing-experienced and hearing-inexperienced rats were analyzed after EIS lasting for different times, with stimulation durations spaced by the factor of 1.6: 45 min, 73 min, 2 h, 3:15 h, and 5 h (Fig. 2 C, D). The electrode used was a CI connected to a communicator both kindly provided by Cochlear GmbH (Hannover, Germany). Bipolar stimulation consisted of 50 Hz biphasic stimuli with a phase width of 50 μs. The electrically evoked brainstem response (EABR) was recorded like the ABR (see below) to determine an appropriate current level. The EABR was visualized using an averager (Multiliner E; Evolution 1.70c), calculating mean amplitudes over 500 sweeps in a frequency band of 0.1 to 10 kHz. We aimed to obtain maximal EABR amplitudes of 10 μV ± 10% by adjusting the current level of EIS to match acoustic stimuli of about 75 dB SPL. Chronic stimulation in the awake rat was done with the same mode using the same electrodes, but implants were connected to the stimulator by way of a swivel and a skull-based interface.

2.4 Auditory and electrically evoked brainstem responses

ABRs and EABRs were measured for hearing-experienced and hearing inexperienced rats. Hearing thresholds were tested acoustically (ABR) and electrically (EABR) by inducing auditory brainstem responses (Fig. 2 A, B). For ABR recording, steel needle electrodes were placed subcutaneously at vertex and mastoids and a 20 Hz train of click stimuli was presented to one side through a brass pipe equipped with a conical plastic tip into the ear canal, while sensations through the other ear were masked by supplying white noise at the same sound pressure level. Sound pressure was stepwise increased, attempting to elicit an ABR visualized by an averager (Multiliner E; Evolution 1.70c; Toennies, Germany). ABR mean amplitudes were determined after 300 sweeps in a frequency band of 0.1 to 3 kHz. If a kanamycin-treated rat showed an ABR at a sound pressure level smaller than 95 dB, recordings were stopped to avoid inducing further sensory stimulation. Following kanamycin treatment, we found ABR thresholds elevated by 75 dB to above 95 dB. These rats consistently failed to show a motor response to a handclap (Preyer's reflex). The absence of Preyer's reflex was taken by Jero et al. (2001) as indicating a rise of ABR threshold beyond 81 dB SPL. This result served as an additionally indication of deafness caused in the kanamycin-treated group.

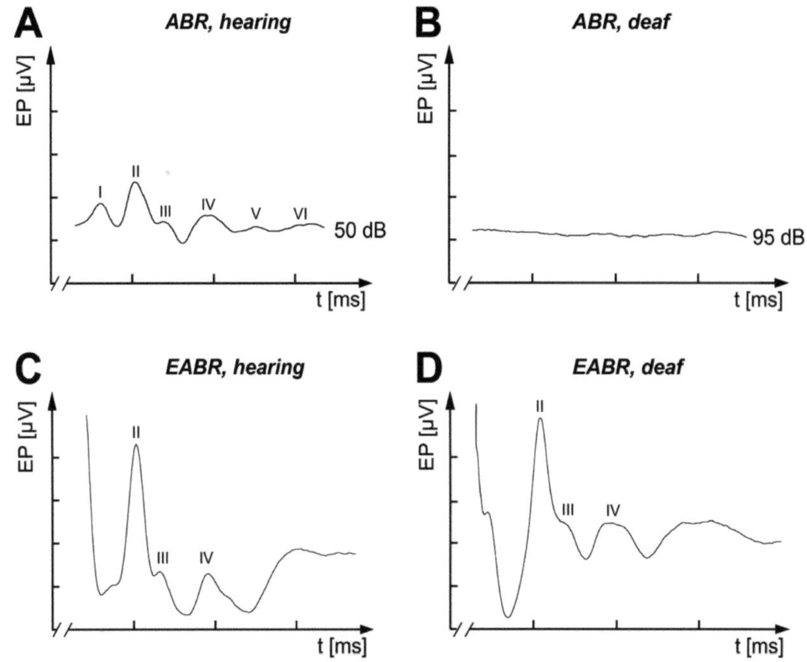

Fig. 2. ABR and EABR in hearing and deaf rats. Representative acoustically (A, B) and electrically (C, D) evoked auditory brainstem responses of hearing (A, C) and deaf (B, D) mature rats. Typically, the ABR of a hearing rat showed six distinguishable peaks (I-VI) and the EABR at least three peaks (II-IV). No ABR was detectable in kanamycin-treated rats up to 95 dB SPL. X-axis: 1 ms per unit; Y-axis: 4 µV per unit; EP: evoked potential.

We localized c-Fos and GAP-43 by several variants of immunocytochemistry and in situ hybridization. Other antigens (p-ATF-2, c-Jun p39, p38 MAPK) were detected by immunocytochemistry based on diaminobenzidine staining or immunfluorescence (cp. Illing & Michler, 2001; Rosskothen et al., 2008; Rosskothen-Kuhl & Illing, 2010).

2.5 Immunohistochemistry (IHC)

After completion of the postoperative survival time or different stimulation periods, animals were killed by sodium-thiopental (i.p., 50 mg/ml per 200 g body weight of Trapanal 2.5 g, Nycomed, Konstanz, Germany) and perfused transcardially with a fixative containing 4% paraformaldehyd and 0% - 0.025% glutaraldehyde in 0.1 M phosphate buffer at pH 7.4. After brains were removed from the skulls and soaked in 30% sucrose overnight, parts containing anteroventral cochlear nucleus (AVCN), DCN, lateral superior olivary complex (LSO), and CIC were cryo-cut into 30 µm thick frontal sections. Following incubation with 0.05% H_2O_2, 1% sodium-borohydride (only for c-Fos and p-ATF-2) and 1% milk powder in 0.02 M phosphate buffer saline (PBS) at pH 7.4 for 30 min each, sections were exposed to a primary antibody either raised in goat against c-Fos (SC-52-G, 1:2000, lot. no. A2810, Santa Cruz Biotechnology Inc., Santa Cruz, USA), or raised in mouse against GAP-43 (MAB347, 1:5000, lot. no. LV1786431, Millipore, California, USA), or raised in rabbit against c-Jun p39 (SC-1694, 1:100–1:500; lot. no. L0606, Santa Cruz Biotechnology Inc.), p38 MAPK (4511S, 1:2000, lot. no. 5, Cell Signaling Technology, Inc., Danvers, USA), p-ATF-2 (5112S, 1:2000, lot. no. 10, Cell Signaling Technology, Inc.) or p-ERK 1/2 (SC-16982, 1:1000, lot. no. K1910, Santa Cruz Biotechnology Inc). After incubation for 48 h at 4° C, visualization of antibody-binding sites was based on DAB staining using biotinylated anti-goat/-mouse/-rabbit (BA-5000/BA2001/BA1000, 1:200, Vector Laboratories, Inc., Burlingame, USA) as secondary antibody and avidin-biotin-technique (Vector Laboratories) for signal intensification. Negative controls were run to verify specificity of the primary and secondary antibodies. Nuclei of the parabrachial region stained for c-Fos immunoreactivity served as positive controls (Illing et al., 2002).

2.6 In Situ Hybridization (ISH)

Thirty micrometer thick cryo-cut frontal brain sections were collected in 2x standard saline citrate (SSC) buffer (Invitrogen, Life Technologies GmbH, Darmstadt, Germany). The sections were washed in 2x SSC buffer for 15 min. Before pre-hybridization sections were pretreated in a 1:1 dilution of 2x SSC and hybridization buffer (50% formamide, Carl Roth GmbH, Karlsruhe, Germany), 4x SSC (Invitrogen), 10% dextransulfate (Sigma, Taufkirchen, Germany), 1x Denhardt's solution (AMRESCO Inc., Ohio, USA), 250 µg/ml heat-denatured cod and herring sperm DNA (Roche Diagnostics GmbH, Mannheim, Germany), 625 µg/ml tRNA from E. coli MRE 600 (Roche)) for 15 min. Pre-hybridization lasted in hybridization buffer for 60 min at 55°C. Hybridization was performed overnight at 55°C in the same solution with the addition of 100 ng/ml digoxigenin (DIG)-labeled c-Fos and 1000 ng/ml DIG-labeled GAP-43 antisense or sense cRNA, respectively. DIG-labeled sense and antisense cRNAs were synthesized by PCR amplification of brain tissue isolated c-Fos/GAP-43 mRNA. Primer design occurred by the use of the NCBI sequences NM_017195.3 (for GAP-43) and NM_022197.2 (for c-Fos). After hybridization, the sections were washed in 2x SSC for 2 x 15 minutes at room temperature, 2x SSC and 50% formamide (MERCK KGAA, Darmstadt, Germany) for 15 min, 0.1x SSC and 50% formamide for 15 min, and 0.1x SSC for 2 x 15 minutes at 65°C each. For immunological detection of DIG-labeled hybrids, brain sections were treated in buffer 1 (100 mM Tris/HCl, pH 7.5) for 2 x 10 min each, blocked in buffer 2 (1% blocking reagent (Roche) in buffer 1) for 60 min at room temperature, and incubated overnight at 4°C with the anti-DIG Fab fragment from sheep tagged with alkaline phosphatase (1:1500, Roche) in buffer 2. For the color reaction, brain sections were equilibrated in buffer 1 for 2 x 10 min each and in buffer 3 (100 mM Tris/HCl, pH 9.5, 100 mM NaCl, 50 mM $MgCl_2$) for 10 min before the addition of nitroblue tetrazolium (0.34 mg/ml, Roche) and 5-bromo-4-chloro-3-indolyl-phosphate, 4-toluidine salt (0.17 mg/ml, Roche) diluted in buffer 3. Development of the color reaction was performed for around 9 hours in the dark at room temperature and stopped by transfer into aqua when the desired staining intensity was reached. Finally, sections were mounted on glass slides, dehydrated in increasing grades of alcohol, cleared in xylene, and coverslipped with DPX (Sigma).

2.7 Electron microscopy

After perfusion as described above, brains were postfixed in the same fixative for 2 h and stored overnight in PBS. Cutting was done on a microtome with vibrating blade (Leica VT 1000S, Bensheim, Germany) at 50 μm and collected in PBS containing 0.05 M glycine. Sections were permeabilized by a treatment with 5% and 10% dimethyl sulphoxide (DMSO), each for 10 min, and 20 min in 20% and 40% DMSO, all in PBS. Following washing in PBS, tissue was successively exposed to 0.05% H_2O_2, 0.05% sodium-borohydride, and 5% normal rabbit or goat serum in PBS each for 30 min, and incubated with antibodies raised against c-Fos (1:2000), p-ATF-2 (1:2000), or p-ERK-1/2 (1:1000). After incubation for 24 h at 4° C, visualization of antibody-binding sites occurred as described before for the IHC protocol (see. 2.5). Afterward, brain sections were incubated with 0.1% osmium-tetroxide in 0.1 M cacodylic acid buffer (pH 7.4), dehydrated in ethanol and embedded in EMbed-812 (Science Services, München, Germany).

3. Results and discussion

3.1 Effectiveness of EIS to induce gene expression

EIS is an effective way to activate neuronal networks in the central auditory system, including the induction of c-Fos expression throughout the brainstem of hearing-experienced rats (Fig. 3).

We monitored c-Fos expression on the transcriptional level by detecting c-Fos mRNA as well as on the translational level by c-Fos immunoreactivity (Illing et al., 1999). In both cases we detected staining in neuronal nuclei that closely matched in space and time (Fig. 4).

Attempting to understand the laws according to which neurons express c-Fos as a consequence of EIS we, first, identified the cell types in which c-Fos emerged. Following 2 h of EIS we found that only distinct subpopulations of neurons in VCN, DCN, LSO, and CIC express c-Fos (Reisch et al., 2007) (Fig.5). Whereas sub-populations of glutamatergic and glycinergic cells responded in all four regions, GABAergic neurons failed to do so except in marginal zones of AVCN and in DCN (but cp. Ishida et al., 2002). Combining immunocytochemistry with axonal tracing, neurons participating in major ascending pathways, commissural cells of VCN and certain types of neurons of the descending auditory system were seen to respond to EIS with early response gene expression. By contrast, principal LSO cells projecting to the contralateral CIC as well as collicular efferents of the DCN did not.

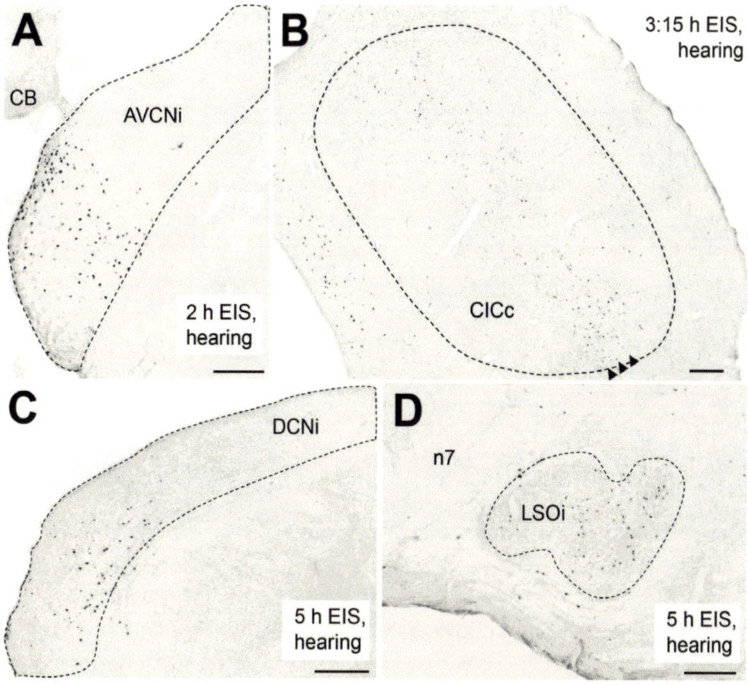

Fig. 3. Effectiveness of EIS to induce c-Fos expression throughout the brainstem of hearing rats. (A) Tonotopic c-Fos expression (black dots) in AVCNi after 2 h of EIS. (B) Tonotopic band (arrowheads) of c-Fos positive nuclei (black dots) in CICc after 3:15 h of EIS. (C) Tonotopic c-Fos expression (black dots) in the deep layers of DCNi after 5 h of EIS. (D) c-Fos expression (black dots) in LSOi following 5 h of sustained EIS. The dashed lines correspond to the borders of the respective auditory regions. Scale bars: 0.2 mm. i: ipsilateral; c: contralateral; CB: cerebellum; n7: facial nerve.

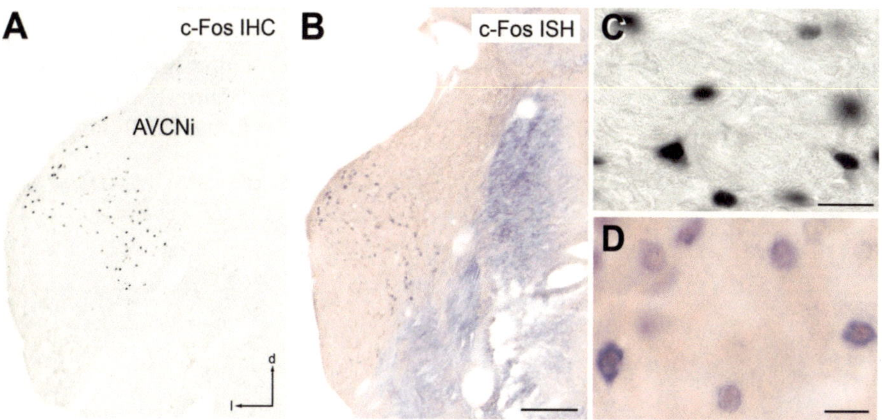

Fig. 4. Comparison of c-Fos immunoreactivity (A, C) vs. c-Fos in situ hybridization (B, D) in AVCNi of a hearing-experienced rat after 73 min EIS. (A, B) The pattern of c-Fos protein (black dots) and c-Fos mRNA (blue dots) of 2 adjacent sections is nearly identical. Scale bar: 0.2 mm. (C, D) Higher magnification of c-Fos protein positive nuclei (C) and c-Fos mRNA positive neurons (D) in AVCNi. Scale bars: 20 µm. i: ipsilateral; d: dorsal; l: lateral.

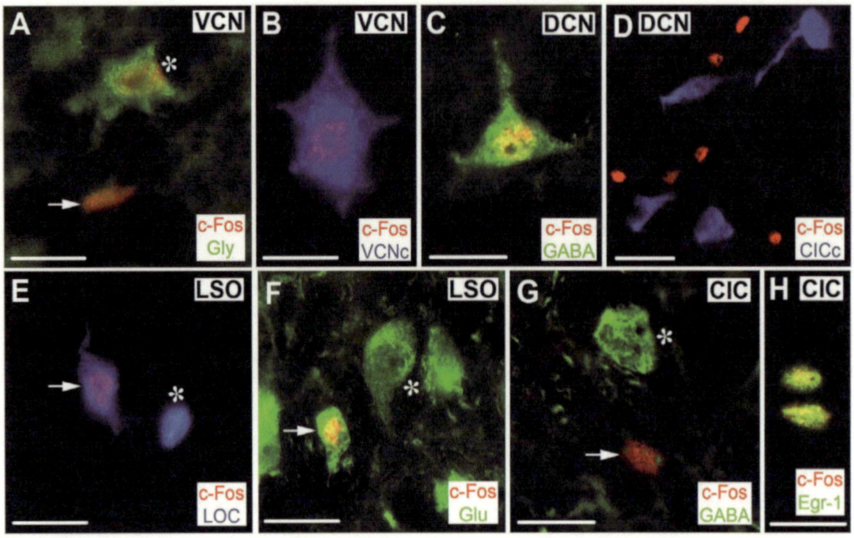

Fig. 5. EIS-dependent c-Fos expression in neurons of the auditory brainstem of hearing-experienced rats (Illing et al., 2010). (A) In VCN, half of the c-Fos positive nuclei were localized in glycinergic cells (Gly, yellow, asterisk), the other half showed no double labeling with glycine (arrow). (B) c-Fos in a large VCN commissural neuron after injection of the tracer Fast Blue into VCNc. (C) c-Fos in a GABAergic neuron of DCN. (D) c-Fos positive nuclei were never observed in neurons of DCN projecting to the contralateral CICc. (E) Some (arrow) but not all (asterisk) lateral olivocochlear (LOC) neurons labeled from the cochlea by axonal tracing showed co-localization with c-Fos. (F) c-Fos positive nuclei in small glutamatergic cells of LSOi (Glu, arrow), large glutamatergic cells lacked c-Fos immunoreactivity (asterisk). (G) CIC lacking c-Fos positive GABAergic cells. (H) Immunoreactivity for Egr-1 coincided with c-Fos immunoreactivity. i: ipsilateral, c: contralateral. Scale bars: 20 µm in D, 10 µm for all others.

Second, following continuous stimulation of hearing-experienced anesthetized rats for various durations from 45 min to 5 hours, we observed a non-linear increase of the population of c-Fos positive neurons, with a rise followed by a decline, followed by a second rise of the number of stained cells in VCN (Rosskothen-Kuhl & Illing, 2010) (Fig. 6).

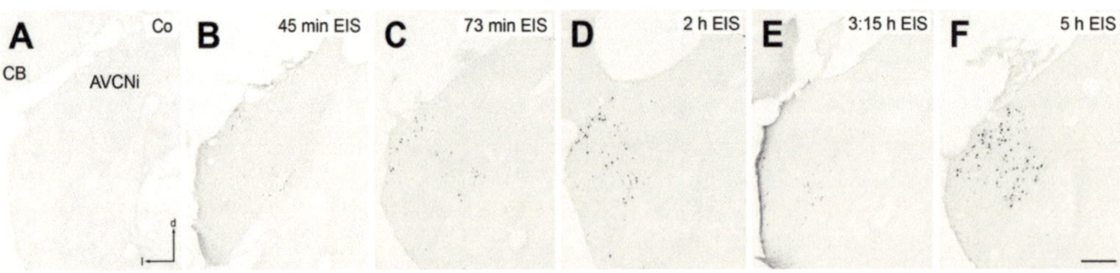

Fig. 6. Pattern of c-Fos expression with increasing stimulation time in AVCNi of hearing-experienced rats. (A) In control rats, AVCNi is devoid of c-Fos staining. (B-D) Typically, the number of c-Fos positive cells (black dots) increased from 45 min to 2 h in a region tonotopically corresponding to the stimulation position. (E-F) By 3:15 h of unilateral EIS, the c-Fos level transiently decreases before it rose again by 5 h (F). Scale bar: 0.2 mm. Co: control; i: ipsilateral; CB: cerebellum; d: dorsal; l: lateral.

Third, we used different temporal patters known to have major significance for central auditory processing (Walton, 2010) for EIS at a constant duration of 2 h (Jakob & Illing, 2008). For each of the major auditory brainstem nuclei and some of their subregions we found specific patterns of the immunoresponsive cell populations reflecting different aspects of the stimulation site and stimulation parameters (Table 1).

	lateralization	intensity	frequency	duration
AVCNi	+	+	0	+
DCNi,upper layers	+	0	+	+
DCNi, deep layers	+	0	+	+
LSOi, medial	+	+	0	0
LSOi, total	+	+	0	0
CICc, dorsolat.	+	+	+	+
CICc, ventromed.	+	+	+	0
MGBc	0	+	0	0

Table 1. Expression pattern of c-Fos across the auditory brainstem depends on stimulation parameters. Each of the major auditory brainstem regions, and some of their subregions, showed a unique fingerprint of c-Fos expression (cp. rows) with respect to reflecting laterality, intensity, frequency (Jakob & Illing, 2008), and duration of EIS. MGB: medial geniculate nucleus, i: ipsilateral, c: contralateral.

3.2 Pharmacology

Apart from the duration of EIS and the particular stimulation parameters used, the possibility exists that the consequences of activating the central auditory system may also be

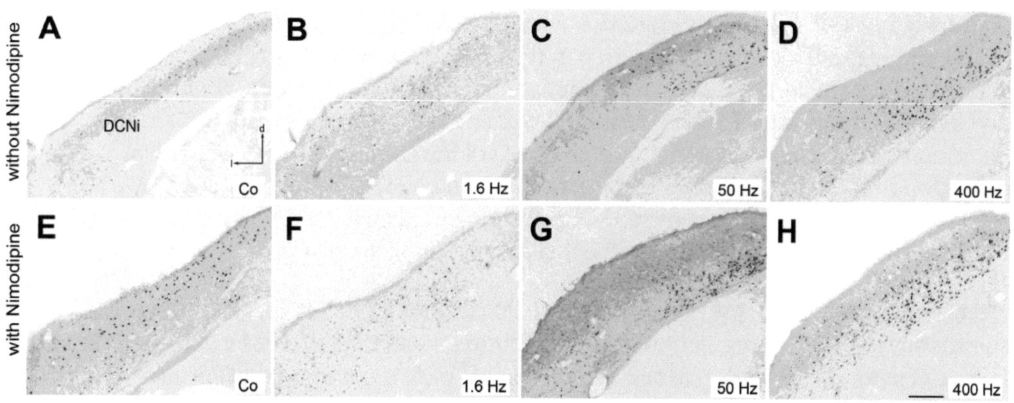

Fig. 7. Effect of Nimodipine on the pattern of c-Fos expression in the DCNi with different stimulation parameters. (B-D, F-H) For both experimental groups a shift of c-Fos positive nuclei (black dots) from the upper to the deep layers of DCN exist with increasing stimulation frequency, after 2 h of EIS. However, the Nimodipine treatment (E-H) resulted in a significant increase in number of c-Fos expressing neurons compared to non-treated (A-D) rats. Scale bar: 0.2 mm. Co: control; i: ipsilateral; d: dorsal; l: lateral.

influenced by pharmacological manipulations. Here we illustrate one example, the impact of Nimodipine systemically administered before EIS. In DCN, the pattern of neurons expressing c-Fos is dramatically different depending on the presence or absence of Nimodipine (Fig. 7).

3.3 Molecules upstream of c-Fos expression

In order to understand the functional relevance of c-Fos expression under any particular mode of stimulation, it is mandatory to co-localize it with other molecular actors of neuroplastic change in space and time. Therefore, we studied the spatio-temporal relationship of c-Fos expression with the expression pattern of molecules known to be involved directly or indirectly in the regulation of c-Fos expression. Upstream of c-Fos expression, p-CREB, ATF-2, p-ERK-1/2, and p38 MAPK unfold their activity. We discovered that their expression is modulated either positively or negatively under EIS (Fig. 8).

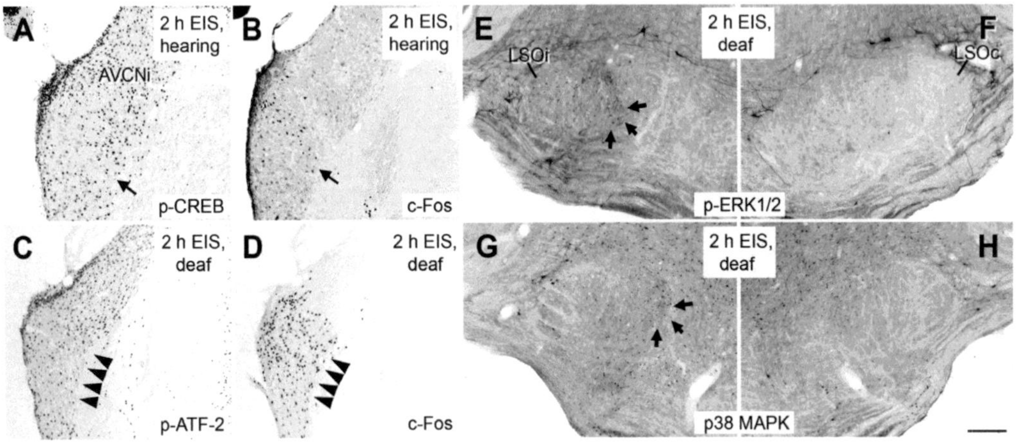

Fig. 8. Modulation of regulatory molecules upstream of c-Fos expression. (A-B) 2 h after EIS of hearing rats p-CREB positive neurons were rare in a middle band of AVCNi (A, arrow) corresponding to the c-Fos positive area in the adjacent section (B, arrow). (C-D) A similar pattern existed for p-ATF-2 (C, arrowheads) and c-Fos (D, arrowheads) positive nuclei in the AVCNi of deaf rats after 2 h of EIS. (E-H) 2 h after EIS of deaf rats p-ERK-1/2 immunoreactivity was detected only in the LSO of the stimulated side (E, arrows) corresponding to the c-Fos expression pattern (not shown). Like for p-ERK-1/2 the p38 MAPK immunoreactivity was increased in the medial LSOi (G, arrows) compared to the contralateral side (H). c: contralateral; i: ipsilateral. Scale bar: 0.2 mm.

Next, we looked for the ultrastructural localizations of molecules involved in the stimulation-dependent regulation of transcription factors (Fig. 9). Under EIS, c-Fos emerged in nuclei and rough endoplasmic reticulum of VCN neurons. p-ATF-2 and p-ERK-1/2 showed specific regional and intracellular staining patterns of their own.

Directly interacting with c-Fos is c-Jun p39. We found that, similar to the immediate early gene *egr-1* (De et al., 2003) but unlike its stimulation-dependent expression in the inner ear (Ruan et al., 2007), c-Jun is present in most of the auditory brainstem in normal brains without specific stimulation (Fig. 10). Upon EIS and ensuing c-Fos expression, c-Fos and c-Jun may dimerize to form AP-1 in a highly active variant (Rosskothen et al., 2008) (Fig. 10 B-D).

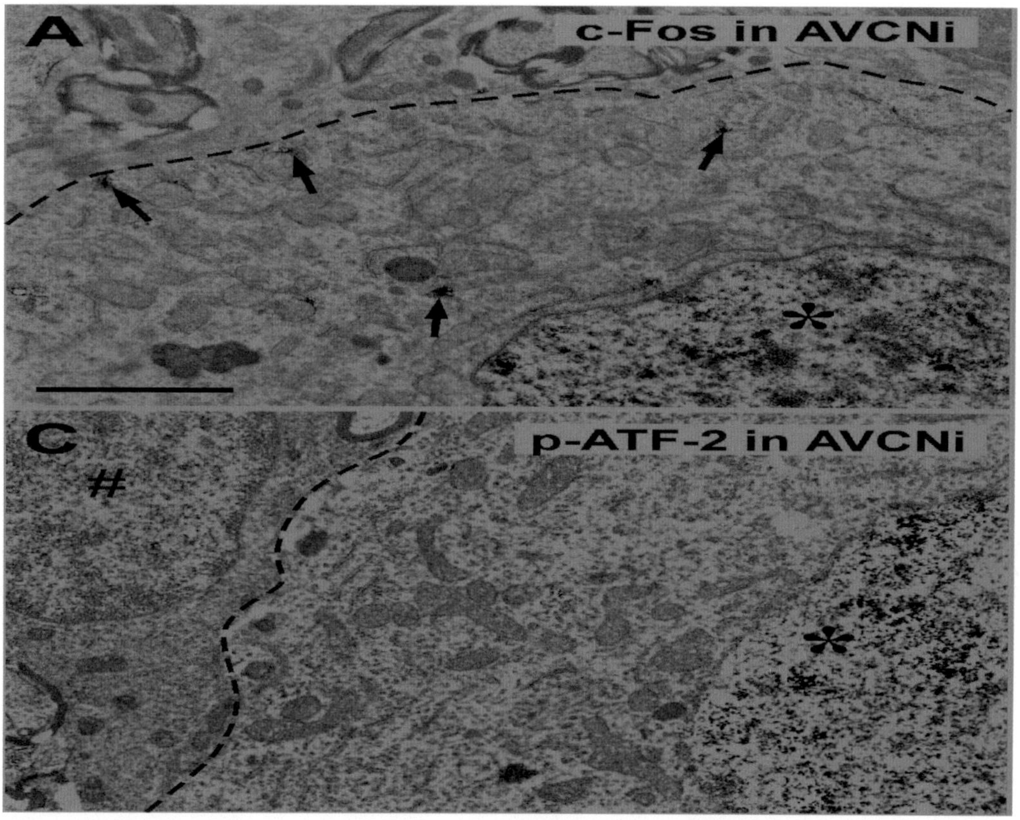

Fig. 9. Modulation of transcription factor regulators by EIS. (A) Ultrastructural localization of c-Fos immunoreactivity in nucleus (asterisk) and cytoplasm (arrows) of a neuron in AVCNi. (B) Contralaterally, no such staining was seen. (C) p-ATF-2 immunoreactivity in the nucleus of an AVCNi neuron; upon EIS, this staining declines. (D) p-ERK-1/2 staining in nucleus (asterisk) and cytoplasm (arrows) in a DCN neuron next to an unstained neuron after EIS. Dashed lines indicate cell boundaries. c: contralateral; i: ipsilateral. Scale bar: 2 μm.

3.4 Molecules downstream of c-Fos expression

Downstream of c-Fos lie many genes regulated by an AP-1 binding site in their promoter, among them the gene encoding GAP-43. We observed an emergence of GAP-43 in fibers and boutons of VCN on the side of chronic EIS (Fig. 11). At the same time, GAP-43 mRNA is strongly up-regulated in neurons of LSO (Fig. 11 C-F).

The LSO is known to be involved in relearning sound localization during unilateral conductive hearing loss (Irving et al., 2011), suggesting that its neurons receive a growth signal by unilateral EIS that, in turn, causes axonal sprouting in VCN on the stimulated side. This scenario poses a remarkable contrast to GAP-43 expression in VCN one week after its total sensory deafferentation by cochlear ablation (Illing et al., 1997). Under these circumstances, GAP-43 in VCN is supplied by neurons of the ventral nucleus of the trapezoid body (VNTB), source of the medial olivocochlear pathway, rather than of LSO, source of the lateral olivocochlear pathway.

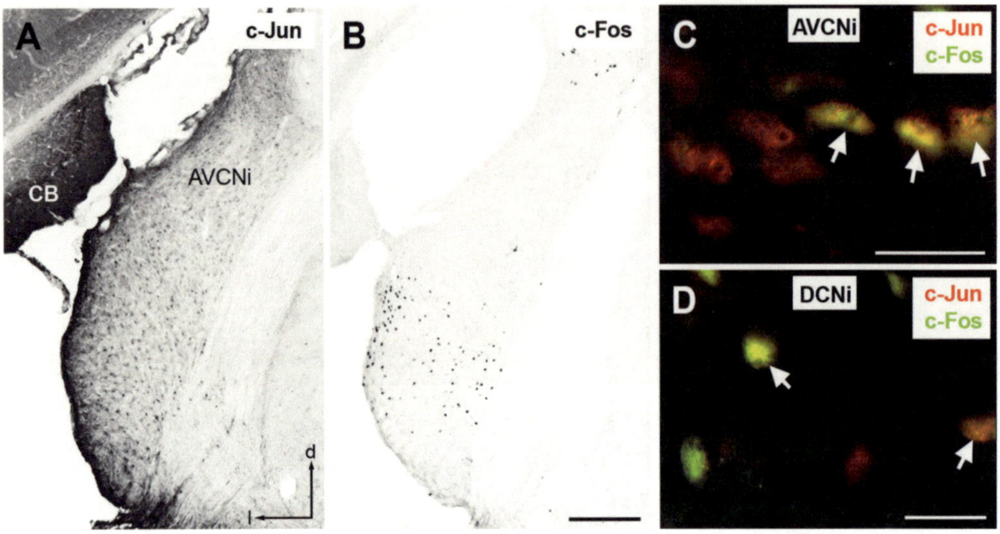

Fig. 10. The molecular environment of c-Fos expression includes the availability of c-Jun p39. (A) Numerous c-Jun positive nuclei (black dots) in the entire AVCNi of an unstimulated, hearing control rat. (B) c-Fos positive nuclei appear after EIS in a band corresponding tonotopically to intracochlear stimulation site. Scale bar: 0.2 mm. (C, D) Following EIS, c-Fos (green) and c-Jun (red) are co-expressed (yellow/orange, arrows) in some but not all cells of AVCNi (C) and DCNi (D). i: ipsilateral; CB: cerebellum; d: dorsal; l: lateral. Scale bars: 20 µm.

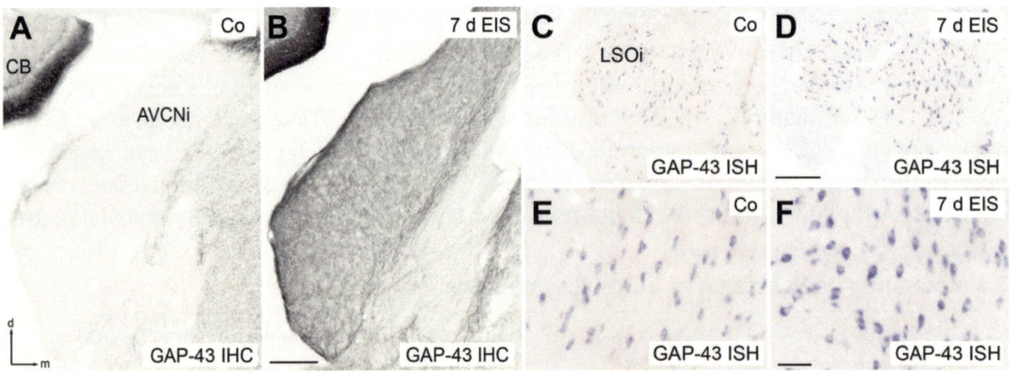

Fig. 11. Emergence of GAP-43 in the AVCNi after chronic EIS for 7 days. (A) AVCNi of a hearing control rat devoid of GAP-43 immunoreactivity. (B) GAP-43 immunoreactivity appears in the entire AVCNi of a 7 days (7 d) chronically stimulated hearing rat. (C-D) GAP-43 mRNA level in the LSOi of a hearing control rat (C) and a 7 days stimulated hearing rat (D). Scale bars (A-D): 0.2 mm. (E-F) GAP-43 mRNA in neurons of the LSOi at higher magnification. Scale bar: 50 µm. CB: cerebellum; Co: control; i: ipsilateral; d: dorsal; m: medial.

3.5 EIS induces c-Fos expression in deaf rats

The absence of hearing experience has far-reaching consequences for the interneuronal communication within networks of the auditory brainstem. First, when hearing fails, EIS entails expression of c-Fos in populations of neurons that are much larger than normally, essentially disregard tonotopic order, and lack much of spatio-temporal variations as seen in hearing-experienced rats (Rosskothen-Kuhl & Illing, 2012) (Fig. 12).

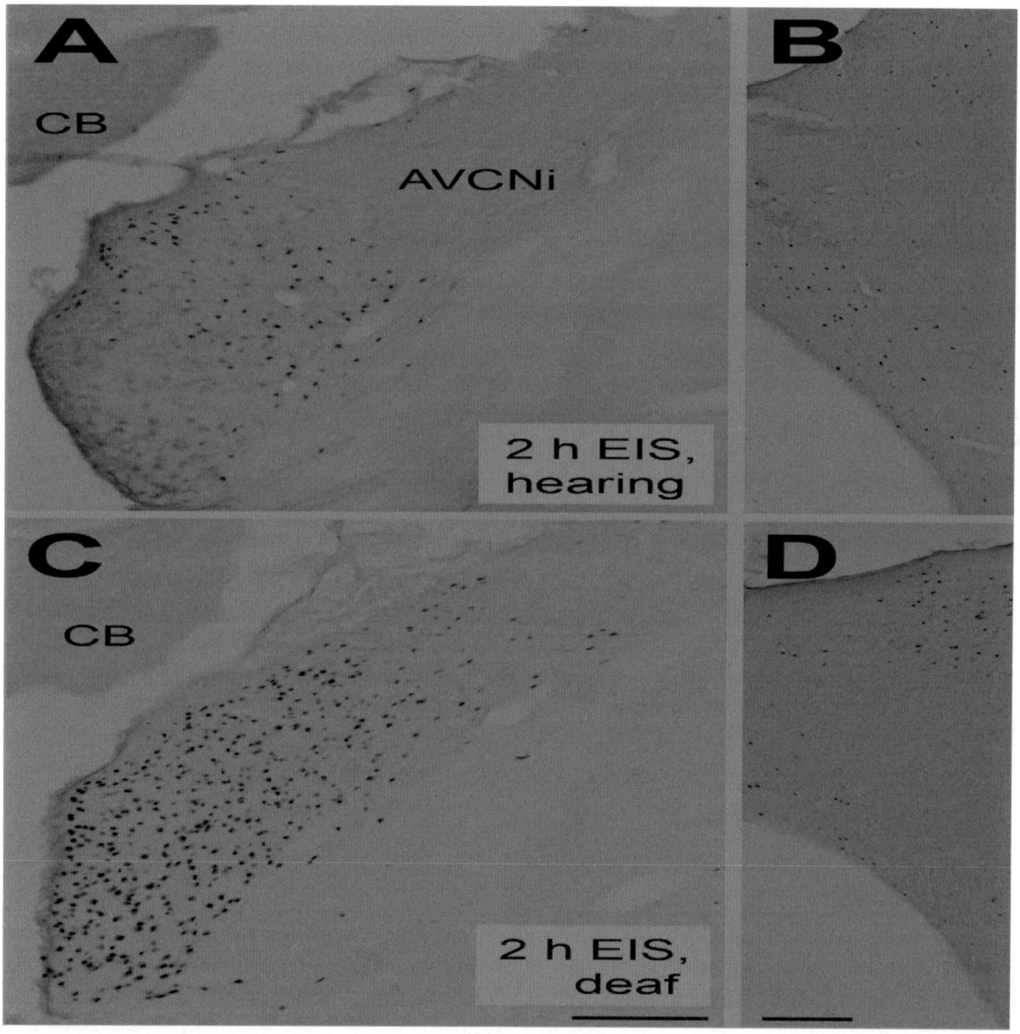

Fig. 12. Differences of c-Fos expression pattern in hearing vs. deafened rats. (A) Tonotopic c-Fos expression (black dots) in AVCNi of a hearing rat after 2 h of EIS. (B) Tonotopic band (arrowheads) of c-Fos positive nuclei (black dots) in CICc of a hearing rat after 3:15 h of EIS. (C) Non-tonotopic c-Fos expression (black dots) in AVCNi of a deaf rat after 2 h of EIS. (D) Strong and extended c-Fos expression (black dots) in the dorsolateral part of the CICc of a deaf rat after 3:15 h of EIS. i: ipsilateral; c: contralateral; CB: cerebellum; CX: Neocortex. Scale bars: 0.2 mm.

Second, the composition of c-Fos expressing subpopulation changed with the preceding hearing experience (Fig. 13).

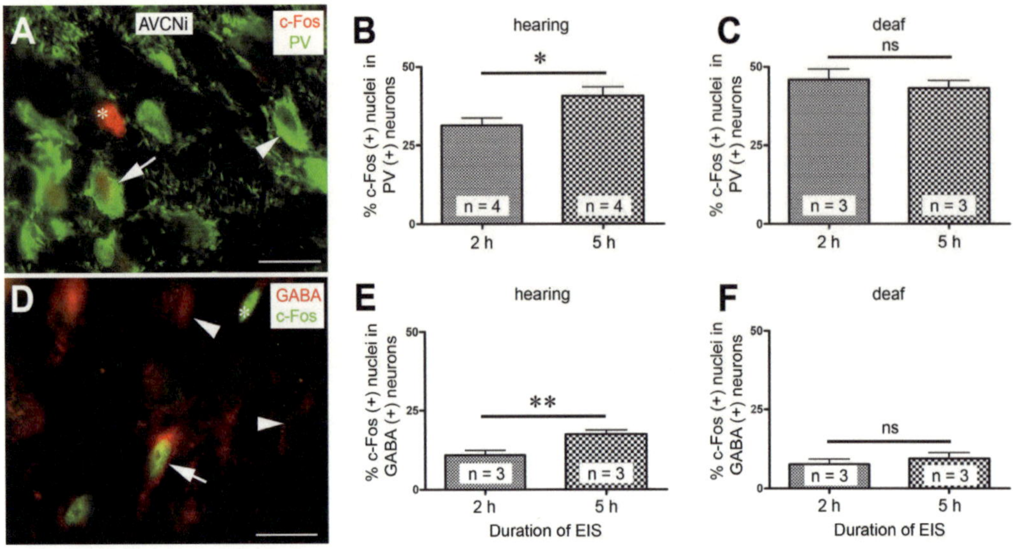

Fig. 13. Composition of c-Fos expressing subpopulations changed depending on preceding hearing experience and stimulation time. (A) Co-localization (arrow) of c-Fos positive nuclei (red, asterisk) and parvalbumin (PV)-positive neurons (green, arrowhead) in the AVCNi after EIS. (B, C) Statistic evaluation of co-localization of c-Fos positive nuclei and PV-positive neurons resulted only for hearing rats (B, $p=0.018$) but not for deaf rats (C) in a significant increase of double-labeling from 2 to 5 h of stimulation. (D) Following EIS, c-Fos expression (green, asterisk) was also co-localized (arrow) with GABAergic somata (red, arrowhead) in marginal zones of AVCNi. Scale bar: 20 µm. (E, F) The statistic evaluation of co-localization of c-Fos positive nuclei and GABA-positive neurons resulted only for hearing rats (E, $p= 0.006$) and not for deaf rats (F) in a significant increase of double-labeling from 2 to 5 h of EIS. i: ipsilateral; ns: non-significant.

4. Conclusions and outlook

The brain is responsive to changes of activity in sensory nerves by forming memory traces on all its levels, from forebrain to hindbrain, and from molecules to neuronal networks. A successful therapy for patients with dysfunctional ears requires a CI that plays patterns of electrical activity corresponding to patterns of sound to the auditory nerve, and a moldable brain responding to this pattern. This response must include the initiation of molecular and synaptic reorganization to make optimal use of sensory-evoked activity, specifically to identify and categorize temporal patterns in spoken language (Munro, 2008; Anderson et al., 2010; Skoe & Kraus 2010). Obviously, then, it is fundamentally important to run the CI in a way that fully exploits the neuroplastic potential of the central auditory system. It is therefore essential to detect short and long term molecular and cellular changes in the central nervous system in response to EIS equivalent to CI stimulation to understand which stimulation parameters are more important than others to elicit a full and focused plasticity response.

As we showed, specific conditions of afferent activity prompt specific populations of neurons in specific regions of the auditory brainstem to prepare for a molecular, structural, and functional remodeling within hours. Laterality, frequency, duration, and intensity of the stimulus each affect different neuronal populations across different regions. Coding of laterality takes place below the midbrain, but appears to be integrated in network activity from the inferior colliculus upwards. Each major brainstem region involved in the analysis of auditory stimuli respond to specific stimulation parameters by a unique dynamic pattern of c-Fos expression. With our studies we have made a first and perhaps a second and third step to understand central auditory plasticity, and there is reason to consider much of our data obtained from a mammalian brain transferable to man. However, our studies are not yet comprehensive in the sense that they already provide binding recommendations to CI programmers or users. Instead, it provides data showing for the first time that the parameters of running a CI bear a very real potential for neuroplastic remodeling of the central auditory system, and that the brain is certain to show a wealth of molecular and cellular responses to CI stimulation.

More stimulation parameters must be tested and more molecular markers monitored in order to delineate robust relationships between modes of stimulation, molecular processes, cellular growth, network remodeling, and the efficiency of signal processing. The knowledge so obtained will set the stage for the development of CIs in the future.

5. Acknowledgements

It is a pleasure to express our gratefulness to many co-workers for help: Heika Hildebrandt, Ann-Kathrin Rauch, Peter Bischoff, Till Jakob, Ulrike Doering, Michaela Fredrich, Eike Michalk, Peter Pedersen, Jürgen John, Alexander Huber, Ralf Birkenhäger, and Sigrid Weis. Moreover, thanks go to Cochlear Deutschland GmbH for kindly providing hard- and software used for EIS, and to Roland Laszig for continuous support.

6. List of abbreviations

2DG, 2-desoxy-D-glucose
ABR, auditory brainstem response
AP-1, activator protein-1
Arc, activity-regulated cytoskeleton-associated protein
ATF-2, activating transcription factor-2
AVCN, anteroventral cochlear nucleus
AVCNc, AVCN contralateral to stimulation
AVCNi, AVCN ipsilateral to stimulation
B50, synonym for GAP-43
BDNF, brain derived neurotrophic factor
bFGF, basic fibroblast growth factor, same as FGF2
c, contralateral
CaMKIV, Ca^{2+}/calmodulin-dependent protein kinases IV
cAMP, cyclic adenosine monophosphate
CB, cerebellum
c-fos, Finkel-Biskin-Jinkins murine osteosarcoma viral oncogene
c-Fos, protein encoded by proto-oncogene *c-fos*
CI, cochlear implant

CIC, central nucleus of the inferior colliculus
CICc, CIC contralateral to stimulation
c-jun, avian sarcoma virus 17, 'Jun' being derived from Japanese 'ju-nana' for '17'
c-Jun, protein encoded by immediate-early gene *c-jun*
Co, control
CRE, cAMP response element
CREB, cAMP response element-binding protein
cRNA, coding ribonucleic acid
CX, neocortex
d, dorsal
DAB, 3,3'-diaminobenzidine tetrahydrochloride
dB, decibel
DCN, dorsal cochlear nucleus
DCNi, DCN ipsilateral to stimulation
DIG, digoxigenin
DMSO, dimethyl sulphoxide
DNA, deoxyribonucleic acid
EABR, electrical auditory brainstem response
Egr-1, early growth response protein-1
EIS, electrical intracochlear stimulation
EP, evoked potential
EphA4, ephedrine A4
ERK, extracellular signal regulated kinase, mitogen-activated protein (MAP) kinases, variants 1 and 2
F1, synonym for GAP-43
FAP, activator protein-1 (AP-1)-like sequence
GABA, gamma amino butyric acid
GAP-43, growth-associated protein-43
Glu, glutamate
Gly, glycine
HuD, member of human Hu proteins identified as target antigens in autoimmune paraneoplastic encephalomyelitis-sensory neuronopathy, RNA-binding and stabilizing protein.
Hz, Hertz
i, ipsilateral
i.p., intraperitoneal
IC, inferior colliculus
IHC, immunhistochemistry
ISH, in situ hybridization
Krox-24, synonym for Egr-1
l, lateral
LOC, lateral olivocochlear
LSO, lateral superior olivary complex
LSOc, LSO contralateral to stimulation
LSOi, LSO ipsilateral to stimulation
m, medial
MAPK, mitogen-activated protein kinase
MGB, medial geniculate body

MGBc, MGB contralateral to stimulation
mRNA, messenger ribonucleic acid
n7, facial nerve
NGF, nerve growth factor
NGFI-A, nerve growth factor-induced protein 1, synonym for Egr-1
NMDA, N-methyl-D-aspartic acid
ns, non-significant
P, postnatal day
p38, protein phosphorylating specific MAPKs
P-57, synonym for GAP-43
p75(NTR), p75 neurotrophin receptor
p-ATF-2, phosphorylated activating transcription factor-2
PBS, phosphate-buffered saline
PCR, polymerase chain reaction
p-CREB, phosphorylated cAMP response element binding protein
p-ERK, phosphorylated ERK
pp46, synonym for GAP-43
PV, parvalbumin
SIE, sis inducible element associated to retroviral DNA sequences (v-sis) originally isolated from simian sarcoma virus
SPL, sound pressure level
SRE, serum response element
SSC, standard saline citrate
Syngr-1, Synaptogyrin-1
Tis8, synonym for Egr-1
TrkA, neurotrophic tyrosine kinase receptor type 1
TrkB, neurotrophic tyrosine kinase receptor type 2
tRNA, transfer ribonucleic acid
VCN, ventral cochlear nucleus
VCNc, VCN contralateral to stimulation
VNTB, ventral nucleus of the trapezoid body
Zenk, synonym for Egr-1
Zif268, synonym for Egr-1

7. References

Ackermann, J.; Ashton, G.; Lyons, S.; James, D.; Hornung, J.P.; Jones, N. & Breitwieser W. (2011). *Loss of ATF2 function leads to cranial motoneuron degeneration during embryonic mouse development.* PLoS One, Vol.6, No.4, e19090.

Adams, J.C. (1995). *Sound stimulation induces Fos-related antigens in cells with common morphological properties throughout the auditory brainstem.* Journal of Comparative Neurology, Vol. 361, No. 4, pp. 645-668.

Aigner, L.; Arber, S.; Kapfhammer, J.P.; Laux, T.; Schneider, C.; Botteri, F.; Brenner, H.R. & Caroni, P. (1995). *Overexpression of the neural growth-associated protein GAP-43 induces nerve sprouting in the adult nervous system of transgenic mice.* Cell, Vol. 83, No. 2, pp. 269–278.

Anderson, S.; Skoe, E.; Chandrasekaran, B. & Kraus, N. (2010). *Neural timing is linked to speech perception in noise.* Journal of Neuroscience Vol. 30, No. 14, pp. 4922-4926.

Benowitz, L.I. & Perrone-Bizzozero, N.I. (1991). *The expression of GAP-43 in relation to neuronal growth and plasticity: When, where, how, and why?* Progress in Brain Research, Vol. 89, pp. 69–87.

Benowitz, L.I. & Routtenberg, A. (1997). *GAP-43: an intrinsic determinant of neuronal development and plasticity.* Trends in Neuroscience, Vol.20, No. 2, pp. 84-91.

Benowitz, L.I.; Apostolides, P.J.; Perrone-Bizzozero, N.; Finklestein, S.P. & Zwiers, H. (1988). *Anatomical distribution of the growth-associated protein GAP-43/B-50 in the adult rat brain.* Journal of Neuroscience, Vol. 8, No. 1, pp. 339–352.

Black, J.E.; Isaacs, K.R.; Anderson, B.J.; Alcantara, A.A. & Greenough, W.T. (1990). *Learning causes synaptogenesis, whereas motor activity causes angiogenesis, in cerebellar cortex of adult rats.* Proceedings of the National Academy of Science USA, Vol. 87, No. 14, pp. 5568-5572.

Brami-Cherrier, K.; Roze, E.; Girault, J.A.; Betuing, S. & Caboche, J. (2009). *Role of the ERK/MSK1 signalling pathway in chromatin remodelling and brain responses to drugs of abuse.* Journal of Neurochemistry, Vol. 108, No. 6, pp. 1323-1335.

Brown, M.C. & Liu, T.S. (1995). *Fos-like immunoreactivity in central auditory neurons of the mouse.* Journal of Comparative Neurology, Vol. 357, No. 1, pp. 85–97.

Campeau, S.; Dolan, D.; Akil, H. & Watson, S.J. (2002). *c-fos mRNA induction in acute and chronic audiogenic stress: possible role of the orbitofrontal cortex in habituation.* Stress, Vol.5, No. 2, pp. 121-130.

Campeau, S.; Watson, S.J. (1997). *Neuroendocrine and behavioral responses and brain pattern of c-fos induction associated with audiogenic stress.* Journal of Neuroendocrinology, Vol.9, No. 8, pp. 577-588.

Carretta, D.; Hervé-Minvielle, A.; Bajo, V.M.; Villa, A.E. & Rouiller, E.M. (1999). *c-Fos expression in the auditory pathways related to the significance of acoustic signals in rats performing a sensory-motor task.* Brain Research, Vol. 841, No. 1-2, pp. 170–183.

Chung, S.; Jiang, L.; Cheng, S. & Furneaux, H. (1996). *Purification and properties of HuD, a neuronal RNA-binding protein.* Journal of Biological Chemistry, Vol. 271, No. 19, pp. 11518-11524.

Clarkson, C.; Juíz, J.M. & Merchán, M.A. (2010). *Transient down-regulation of sound-induced c-Fos protein expression in the inferior colliculus after ablation of the auditory cortex.* Frontiers in Neuroanatomy, Vol. 4, Article 141.

Curran, T.; Miller, A.D.; Zokas, L. & Verma, I.M. (1984). *Viral and cellular fos proteins: a comparative analysis.* Cell, Vol.36, No. 2, pp. 259-268.

De Graan, P.N.; Van Hooff, C.O.; Tilly, B.C.; Oestreicher, A.B.; Schotman, P. & Gispen, W.H. (1985). *Phosphoprotein B-50 in nerve growth cones from fetal rat brain.* Neuroscience Letters, Vol. 61, No. 3, pp. 235–241.

De, S.; Shuler, C.F. & Turman, J.E. Jr. (2003). *The ontogeny of Krox-20 expression in brainstem and cerebellar neurons.* Journal of Chemical Neuroanatomy, Vol. 25, No. 3, pp. 213-226.

Diolaiti, D.; Bernardoni, R.; Trazzi, S.; Papa, A.; Porro, A.; Bono, F.; Herbert, J.M.; Perini, G. & Della Valle, G. (2007). *Functional cooperation between TrkA and p75(NTR) accelerates neuronal differentiation by increased transcription of GAP-43 and p21(CIP/WAF) genes via ERK1/2 and AP-1 activities.* Experimental Cell Research, Vol. 313, No. 14, pp. 2980-2992.

Edling, Y.; Ingelman-Sundberg, M. & Simi, A. (2007). *Glutamate activates c-fos in glial cells via a novel mechanism involving the glutamate receptor subtype mGlu5 and the transcriptional repressor DREAM.* Glia, Vol. 55, No. 3, pp. 328-340.

Edsjö, A.; Hallberg, B.; Fagerström, S.; Larsson, C.; Axelson, H. & Påhlman, S. (2001). *Differences in early and late responses between neurotrophin-stimulated trkA- and trkC-transfected SH-SY5Y neuroblastoma cells.* Cell Growth Differentiation, Vol. 12, No. 1, pp. 39-50.

Ehret, G. & Fischer, R. (1991). *Neuronal activity and tonotopy in the auditory system visualized by c-fos gene expression.* Brain Research, Vol. 567, No. 2, pp. 350-354.

Fichtel, I. & Ehret, G. (1999). *Perception and recognition discriminated in the mouse auditory cortex by c-Fos labeling.* Neuroreport, Vol. 10, No. 11, pp. 2341-2345.

Friauf, E. (1995). *C-fos immunocytochemical evidence for acoustic pathway mapping in rats.* Behavioral Brain Research, Vol. 66, No. 1-2, pp. 217-224.

Fujii, K.; Saika, T.; Yamamoto, K.; Doi, K. & Kubo, T. (1997). *Electrically evoked auditory brainstem response and Fos-immunoreactivity in kanamycin-deafened rats.* Advances in Otorhinolaryngology, Vol. 52, pp. 27-29.

Gao, Y.J. & Ji, R.R. (2009). *c-Fos and pERK, which is a better marker for neuronal activation and central sensitization after noxious stimulation and tissue injury?* Open Pain Journal Vol. 2, pp. 11-17.

Geissler, D.B. & Ehret, G. (2004). *Auditory perception vs. recognition: representation of complex communication sounds in the mouse auditory cortical fields.* European Journal of Neuroscience, Vol. 19, No. 4, pp. 1027-40.

Gil-Loyzaga, P.; Carricondo, F.; Bartolomé, M.V.; Iglesias, M.C.; Rodríguez, F. & Poch-Broto, J. (2010). *Cellular and molecular bases of neuroplasticity: brainstem effects after cochlear damage.* Acta Otolaryngologica, Vol. 130, No. 3, pp. 318-325.

Ginty, D.D.; Bonni, A. & Greenberg, M.E. (1994). *Nerve growth factor activates a Ras-dependent protein kinase that stimulates c-fos transcription via phosphorylation of CREB.* Cell, Vol. 77, No. 5, pp. 713–725.

Gispen, W.H.; Nielander, H.B.; De Graan, P.N.E.; Oestreicher, A.B.; Schrama, L.H. & Schotman P. (1991). *Role of the growth-associated protein B-50/GAP-43 in neuronal plasticity.* Molecular Neurobiology, Vol. 5, No. 2-3, pp. 61–85.

Harris, J.A.; Hardie, N.A.; Bermingham-McDonogh, O. & Rubel. E.W. (2005). *Gene expression differences over a critical period of afferent-dependent neuron survival in the mouse auditory brainstem.* Journal of Comparative Neurology, Vol. 493, No. 3, pp. 460-474.

Harris, J.A.; Iguchi, F.; Seidl, A.H.; Lurie, D.I. & Rubel, E.W. (2008). *Afferent deprivation elicits a transcriptional response associated with neuronal survival after a critical period in the mouse cochlear nucleus.* Journal of Neuroscience, Vol. 28, No. 43, pp. 10990-11002.

Herdegen, T. & Leah, J.D. (1998). *Inducible and constitutive transcription factors in the mammalian nervous system: Control of gene expression by Jun, Fos and Krox, and CREB/ATF proteins.* Brain Research Reviews, Vol. 28, No. 3, pp. 370–490.

Hildebrandt, H.; Hoffmann, N.A. & Illing, R.B. (2011). *Synaptic reorganization in the adult rat's ventral cochlear nucleus following its total sensory deafferentation.* PLoS One, Vol. 6, No. 8, e23686.

Illing, R.B. & Horváth, M. (1995). *Re-emergence of GAP-43 in cochlear nucleus and superior olive following cochlear ablation in the rat.* Neuroscience Letters, Vol. 194, No. 1-2, pp. 9-12.

Illing, R.B. & Michler S.A. (2001). *Modulation of P-CREB and expression of c-Fos in cochlear nucleus and superior olive following electrical intracochlear stimulation.* Neuroreport, Vol. 12, No. 4, pp. 875-878.

Illing, R.B. & Reisch, A. (2006). *Specific plasticity responses to unilaterally decreased or increased hearing intensity in the adult cochlear nucleus and beyond.* Hearing Research, Vol. 216-217, pp. 189-197.

Illing, R.B. (2001). *Activity-dependent plasticity in the adult auditory brainstem.* Audiology and Neurootology, Vol. 6, No. 6, pp. 319-345.

Illing, R.B.; Cao, Q.L.; Förster, C.R. & Laszig, R. (1999). *Auditory brainstem: development and plasticity of GAP-43 mRNA expression in the rat.* Journal of Comparative Neurology, Vol. 412, No. 2, pp. 353-372.

Illing, R.B.; Horváth, M. & Laszig, R. (1997). *Plasticity of the auditory brainstem: effects of cochlear lesions on GAP-43 immunoreactivity in the rat.* Journal of Comparative Neurology, Vol. 382, No. 1, pp. 116-138.

Illing, R.B.; Kraus, K.S. & Meidinger, M.A. (2005). *Reconnecting neuronal networks in the auditory brainstem following unilateral deafening.* Hearing Research, Vol. 206, No. 1-2, pp. 185-199.

Illing, R.B.; Michler, S.A.; Kraus, K.S. & Laszig, R. (2002). *Transcription factor modulation and expression in the rat auditory brainstem following electrical intracochlear stimulation.* Experimental Neurology, Vol. 175, No. 1, pp. 226-244.

Illing, R.B.; Rosskothen-Kuhl, N.; Fredrich, M.; Hildebrandt, H. & Zeber, A.C. (2010). *Imaging the plasticity of the central auditory system on the cellular and molecular level.* Audiological Medicine, Vol. 8, No. 2, pp. 63-76.

Irving, S.; Moore, D.R.; Liberman, M.C. & Sumner CJ. (2011). *Olivocochlear efferent control in sound localization and experience-dependent learning.* Journal of Neuroscience, Vol. 31, No. 7, pp. 2493-2501.

Ishida, Y.; Nakahara, D.; Hashiguchi, H.; Nakamura, M.; Ebihara, K.; Takeda, R.; Nishimori, T. & Niki H. (2002). *Fos expression in GABAergic cells and cells immunopositive for NMDA receptors in the inferior and superior colliculi following audiogenic seizures in rats.* Synapse, Vol. 46, No. 2, pp. 100-107.

Jakob, T. & Illing, R.B. (2008). *Laterality, intensity, and frequency of electrical intracochlear stimulation are differentially mapped into specific patterns of gene expression in the rat auditory brainstem.* Audiological Medicine, Vol. 6, No. 3, pp. 215-227.

Jero, J.; Coling, D.E. & Lalwani, A.K. (2001). *The use of Preyer's reflex in evaluation of hearing in mice.* Acta Otolaryngologica, Vol.121, No. 5, pp. 585-589.

Kai, N. & Niki, H. (2002). *Altered tone-induced Fos expression in the mouse inferior colliculus after early exposure to intense noise.* Neuroscience Research, Vol. 44, No. 3, pp. 305-313.

Keilmann, A & Herdegen, T. (1995). *Expression of the c-fos transcription factor in the rat auditory pathway following postnatal auditory deprivation.* European Archive of Otorhinolaryngology, Vol. 252, No. 5, pp. 287-291.

Keilmann, A & Herdegen, T. (1997). *The c-Fos transcription factor in the auditory pathway of the juvenile rat: effects of acoustic deprivation and repetitive stimulation.* Brain Research, Vol. 753, No. 2, pp. 291-298.

Kinney, H.C.; Rava, L.A. & Benowitz, L.I. (1993). *Anatomic distribution of the growth-associated protein GAP-43 in the developing human brainstem.* Journal of Neuropathology and Experimental Neurology, Vol. 52, No. 1, pp. 39-54.

Kleim, J.A.; Lussnig, E.; Schwarz, E.R.; Comery, T.A. & Greenough, W.T. (1996). *Synaptogenesis and Fos expression in the motor cortex of the adult rat after motor skill learning.* Journal of Neuroscience, Vol. 16, No. 14, pp. 4529-4535.

Koponen, E.; Lakso, M. & Castrén, E. (2004). *Overexpression of the full-length neurotrophin receptor trkB regulates the expression of plasticity-related genes in mouse brain.* Molecular Brain Research, Vol. 130, No. 1-2, pp. 81-94.

Kraus, K.S. & Illing, R.B. (2004). *Superior olivary contributions to auditory system plasticity: medial but not lateral olivocochlear neurons are the source of cochleotomy-induced GAP-43 expression in the ventral cochlear nucleus.* Journal of Comparative Neurology, Vol. 475, No. 3, pp. 374-390.

Lu, H.P.; Chen, S.T. & Poon, P.W. (2009). *Nuclear size of c-Fos expression at the auditory brainstem is related to the time-varying nature of the acoustic stimuli.* Neuroscience Letters, Vol. 451, No. 2, pp. 139-143.

Luo, L.; Ryan, A.F. & Saint Marie, R.L. (1999). *Cochlear ablation alters acoustically induced c-fos mRNA expression in the adult rat auditory brainstem.* Journal of Comparative Neurology, Vol. 404, No. 2, pp. 271-283.

Mahalik, T.J.; Carrier, A.; Owens, G.P. & Clayton, G. (1992). *The expression of GAP43 mRNA during the late embryonic and early postnatal development of the CNS of the rat: An in situ hybridization study.* Developmental Brain Research, Vol. 67, No. 1, pp. 75–83.

Matsuda, K.; Ueda, Y.; Doi, T.; Tono, T.; Haruta, A.; Toyama, K. & Komune, S. (1999). *Increase in glutamate-aspartate transporter (GLAST) mRNA during kanamycin-induced cochlear insult in rats.* Hearing Research, Vol. 133, No. 1-2, pp. 10-16.

McNamara, J.O.; Bonhaus, D.W. & Shin, C. (1993). The kindling model of epilepsy. In: *Epilepsy: models, mechanisms, and concepts* , P.A. Schwartzkroin, (Ed.), 27-47. Cambridge, UK: Cambridge UP.

Meidinger, M.A.; Hildebrandt-Schoenfeld, H. & Illing, R.B. (2006). *Cochlear damage induces GAP-43 expression in cholinergic synapses of the rat cochlear nucleus in the adult rat: A light and electron microscopical study.* European Journal of Neuroscience, Vol. 23, No. 12, pp. 3187-3199.

Meiri, K.F.; Saffell, J.L.; Walsh, F.S. & Doherty, P. (1998). *Neurite outgrowth stimulated by neural cell adhesion molecules requires growth-associated protein-43 (GAP-43) function and is associated with GAP-43 phosphorylation in growth cones.* Journal of Neuroscience, Vol. 18, No. 24, pp. 10429–10437.

Metz, G.A. & Schwab, M.E. (2004). *Behavioral characterization in a comprehensive mouse test battery reveals motor and sensory impairments in growth-associated protein-43 null mutant mice.* Neuroscience, Vol. 129, No. 3, pp. 563-574.

Michler, S.A. & Illing, R.B. (2003). *Molecular plasticity in the rat auditory brainstem: Modulation of expression and distribution of phosphoserine, phospho-CREB and TrkB after noise trauma.* Audiology and Neurootology, Vol. 8, No. 4, pp. 190-206.

Miko, I.J.; Nakamura, P.A.; Henkemeyer, M. & Cramer, K.S. (2007). *Auditory brainstem neural activation patterns are altered in EphA4- and ephrin-B2-deficient mice.* Journal of Comparative Neurology, Vol. 505, No. 6, pp. 669-681.

Mobarak, C.D.; Anderson, K.D.; Morin, M.; Beckel-Mitchener, A.; Rogers, S.L.; Furneaux, H.; King, P. & Perrone-Bizzozero, N.I. (2000). *The RNA-binding protein HuD is required for GAP-43 mRNA stability, GAP-43 gene expression, and PKC-dependent neurite outgrowth in PC12 cells.* Molecular Biology of the Cell, Vol. 11, No. 9, pp. 3191-3203.

Müller, R., Bravo, R., Burckhardt, J. & Curran, T. (1984). *Induction of c-fos gene and protein by growth factors precedes activation of c-myc.* Nature, Vol. 312, No. 5996, pp. 716-720.

Munro, K.J. (2008). *Reorganization of the adult auditory system: perceptual and physiological evidence from monaural fitting of hearing aids.* Trends in Amplification, Vol. 12, No. 3, pp. 254-271.

Nagase, S.; Miller, J.M.; Dupont, J.; Lim, H.H.; Sato, K. & Altschuler, R.A. (2000). *Changes in cochlear electrical stimulation induced Fos expression in the rat inferior colliculus following deafness.* Hearing Research, Vol. 147, No. 1-2, pp. 242–250.

Nagase, S.; Mukaida, M.; Miller, J.M. & Altschuler, R.A. (2003). *Neonatal deafening causes changes in Fos protein induced by cochlear electrical stimulation.* Journal of Neurocytology, Vol. 32, No. 4, pp. 353-361.

Nakamura, M.; Rosahl, S.K.; Alkahlout, E.; Gharabaghi, A.; Walter, G.F. & Samii, M. (2003). *C-Fos immunoreactivity mapping of the auditory system after electrical stimulation of the cochlear nerve in rats.* Hearing Research, Vol. 184, No. 1-2, pp. 75-81.

Nakamura, M.; Rosahl, S.K.; Alkahlout, E.; Walter, G.F. & Samii, M.M. (2005). *Electrical stimulation of the cochlear nerve in rats: analysis of c-Fos expression in auditory brainstem nuclei.* Brain Research, Vol. 1031, No. 1, pp. 39-55.

Nedivi, E.; Basi, G.S.; Akey, I.V. & Skene, J.H. (1992). *A neural-specific GAP-43 core promoter located between unusual DNA elements that interact to regulate its activity.* Journal of Neuroscience, Vol. 12, No. 3, pp. 691-704.

Oh, S.H.; Kim, C.S. & Song, J.J. (2007). *Gene expression and plasticity in the rat auditory cortex after bilateral cochlear ablation.* Acta Otolaryngologica, Vol. 127, No. 4, pp. 341-350.

Osako, S.; Tokimoto, T. & Matsuura, S. (1979). *Effects of kanamycin on the auditory evoked responses during postnatal development of the hearing of the rat.* Acta Otolaryngologica, Vol. 88, No. 5-6, 359-368.

Ota, K.T.; Monsey, M.S.; Wu, M.S.; Young, G.J. & Schafe, G.E. (2010). *Synaptic plasticity and NO-cGMP-PKG signaling coordinately regulate ERK-driven gene expression in the lateral amygdala and in the auditory thalamus following Pavlovian fear conditioning.* Learning and Memory, Vol. 17, No. 4, pp. 221-235.

Peña, M.; Maki, A.; Kovacić, D.; Dehaene-Lambertz, G.; Koizumi, H.; Bouquet, F. & Mehler, J. (2003). *Sounds and silence: an optical topography study of language recognition at birth.* Proceedings of the National Academy of Science USA, Vol. 100, No. 20, pp. 11702-11705.

Pierson, M. & Snyder-Keller, A. (1994). *Development of frequency-selective domains in inferior colliculus of normal and neonatally noise-exposed rats.* Brain Research, Vol. 636, No. 1, pp. 55-67.

Pollin, B. & Albe-Fessard, D. (1979). *Organization of somatic thalamus in monkeys with and without section of dorsal spinal tracts.* Brain Research, Vol. 173, No. 3, pp. 431–449.

Racaniello, M.; Cardinale, A.; Mollinari, C.; D'Antuono, M.; De Chiara, G.; Tancredi, V. & Merlo D. (2010). *Phosphorylation changes of CaMKII, ERK1/2, PKB/Akt kinases and CREB activation during early long-term potentiation at Schaffer collateral-CA1 mouse hippocampal synapses.* Neurochemical Research, Vol. 35, No. 2, pp. 239-246.

Reisch, A.; Illing, R.B. & Laszig, R. (2007). *Immediate early gene expression invoked by electrical intracochlear stimulation in some but not all types of neurons in the rat auditory brainstem.* Experimental Neurology, Vol. 208, No. 2, pp. 193-206.

Rekart, J.L.; Meiri, K. & Routtenberg, A. (2005). *Hippocampal-dependent memory is impaired in heterozygous GAP-43 knockout mice.* Hippocampus, Vol. 15, No. 1, pp. 1-7.

Robinson, G.A. (1996). *Changes in the expression of transcription factors ATF-2 and Fra-2 after axotomy and during regeneration in rat retinal ganglion cells.* Molecular Brain Research, Vol. 41, No. 1-2, pp. 57-64.

Rosskothen, N.; Hirschmüller-Ohmes, I. & Illing, R.B. (2008). *AP-1 activity rises by stimulation-dependent c-Fos expression in auditory neurons.* Neuroreport, Vol. 19, pp. 1091-1093.

Rosskothen-Kuhl, N. & Illing R.B. (2010). *Nonlinear development of the populations of neurons expressing c-Fos under sustained electrical intracochlear stimulation in the rat auditory brainstem.* Brain Research, Vol. 1347, No. 11, pp. 33-41.

Rosskothen-Kuhl, N. & Illing R.B. (2012) *The impact of hearing experience on signal integration in the auditory brainstem: A c-Fos study of the rat.* Brain Research, Vol. 1435, No. 1, pp. 40-55.

Rouiller, E.M.; Wan, X.S.; Moret, V. & Liang, F. (1992). *Mapping of c-fos expression elicited by pure tones stimulation in the auditory pathways of the rat, with emphasis on the cochlear nucleus.* Neuroscience Letters, Vol. 144, No. 1-2, pp. 19-24.

Ruan, Q.; Wang, D.; Gao, H.; Liu, A.; Da, C.; Yin, S. & Chi, F. (2007). *The effects of different auditory activity on the expression of phosphorylated c-Jun in the auditory system.* Acta Otolaryngologica, Vol. 127, No. 6, pp. 594-604.

Saint Marie, R.L.; Luo, L. & Ryan, A.F. (1999A). *Spatial representation of frequency in the rat dorsal nucleus of the lateral lemniscus as revealed by acoustically induced c-fos mRNA expression.* Hearing Research, Vol. 128, No. 1-2, pp. 70–74.

Saint Marie, R.L.; Luo, L. & Ryan A.F. (1999B). *Effects of stimulus frequency and intensity on c-fos mRNA expression in the adult rat auditory brainstem.* Journal of Comparative Neurology, Vol. 404, No. 2, pp. 258-270.

Saito, H.; Miller, J.M. & Altschuler, R.A. (2000). *Cochleotopic fos immunoreactivity in cochlea and cochlear nuclei evoked by bipolar cochlear electrical stimulation.* Hearing Research, Vol. 145, No. 1-2, pp. 37-51.

Saito, H.; Miller, J.M.; Pfingst, B.E. & Altschuler, R.A. (1999). *Fos-like immunoreactivity in the auditory brainstem evoked by bipolar intracochlear electrical stimulation: effects of current level and pulse duration.* Neuroscience, Vol. 91, No. 1, pp. 139-161.

Sakamoto, K.M.; Bardeleben, C.; Yates, K.E.; Raines, M.A.; Golde, D.W. & Gasson, J.C. (1991). *5' upstream sequence and genomic structure of the human primary response gene, EGR-1/TIS8.* Oncogene, Vol. 6, No. 5, pp. 867–871.

Sato, K.; Houtani, T.; Ueyama, T.; Ikeda, M.; Yamashita, T.; Kumazawa, T. & Sugimoto T. (1993). *Identification of rat brainstem sites with neuronal Fos protein induced by acoustic stimulation with pure tones.* Acta Otolaryngologica, Supplement, Vol. 500, pp. 18–22.

Schaechter, J.D. & Benowitz, L.I. (1993). *Activation of protein kinase C by arachidonic acid selectively enhances the phosphorylation of GAP-43 in nerve terminal membranes.* Journal of Neuroscience, Vol. 13, No. 10, pp. 4361–4371.

Scheich, H. & Zuschratter, W. (1995). *Mapping of stimulus features and meaning in gerbil auditory cortex with 2-deoxyglucose and c-Fos antibodies.* Behavioral Brain Research, Vol. 66, No. 1-2, pp. 195–205.

Schwachtgen, J.L.; Campbell, C.J. & Braddock M. (2000). *Full promoter sequence of human early growth response factor-1 (Egr-1): Demonstration of a fifth functional serum response element.* DNA Sequencing, Vol. 10, No. 6, pp. 429–432.

Sharp, F.R.; Sagar, S.M. & Swanson, R.A. (1993). *Metabolic mapping with cellular resolution: c-fos vs. 2-deoxyglucose.* Critical Reviews in Neurobiology, Vol. 7, No. 3-4, pp. 205-228.

Shea, T.B.; Perrone-Bizzozero, N.I.; Beermann, M.L. & Benowitz, L.I. (1991). *Phospholipid-mediated delivery of anti-GAP-43 antibodies into neuroblastoma cells prevents neuritogenesis.* Journal of Neuroscience, Vol. 11, No. 6, pp. 1685–1690.

Sheng, M. & Greenberg, M.E. (1990). *The regulation and function of c-fos and other immediate early genes in the nervous system.* Neuron, Vol. 4, No. 4, pp. 477-485.

Shibata, F.; Baird, A. & Florkiewicz, R.Z. (1991). *Functional characterization of the human basic fibroblast growth factor gene promoter.* Growth Factors, Vol. 4, No. 4, pp. 277-287.

Skene, J.H. & Willard, M. (1981). *Characteristics of growth-associated polypeptides in regenerating toad retinal ganglion cell axons.* Journal of Neuroscience, Vol. 1, pp. 419–426.

Skene, J.H. (1989). *Axonal growth-associated proteins.* Annual Reviews of Neuroscience, Vol. 12, pp. 127–56.

Skoe, E & Kraus, N. (2010). *Hearing it again and again: on-line subcortical plasticity in humans.* PLoS One, Vol. 5, No. 10, e13645.

Smith, C.L.; Afroz, R.; Bassell, G.J.; Furneaux, H.M.; Perrone-Bizzozero, N.I. & Burry, R.W. (2004). *GAP-43 mRNA in growth cones is associated with HuD and ribosomes.* Journal of Neurobiology, Vol. 61, No. 2, pp. 222-235.

Strittmatter, S.M.; Fankhauser, C.; Huang, P.L.; Mashimo, H. & Fishman, M.C. (1995). *Neuronal pathfinding is abnormal in mice lacking the neuronal growth cone protein GAP-43.* Cell, Vol. 80, No. 3, pp. 445–452.

Sun, X.; Guo, Y.P. & Shum, D.K.; Chan, Y.S. & He J. (2009). *Time course of cortically induced fos expression in auditory thalamus and midbrain after bilateral cochlear ablation.* Neuroscience, Vol. 160, No. 1, pp. 186-197.

Suneja, S.K. & Potashner, S.J. (2003). *ERK and SAPK signaling in auditory brainstem neurons after unilateral cochlear ablation.* Journal of Neuroscience Research, Vol. 73, No. 2, pp. 235-245.

Takagi, H.; Saito, H.; Nagase, S. & Suzuki M. (2004). *Distribution of Fos-like immunoreactivity in the auditory pathway evoked by bipolar electrical brainstem stimulation.* Acta Otolaryngologica, Vol. 124, No. 8, pp. 907-913.

Tanabe, Y.; Hashimoto, M.; Sugioka, K.; Maruyama, M.; Fujii, Y.; Hagiwara, R.; Hara, T.; Hossain, S.M. & Shido, O. (2004). *Improvement of spatial cognition with dietary docosahexaenoic acid is associated with an increase in Fos expression in rat CA1 hippocampus.* Clinical and Experimental Pharmacology and Physiology, Vol. 31, No. 10, pp. 700-703.

Tao, X.; Finkbeiner, S.; Arnold, D.B.; Shaywitz, A.J. & Greenberg, M.E. (1998). *Ca2+ influx regulates BDNF transcription by a CREB family transcription factor-dependent mechanism.* Neuron, Vol. 20, No. 4, pp. 709–726.

van Dam, H. & Castellazzi, M. (2001). *Distinct roles of Jun:Fos and Jun:ATF dimers in oncogenesis.* Oncogene, Vol. 20, No. 19, pp. 2453-2464.

Verhaagen, J.; Hermens, W.T.; Oestreicher, A.B.; Gispen, W.H.; Rabkin, S.D.; Pfaff, D.W. & Kaplitt, M.G. (1994). *Expression of the growth-associated protein B-50/GAP43 via a defective herpes-simplex virus vector results in profound morphological changes in non-neuronal cells.* Molecular Brain Research, Vol. 26, No. 1-2, pp. 26–36.

Vischer, M.W.; Bajo-Lorenzana, V.; Zhang, J.; Häusler, R. & Rouiller, E.M. (1995). *Activity elicited in the auditory pathway of the rat by electrical stimulation of the cochlea.* Journal of Otorhinolaryngology, Vol. 57, No. 6, pp. 305-309.

Vischer, M.W.; Häusler, R. & Rouiller E.M. (1994). *Distribution of Fos-like immunoreactivity in the auditory pathway of the Sprague-Dawley rat elicited by cochlear electrical stimulation.* Neuroscience Research, Vol. 19, No. 2, pp. 175-185.

Wall, P.D. & Egger, M.D. (1971). *Formation of new connexions in adult rat brains after partial deafferentation.* Nature, Vol. 232, No. 5312, pp. 542–545.

Walton, J.P. (2010). Timing is everything: temporal processing deficits in the aged auditory brainstem. Hearing Research, Vol. 264, No. 1-2, pp. 63-69.

Wan, H.; Warburton, E.C.; Kuśmierek, P.; Aggleton, J.P.; Kowalska, D.M. & Brown M.W. (2001). *Fos imaging reveals differential neuronal activation of areas of rat temporal cortex by novel and familiar sounds.* European Journal of Neuroscience, Vol. 14, No. 1, pp. 118-124.

Watanabe, Y.; Johnson, R.S.; Butler, L.S.; Binder, D.K.; Spiegelman, B.M.; Papaioannou, V.E. & McNamara, J.O. (1996). *Null mutation of c-fos impairs structural and functional plasticities in the kindling model of epilepsy.* Journal of Neuroscience, Vol. 16, No. 12, pp. 3827-3836.

Weber, J.R. & Skene J.H. (1998). *The activity of a highly promiscuous AP-1 element can be confined to neurons by a tissue-selective repressive element.* Journal of Neuroscience, Vol. 18, No. 18, pp. 5264-5274.

Widmer, F. & Caroni, P. (1993). *Phosphorylation-site mutagenesis of the growth-associated protein GAP-43 modulates its effects on cell spreading and morphology.* Journal of Cell Biology, Vol. 120, No. 2, pp. 503–512.

Williams, S.; Evan, G. & Hunt S.P. (1991). *C-fos induction in the spinal cord after peripheral nerve lesion.* European Journal of Neuroscience, Vol. 3, No. 9, pp. 887-894.

Wisdom, R. (1999). *AP-1: One switch for many signals.* Experimental Cell Research, Vol. 253, No. 1, pp. 180–185.

Woolf, C.J.; Reynolds, M.L.; Molander, C.; O'Brien, C.; Lindsay, R.M. & Benowitz, L.I. (1990). *The growth-associated protein GAP-43 appears in dorsal root ganglion cells and in the dorsal horn of the rat spinal cord following peripheral nerve injury.* Neuroscience, Vol. 34, No. 2, pp. 465 -478.

Wu, J.L.; Chiu, T.W. & Poon P.W. (2003). *Differential changes in Fos-immunoreactivity at the auditory brainstem after chronic injections of salicylate in rats.* Hearing Research, Vol. 176, No. 1-2, pp. 80-93.

Xu, B.; Gottschalk, W.; Chow, A.; Wilson, R.I.; Schnell, E.; Zang, K.; Wang, D.; Nicoll, R.A.; Lu, B. & Reichardt L.F. (2000). *The role of brain-derived neurotrophic factor receptors in the mature hippocampus: Modulation of long-term potentiation through a presynaptic mechanism involving TrkB.* Journal of Neuroscience, Vol. 20, No. 18, pp. 6888–6897.

Yang, H.; Xia, Y.; Lu, S.Q.; Soong, T.W. & Feng, Z.W. (2008). *Basic fibroblast growth factor-induced neuronal differentiation of mouse bone marrow stromal cells requires FGFR-1, MAPK/ERK, and transcription factor AP-1.* Journal of Biological Chemistry, Vol. 283, No. 9, pp. 5287-5295.

Yankner, B.A.; Benowitz, L.I.; Villa-Komaroff, L. & Neve, R.L. (1990). *Transfection of PC12 cells with the human GAP-43 gene: Effects on neurite outgrowth and regeneration.* Molecular Brain Research, Vol. 7, No. 1, pp. 39–44.

Yuan, Z.; Gong, S.; Luo, J.; Zheng, Z.; Song, B.; Ma, S.; Guo, J.; Hu, C.; Thiel, G.; Vinson, C.; Hu, C.D.; Wang, Y. & Li, M. (2009). *Opposing roles for ATF2 and c-Fos in c-Jun-mediated neuronal apoptosis.* Molecular and Cellular Biology, Vol. 29, No. 9, pp. 2431-2442.

Zhang, J. & Zhang, X. (2010). *Electrical stimulation of the dorsal cochlear nucleus induces hearing in rats.* Brain Research, Vol. 1311, pp. 37-50.

Zhang, J.S.; Haenggeli, C.A.; Tempini, A.; Vischer, M.W.; Moret, V. & Rouiller, E.M. (1996). *Electrically induced fos-like immunoreactivity in the auditory pathway of the rat: effects of survival time, duration, and intensity of stimulation.* Brain Research Bulletin, Vol. 39, No. 2, pp. 75-82.

Zhang, J.S.; Vischer, M.W.; Moret, V.; Roulin, C. & Rouiller, E.M. (1998). *Antibody-dependent Fos-like immunoreactivity (FLI) in the auditory pathway of the rat in response to electric stimulation of the cochlea.* Journal für Hirnforschung, Vol. 39, No. 1, pp. 21–35.

Zuschratter, W.; Gass, P.; Herdegen, T. & Scheich, H. (1995). *Comparison of frequency-specific c-Fos expression and fluoro-2-deoxyglucose uptake in auditory cortex of gerbils (Meriones unguiculatus).* European Journal of Neuroscience, Vol. 7, No. 7, pp. 1614-1626.

9

Cochlear Implantation, Synaptic Plasticity and Auditory Function

Jahn N. O'Neil[1] and David K. Ryugo[1,2]
[1]*Johns Hopkins University, Dept. of Otolarygology, Head and Neck Surgery, Center for Hearing and Balance, Baltimore, MD*
[2]*Garvan Institute of Medical Research, Hearing Research, Sydney, NSW*
[1]*USA*
[2]*AU*

1. Introduction

The ability to hear, our perception of sound, is fundamental to how we perceive our external environment and interact with others using spoken language. Sound also plays a critical role in the normal development of the auditory system. In this review, we will discuss sound, hearing, and the role of hearing in brain development. We will examine the effect of deafness and the impact of cochlear implants on neuronal plasticity and auditory function.

It is speculated that hearing evolved as a distance sense so that organisms could detect potential dangers that were not visible, such as during the dark of night or where grass or forests were too dense (Jerison, 1973). All animals have the ability to sense mechanical perturbations in the air, and in vertebrates, the inner ear is a highly developed structure that solves this problem. This sense organ consists of specialized cellular structures that transduce (or convert) sound stimuli into neural signals.

Sound is created by vibrations within a plastic medium (air, water, gas etc.) caused by the movement of molecules. The oscillations of these sound waves can be described by their rate, which is defined in cycles per second, also known as frequency. The sensation of pitch is positively correlated to the frequency of sound. The pressure (or intensity) of these vibrations is perceived as loudness. Sound in air is captured by the auricle, the external portion of the ear, and funneled through the external auditory canal to the tympanic membrane, also known as the eardrum. The tympanic membrane is mechanically coupled to the middle ear ossicles (malleus, incus and stapes) where the vibrations are amplified and delivered to the cochlea. The vibrations in air become vibrations in fluid and are transmitted to the sensory hair cells of the organ of Corti. This mechanical signal is converted to neural signals and relayed to the brain by the auditory nerve. The brain receives and interprets these signals and the result is what we perceive as hearing.

In humans, the range of hearing that is audible contains frequencies between approximately 20 to 20,000 Hz. Hearing range is variable between individuals as well as species (Figure 1). Mammals in particular have developed high frequency hearing and have the largest frequency range among vertebrates. The ear is the structural organ that detects sounds, however, the brain is the organ that perceives sound through the firing of nerve cell impulses. This neural activity is important for the normal construction and maintenance of the auditory structure and function. The brain combines auditory input received from both ears to determine the level, direction and distance of the sound. The inability of the brain to perceive auditory information from one or both ears is termed hearing loss. Hearing loss is the most common sensory loss, affecting millions worldwide. In the U.S., the National Institute of Deafness and Other Communications Disorders, (NIDCD) has determined that 2-3 out of 1,000 newborns, and 36 million adults are affected by hearing loss (http://www.nidcd.nih.gov/health/statistics/Pages/quick.aspx). Hearing loss or deafness can be defined as congenital or acquired. Congenital hearing loss occurs at birth, whereas acquired deafness occurs after birth. The type of hearing loss is classified as sensorineural, conductive or mixed. Sensorineural hearing loss is defined as being caused by an abnormality in the inner ear, cranial nerve VIII (auditory nerve), or the central processing auditory centers of the brain. Conductive hearing loss occurs when sound is not being conducted efficiently throughout the ear canal, eardrum and the middle ear.

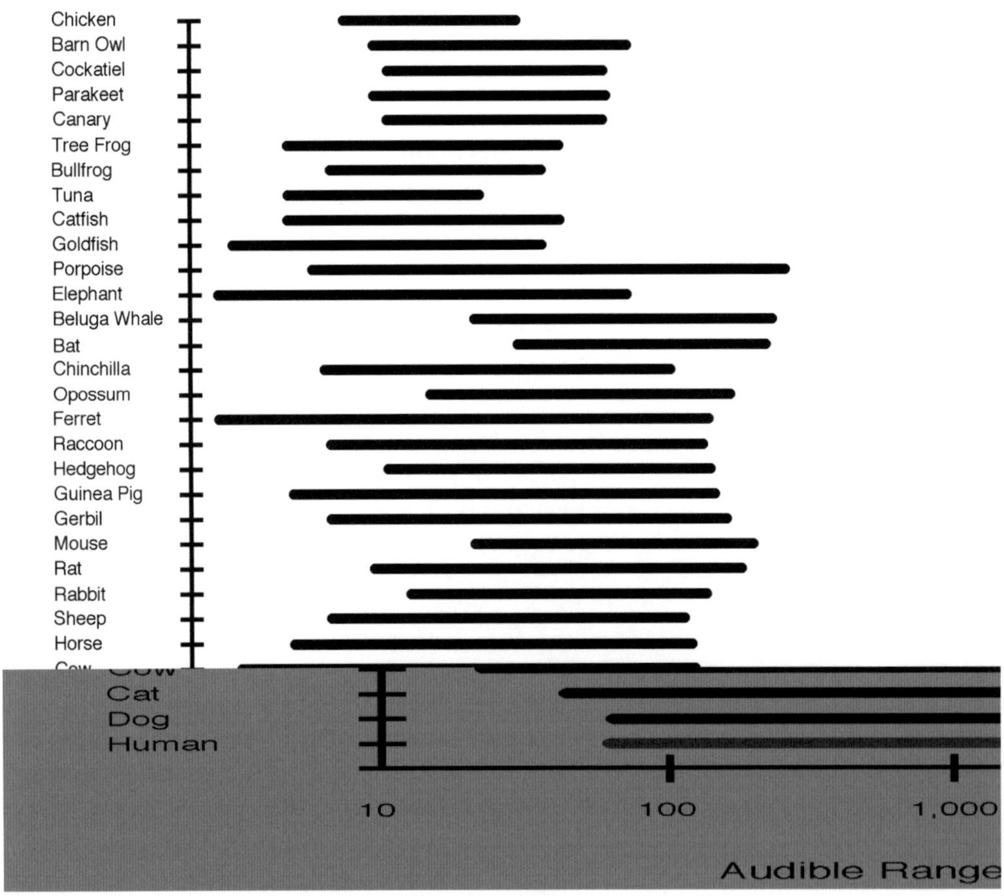

Fig. 1. Hearing Range * approximate values, not drawn to scale (adapted from Fay, R.R. (1988). *Hearing in vertebrates: a psychophysics databook*, Hill-Fay Associates, Winnetka, IL).

For many individuals affected by hearing loss, depending on the severity of hearing impairment, listening needs, and lifestyle, several options are available. Current treatment of sensorineural hearing loss is available via acoustic hearing aids, implantable middle ear hearing devices, and cochlear implants. Hearing aids are widely used to amplify and modulate sound enabling an individual with damaged hearing to communicate and participate more fully in daily activities. Cochlear implants, however, provide a sense of sound to individuals profoundly deaf or severely hard of hearing. Implants work to bypass the sensory hair cells within the organ of Corti. Conversely, hearing aids amplify sound. Cochlear implants do not restore normal hearing but rather provides the individual with a useful representation of sounds in the environment. Other acoustic aids such as middle ear implants work to remedy ossicular dysfunction and auditory brainstem implants work by bypassing the auditory nerve and is implanted directly into the midbrain. The biggest and still outstanding problem with listening aid devices is their inability to function optimally in the presence of background noise.

The improved quality of cochlear implants over the last several decades have restored hearing to more than 200,000 deaf patients worldwide, in the US alone, over 42,000 adults and 28,000 kids (http://www.nidcd.nih.gov/health/hearing/pages/coch.aspx.) Cochlear implants have become the most successful neural prostheses to date. Cochlear implants have been found to be most beneficial to post-lingually deafened adults and young children (Waltzman & Roland, 2005; Niparko et al., 2009). The use of auditory training has been found to induce post-implantation synaptic plasticity and to enhance post-implantation performance. Auditory function with cochlear implantation has achieved enormous success in the past several years. The robust outcomes and satisfaction of cochlear implant patients have contributed to the widespread acceptance of implant use.

2. Historical origin of cochlear implants

Cochlear implants work by directly stimulating the auditory nerve. It requires both a surgical approach and significant post-surgical training. The earliest example of electrical stimulation to the auditory system was by an Italian physicist, Alessandro Volta in 1790. Volta is famous for discovering the first practical method of generating electricity, the electrolytic cell. By placing the ends of metal rods in his ears connected to an electrical supply (approx. 50 V), he discovered that the initial "boom in the head" was followed by a resultant electronic sound similar to "a thick boiling soup"—what we know now to be electronic static. Over the next several decades, it was surmised that since sound is more of an alternating sinusoidal signal, stimulation via direct current (DC) would probably not produce an adequate hearing sensation. In the early 19th century, the Frenchman Duchenne used an alternating current to stimulate hearing. His observation was described "as a sound similar to an insect trapped between a glass pane and a curtain."

Wever & Bray, (1930) went on to discover that an electrical response recorded near the auditory nerve of a cat was similar in frequency and amplitude to the stimulating sound. Gersuni & Volokhov, (1936) are credited for observing the effects of an alternating electrical stimulus on hearing. Another important discovery made by these investigators was that hearing could persist even after surgical removal of the tympanic membrane and middle ossicles, and thus hypothesized that the cochlea was the site of stimulation. Stevens & Jones, (1939), observed that several mechanisms produced hearing when the cochlea was stimulated electrically. Direct stimulation of the auditory nerve in a human was performed by Lundberg in 1950 and resulted in the patient hearing noise. In 1957, French-Algerian surgeons Andre Djourno and Charles Eyries directly stimulated exposed acoustic nerves and reported the patients' experience when current was applied (Djourno et al., 1957). It became distinctly apparent to researchers during the 1940's and 1950's that if precise hearing sensations were to be produced it would be more beneficial for current to be applied locally rather than widespread.

In 1961, William House developed a device to stimulate auditory function based in part on notes made by Djourno and colleagues. Together with Jack Urban, an engineer, he developed a single channel electrode implant device to assist with lip reading. Three deaf patients received this implant, with all reporting some benefit. Doyle et al., (1964), is credited for designing a four-electrode implant to try to limit the spread of the electrical current within the cochlea. Results obtained from a singular patient were only satisfactory, the most significant finding being the patients' new ability to repeat phrases. Simons, (1966) went on to perform a more extensive study by placement of electrodes throughout the promontory and vestibule areas and into the modiolar section of the auditory nerve. This approach allowed for stimulation of auditory fibers representing different frequencies. Results from testing showed the patient was able to discern the length of the stimulus duration and tonality could be achieved.

Cochlear implantation was tested and refined by use of scala tympani implantation of electrode arrays driven by an implantable receiver-stimulator by House, (1976) and Michelson, (1971). The House 3M single channel cochlear implant was the first to be commercially available in the US receiving FDA approval in 1984. Several hundred of these were implanted in patients beginning in 1972 and throughout the mid 1980's.

Meanwhile, outside the US, progress was being made by Graeme Clark in Australia. Professor Graeme Clark and colleagues developed a multi-channel cochlea implant, which enhanced the spectral perception and speech recognition capabilities in adult patients. This device was implanted in Rod Saunders in 1978, the first multi-channel cochlear implant recipient in the world. By the late eighties this implant marketed under the name "Nucleus Multi-channel Cochlear Implant" by Cochlear Pty Ltd. became the most widely used. This device received FDA approval in 1984 for use in adults, however by 1990 the age was reduced to 2, by 1998 to age 18 months, and by 2002 age 12 months. In some cases special approval have been obtained from the FDA for cochlear implantation of babies as young as 6 months of age (Eisen, 2009).

Today, due to advancement of technical and electronic development over the last few years, the size of the external components has been decreased in all commercially available cochlear implants. Companies such as Advanced Bionics and Neurelec provide only cochlear implants. Med El and Cochlear Corp., in addition to cochlear implants offer the middle ear implant system and Baha® bone conduction system respectively. As recently as last year, 2010, the FDA approved the Esteem® Totally Implantable Hearing System by Envoy Medical --intended to alleviate moderate to severe hearing loss in adults. The Esteem system, functions by sensing vibrations from the eardrum and the middle ear and converts these mechanical vibrations into electrical signals thereby replicating the ossicular chain and providing addition gain.

3. Animal models of deafness

Many different models of congenital deafness have been studied and include, cochlear ablation, acoustic trauma, ototoxic drugs, and hereditary deafness. The power of experimental animal models is that they enable researchers to study the effects of deafness in the auditory system and to infer mechanisms of pathophysiology in highly invasive preparations that would not be possible in human subjects. The consequences of congenital versus acquired deafness often reveal the importance of features involved in development. Neural activity is critical for normal construction and maintenance of auditory structure and function (Parks et al., 2004; Shepherd et al., 2006) with its lack having important implications on the auditory pathway. Neural activity influences the refinement of the genetic blueprint for circuitry including axonal distribution and synapse formation within the auditory system (Leake et al., 2006; Baker et al., 2010). In the absence of auditory stimulation, a series of pathological and atrophic changes is introduced that include more widespread distributions of axonal projections (Leake & Hradek, 1988), abnormal projections (Nordeen et al., 1983) delayed maturation (Kandler, 2004), and language impairments (Robbins, 2006).

The developing animal highlights the importance of auditory stimulation. Lack of auditory stimulation early in the postnatal period produces severe abnormalities in the auditory pathways, whereas, in mature animals with previous auditory experience, these effects are diminished (Rubel & Parks, 1988). These observations have been associated with the age related benefits of cochlear implantation in congenitally deaf humans (Waltzman et al., 1991; Gantz et al., 1994) because younger children typically gain more benefit from a cochlear implantation than older children. Data imply that deafness causes change in the central nervous system that, if not corrected, interferes with implant effectiveness.

For the purpose of this chapter we will focus primarily on the congenitally deaf white cat model of deafness. The congenitally deaf white cat model manifests a type of cochleosaccular degeneration that causes sensorineural hearing loss, mimicking the Scheibe deformity in humans (Scheibe, 1882; Suga & Hattler, 1970). Deafness in these animals is manifest by a collapse of Reissner's membrane, which obliterates the scala media and the organ of Corti (Figure 2).

It is not possible to conclude that deafness is solely due to the collapse of Reissner's membrane. First, these kittens are all born with normal looking cochlear morphology (Baker et al., 2010). It is only after the end of the first postnatal week that the pathology begins to emerge. The stria vascularis is pathologically thin, and this abnormality accompanies an irregular lengthening of Reissner's membrane that causes it to undulate. In addition, there is shrinkage of the tectorial membrane and it begins to curl upon itself and roll against the spiral ligament. This lengthening of Reissner's membrane proceeds rather rapidly such that it collapses by the end of the second postnatal week. By this time, the tectorial membrane is tightly curled against the spiral ligament. At the start of the third postnatal week of life, those kittens that are destined to become deaf exhibit a completely pathologic inner ear with no cochlear duct and no organ of Corti. Hair cell receptors are completely absent.

4. Synaptic morphology

Surprisingly, there are abnormalities in auditory nerve synapses in the cochlear nucleus that are evident at birth. The surprise is because it occurs well before the onset of hearing, and the idea had been that the effects of deafness wouldn't appear until after the normal onset of hearing. The delayed effect was presumed to occur because a lack of sound-evoked activity was hypothesized to underlie the abnormal synapses. The occurrence of abnormal synapses prior to the lack of activity implies that the system knows that it is deaf before there is evidence that the animal can hear or not.

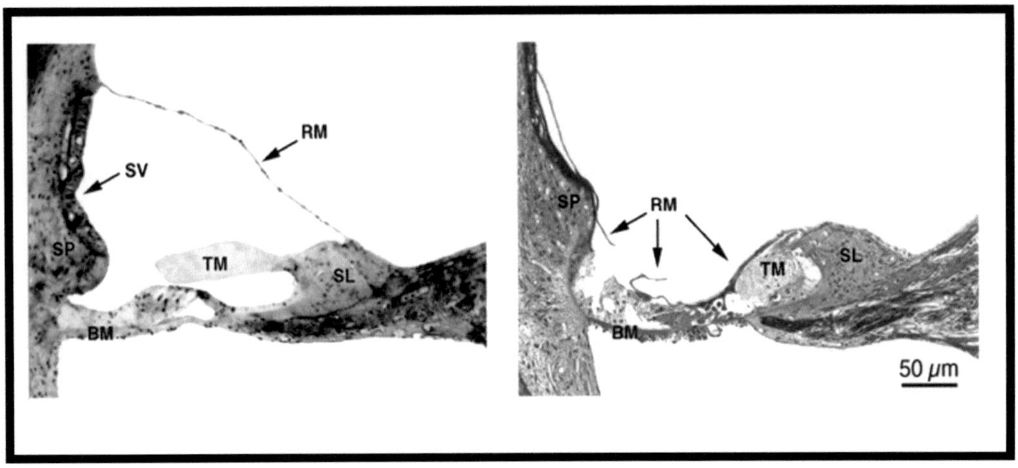

Fig. 2. Light micrographs of mid-modioloar sections showing the organ of Corti from a normal hearing (left) and deaf cat (right). RM= Reissners membrane, SP= spiral prominence, BM= basilar membrane, TM= tectorial membrane, SL= spiral limbus, SV=Stria vascularis.

Synapses are definable not only by presynaptic characteristics at the release site such as synaptic vesicle size and shape, transmitter chemicals, neuromodulators, and transporter molecules but also by the postsynaptic composition of transmitter receptor subunits, shape and curvature of the postsynaptic density (PSD), ion channels, and associated second messenger and retrograde signaling systems. Moreover, there must also be consideration of size and distribution of the terminal, target compartment (e.g., cell body, dendritic shaft, spine), and location of the cell bodies that give rise to the projection. Proper transmission of acoustic signals from neuron to neuron depends in large part on the precise spatial arrangement of these factors at the release site. The corollary to this notion is that abnormalities of synaptic structure will impair signal transmission, thereby corrupting the neural representation of the acoustic stimulus.

For the processing of sound, neural activity in the central nervous system must be tightly coupled in time to acoustic events. Sound, perhaps more than any other sensory stimuli, conveys meaning by the time-varying nature of frequency and level (or loudness). By virtue of the time-dependence of sound for information significance, neural activity pertaining to sound must be synchronized to time-dependent variables of the physical stimulus. Different sounds are revealed by distinctive characteristics in their time-varying features. It is accepted that different features of the physical components of sound are parsed and sent along separate and distinct pathways. Eventually, the information conveyed down the various circuits must reconvene with precise timing to produce a conscious percept of the stimulus. It is for these reasons that timing is so important to the auditory system. As a corollary, aberrations in these pathways will corrupt processing and disturb how sound is perceived.

The hair cell receptors within the cochlea transduce sound energy into neural signals in auditory nerve fibers that are conveyed to the cochlear nucleus (Kiang et al., 1965). The cochlear nucleus receives all incoming auditory information and gives rise to the ascending auditory pathways. The relatively homogeneous responses of incoming auditory nerve fibers are transformed into a variety of different response patterns by the different classes of resident neurons in the cochlear nucleus. These signals are in turn transmitted to higher centers by the ascending pathways. The spectrum of the responses depends not only upon the synaptic organization of the auditory nerve but also on intrinsic neurons and descending inputs; the types and distribution of receptors, ion channels, and G proteins; and second messengers. These features form the signaling capabilities for each cell class. In order to understand how sound is processed, there is a need to study identified cell populations, to analyze their synaptic connections, and to reveal features of their signal processing capabilities.

Auditory nerve fibers are the major source of excitation to cells of the ventral cochlear nucleus (Koerber et al., 1966). In the anteroventral cochlear nucleus (AVCN), myelinated auditory nerve fibers give rise to large, axosomatic synaptic endings known as endbulbs of Held (Held, 1893; Lorente de Nó, 1981). Endbulbs have a calyx-like appearance where the end of the fiber is marked by the emergence of several thick, gnarled branches that divide repeatedly to form an elaborate arborization of *en passant* and terminal swellings to embrace

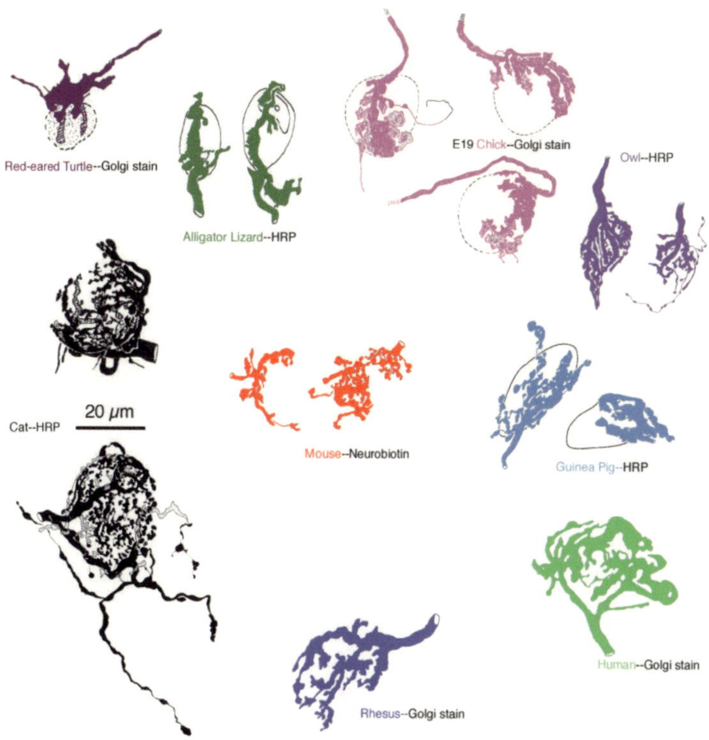

Fig. 3. Photomicrographs of the Endbulb of Held in different vertebrate species showing the evolutionary conservation of this synapse. (Adapted from Ryugo, D.K. & Parks, T.N. (2003). *Brain Res Bull*, Vol. 60, No. 5-6, pp. 435-456).

the postsynaptic spherical bushy cell (SBC, Ryugo & Fekete, 1982). These endbulbs are among the largest synaptic endings in the brain (Lenn & Reese, 1966), and one-to-three endbulbs selectively contact a single SBC (Ryugo & Sento, 1991; Nicol & Walmsley, 2002). They contain up to 2,000 release sites (Ryugo et al., 1996) and transmit activity with high-fidelity to the postsynaptic SBC (Babalian et al., 2003). The size and evolutionary conservation of endbulbs among vertebrates emphasize its importance in enabling spike activity to be yoked in time to acoustic events (see Figure 3).

4.1 Normal hearing animals

During postnatal development, the endbulb of Held begins with the formation of a solid, spoon-shaped growth cone and culminates in a highly branched axosomatic arborization. Each endbulb can form hundreds of synapses onto the postsynaptic SBC (Ryugo et al., 1996). This feature in particular suggests a highly secure synaptic interface to maintain the temporal fidelity of all incoming signals to the SBC (Manis & Marx, 1991). The structure of this giant synaptic terminal has been extensively studied to learn about synapse formation, its target specificity, and its reaction to deafness (Limb & Ryugo, 2000; Ryugo et al., 1997, 1998; Oleskevich et al., 2004, see Figure 4).

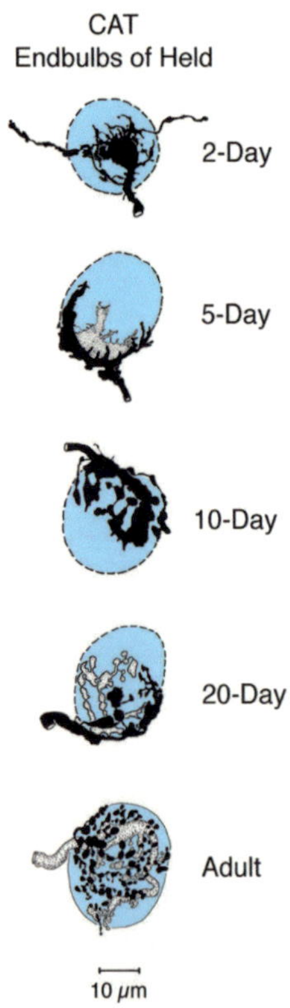

Fig. 4. Development of the endbulb of Held in a normal hearing cat from birth to adulthood. (Adapted from from Ryugo, D.K. & Spirou, G.A. (2009). Auditory System: Giant Synaptic Terminals, Endbulbs and Calyces. In: *New Encyclopedia of Neuroscience,* Vol. 1, Squire, L.R. (Ed.), pp. 759-770, Academic Press, Oxford).

In normal hearing cats, the endbulb arborization onto the SBC have been shown to vary systematically with respect to the average level of spike discharges received from auditory nerve fibers having low or high levels of activity. Endbulbs from fibers having high levels of activity (e.g., high (>18 s/s) spontaneous discharge rates and low thresholds for evoked responses) exhibit modest levels of branching with relatively large *en passant* and terminal swellings. In contrast, endbulbs from fibers having relatively low levels of activity (e.g., low (<18 s/s) spontaneous discharge rates and high thresholds for evoked responses) exhibit highly elaborate branching with relatively small *en passant* and terminal swellings (Figure 5). The differences in branching complexity were confirmed by statistically significant differences in fractal values. Moreover, the larger swellings on the highly active endbulbs resembled the swollen endings of overactive terminals where it was speculated that the swelling was caused by the fusion of synaptic vesicles (Burwen & Satir, 1977). Using electron microscopy to study synaptic ultrastructure, endbulbs receiving relatively low levels of spike discharges were associated with larger PSDs, whereas those exhibiting high rates of spike discharges exhibited smaller PSDs (Ryugo et al., 1996). These data are consistent with observations from rats exposed to repetitive tones or silence; stimulated animals exhibited endbulbs with smaller PSDs compared to those of animals exposed to silence (Rees et al., 1985). The synapse structure of endbulbs is clearly plastic and subject to activity-related change.

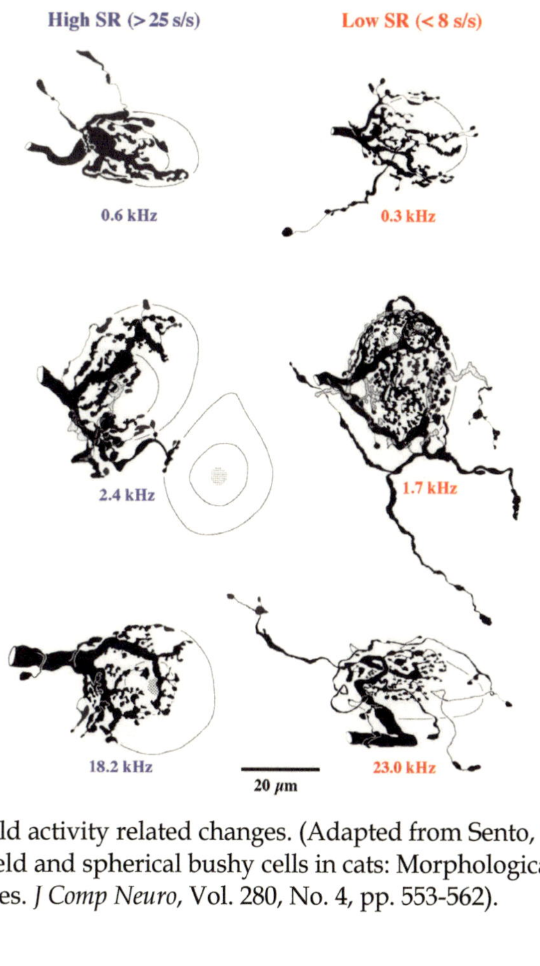

Fig. 5. Endbulbs of Held activity related changes. (Adapted from Sento, S. & Ryugo, D.K. (1989). Endbulbs of Held and spherical bushy cells in cats: Morphological correlates with physiological properties. *J Comp Neuro*, Vol. 280, No. 4, pp. 553-562).

4.2 Congenitally deaf animals

The endbulb synapse has been studied in congenitally deaf white cats to infer the extent to which sound influences its growth (Ryugo et al., 1997, 1998). Due to the elaborate form of the endbulb, changes in morphology should be evident and quantifiable. Moreover, given that variations in endbulb morphology were already apparent in normal hearing cats where differences could be attributed to disparities in spike discharge rates, it was predicted that in the extreme case of congenital deafness, there should be definable and obvious abnormalities.

Single unit recordings in the auditory nerve of congenitally deaf white cats revealed several important features. First, in completely deaf cats, there was little spontaneous activity and no evoked activity. Second, in hard of hearing cats (thresholds >60 dB), there was spontaneous activity, but elevated in distribution. Spontaneous activity in general was similar to that of normal hearing cats, but the upper range of spontaneous activity was extended (>150 s/s). In some auditory nerve fibers, spontaneous discharges exceeded 180 s/s. These data on activity were consistent with inner ear histology: deaf animals exhibited no organ of Corti, whereas hard of hearing animals exhibited a full complement of hair cells but showed signs of hydrops with an outward bulging Reissner's membrane (Ryugo et al., 1998).

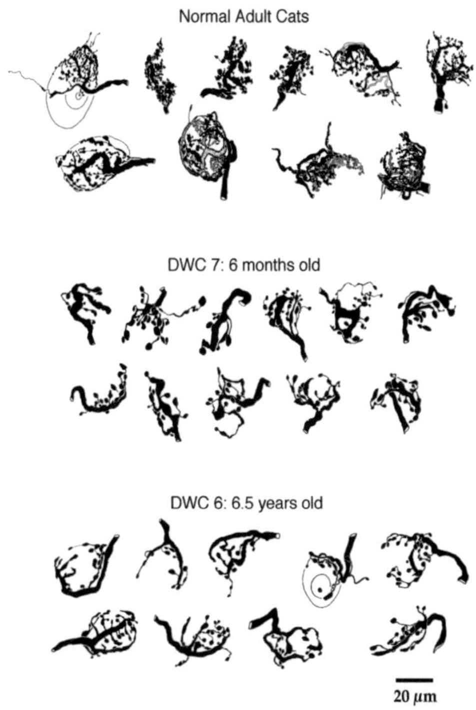

Fig. 6. Three-dimentional reconstruction of HRP-labeled endbulbs. Note the branching complexity is correlated to hearing status. (Adapted from Ryugo, D.K.; Pongstaporn, T.; Huchton, D.M. & Niparko, J.K. (1997). Ultrastructural analysis of primary endings in deaf white cats: Morphologic Alterations in Endbulbs of Held. *J Comp Neurol*, Vol. 385, No. 2, pp. 230-244 and Ryugo, D.K.; Rosenbaum, B.T.; Kim, P.J.; Niparko, J.K. & Saada, A.A. (1998). Single unit recordings in the auditory nerve of congenitally deaf white cats: Morphological correlates in the cochlea and cochlear nucleus. *J Comp Neurol*, Vol. 397, No. 4, pp. 532-548).

The most obvious structural correlate in the cochlear nucleus was that the endbulbs contacted significantly smaller postsynaptic SBCs (Saada et al., 1996; O'Neil et al., 2010; Ryugo et al., 2010). Second, the degree of endbulb arborization was graded in arborization complexity with respect to hearing threshold. In completely deaf cats, the extent and complexity of endbulb branching were less with significantly fewer swellings (Ryugo et al., 1997, 1998). These features were quantified by fractal analysis. Cats with elevated thresholds exhibited statistically different fractal values from completely deaf cats and normal hearing cats. Normal hearing cats displayed the most elaborate and complex endbulb arborizations (see Figure 6).

When these endbulbs were examined at greater resolution with an electron microscope, additional features are affected by hearing loss (Ryugo et al., 1997, 1998). In normal hearing cats, endbulbs give rise to numerous punctate, dome-shaped PSDs. Surrounding the PSD were accumulations of round, clear synaptic vesicles (Figure 7). In contrast, endbulbs of congenitally deaf white cats exhibited a flattening and hypertrophy of the PSDs (see Figure 8). Moreover, there was a striking increase in synaptic vesicle density near the release site (Baker et al., 2010). The endbulb synapses from cats that were not deaf but suffering from hearing loss exhibited features that were intermediate between those of normal hearing and completely deaf cats (Ryugo et al., 1998). That is, the PSDs were intermediate in size and curvature.

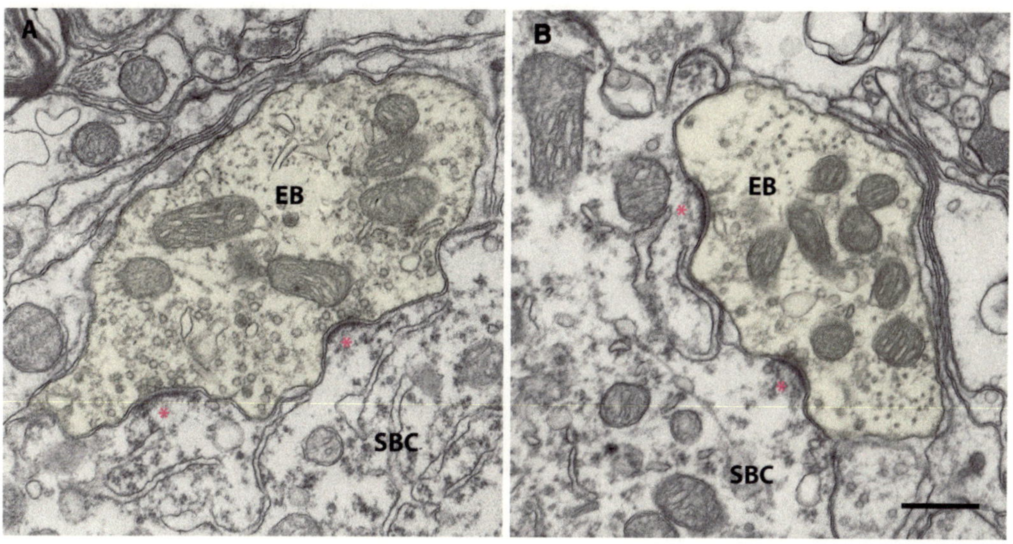

Fig. 7. Electron micrographs showing endbulbs of Held (EB) in normal cats. Note the typical dome-shaped appearance of PSDs marked with asterisk. Scale bar = 0.5 μm. (Adapted from O'Neil, J.N.; Limb, C.J.; Baker, C.A. & Ryugo, D.K. (2010). Bilateral effects of unilateral cochlear implantation in congenitally deaf cats. *J Comp Neuro*, Vol. 518, No. 12, pp. 2382-2404).

Deafness and hearing loss caused abnormalities in endbulb branching, soma size, and synapse morphology that were statistically different between cohorts (Ryugo et al., 1998). Abnormalities in synaptic transmission do not just occur with complete deafness. There has been transmission abnormalities reported in DBA/2J mice with hearing loss (Wang & Manis, 2006). These changes reveal that auditory synapses are highly sensitive to the quantity and quality of simulation. The presence of transmission irregularities from the presynaptic endbulb to the postsynaptic SBC could introduce jitter or perhaps even transmission failure. Such interruptions would diminish the precise processing of timing information. The implication is that even hearing loss will produce difficulties beyond elevated thresholds.

4.3 Chemical (ototoxic), and genetic deafening

The question could be asked whether the synaptic changes observed in the deaf cats are due to loss of neural activity in the auditory nerve, or whether they are part of the genetic syndrome and unrelated to spike activity. Several arguments can be presented to counter this concern. First, ototoxic deafening produces a similar flattening and hypertrophy of the PSD (Ryugo et al., 2010). Second, in *Shaker-2* mice whose deafness is caused by a mutation of the myosin 15 gene that leads to loss of hair cells, changes in endbulb arborization (Limb & Ryugo, 2000) and synaptic morphology (Lee et al., 2003) resemble those of the congenitally deaf white cat. Third, similar pathologic changes in endbulb morphology have been observed in the congenitally deaf guinea pig (Gulley et al., 1978). Because non-feline animals with deafness caused by independent means and cats of normal genetics but deafened by drugs all show these same synaptic anomalies, we can attribute the synaptic pathology to the lack of auditory nerve activity caused by deafness.

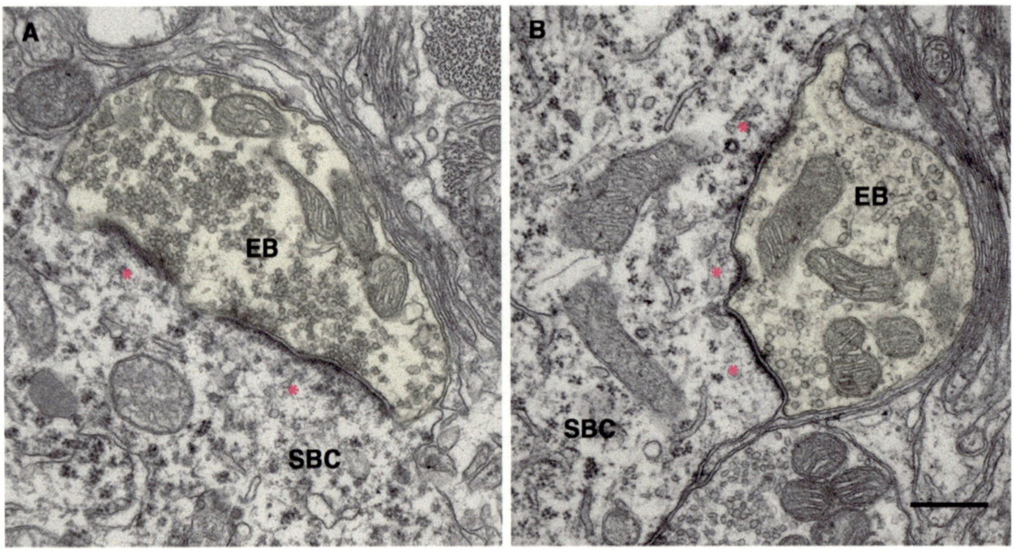

Fig. 8. Electron micrographs showing endbulbs of Held (EB) in deaf cats. Note the typical flat and elongated appearance of PSDs marked with asterisk. Scale bar = 0.5 µm. (Adapted from O'Neil, J.N.; Limb, C.J.; Baker, C.A. & Ryugo, D.K. (2010). Bilateral effects of unilateral cochlear implantation in congenitally deaf cats. *J Comp Neuro*, Vol. 518, No. 12, pp. 2382-2404).

Congenital deafness does not restrict its effects to the auditory nerve and cochlear nucleus (Saada et al., 1996). Alterations in cell size and number, receptive field properties, and laminar organization are expressed at higher nuclei of the auditory system including the superior olivary complex (Schwartz & Higa, 1982), inferior colliculus (Snyder et al., 2000), and auditory cortex (Klinke et al., 2001; Kral et al., 2001). Thus, alterations and plasticity at the endbulb synapse are reflections of a wider range of possible change throughout the central auditory system initiated by hearing loss and deafness.

5. Critical period of development

The concept of the critical period has been applied to explain biological phenomena that occur or are most severely affected over a brief period of time during development. Examples of such developmental events are exemplified by "imprinting" (Lorenz, 1935), cortical barrel plasticity (Weller & Johnson, 1975), birdsong acquisition (Konishi, 1985), and functional maturation of auditory cortex (Chang & Merzenich, 2003; Zhou et al., 2008). Reports that young children receiving cochlear implants gained far superior benefit compared to that of older children and adults also hinted strongly at a critical period (Gantz et al., 1994; Tyler & Summerfield, 1996). In congenitally deaf cats, electrical stimulation was reported to recruit auditory cortical responses contingent upon its commencement before 6 months of age (Klinke et al., 2001; Kral et al., 2002). The structural foundation for these observations may be attributable to the fact that 3-month old cochlear implant recipients exhibited somewhat restored auditory nerve synapses, whereas 6-month old cochlear implant recipients did not (O'Neil et al., 2010). The developmental period preceding puberty (cats reach puberty at six months of age) appears most favorable for implant-induced synaptic plasticity, and the restoration of endbulb synapses is hypothesized to have facilitated the proper delivery of afferent signals to the forebrain in a timely, coherent, and synchronized way.

6. Synaptic plasticity: Implications for cochlear implants

Synaptic strength and plasticity have been studied in other central synapses such as CA1 in the rat hippocampus where it was shown that the size of PSDs increases in response to pharmacological blockade of spike activity (e.g., Qin et al., 2001; Yasui et al., 2005). Quiescent synapses exhibited larger PSDs and increased numbers of synaptic vesicles that were accompanied by increases in synaptic strength. Consistent with this correlation, an increase in synaptic strength is seen in the AVCN of the congenitally deaf mouse when compared to that of normal hearing mice (Oleskevich & Walmsley, 2002; Oleskevich et al., 2004). This increase in synaptic strength may be related to an increase in transmitter receptors that become distributed in the enlarged PSDs.

Several abnormalities have been demonstrated in the auditory system following deafness including reduced numbers of spiral ganglion neurons (Leake & Hradek, 1988; Ryugo et al., 1998), abnormal synaptic structure (Ryugo et al., 1997), physiological alterations of auditory nerve responses in the cochlear nucleus (Oleskevich & Walmsley, 2002; Wang & Manis, 2006), and ectopic projections in the ascending pathways (Franklin et al., 2006). These changes undoubtedly affected synaptic transmission where degraded responses in the inferior colliculus (Vale & Sanes, 2002; Vollmer et al., 2005) and auditory cortex (Kral et al., 2006) have been observed. Endbulbs are implicated in mediating the precise temporal processing of sound (Molnar & Pfeiffer, 1968) and are known to transmit from auditory nerve to postsynaptic cell with a high degree of fidelity (Babalian et al., 2003). Detection and identification of some sounds are not nearly as demanding as the processing of temporal cues needed for sound localization, pattern recognition or speech comprehension. The introduction of synaptic jitter, delay, or failure by congenital deafness at the endbulb synapse appears to compromise such processing. If deafness-induced abnormalities go uncorrected, a cochlear implant may not be able to overcome the degraded signals, resulting in decreased benefit. The contribution of electrical activity to synaptic ultrastructure demonstrates that a cochlear implant can reverse some morphologic abnormalities in the auditory pathway when stimulation is started early.

6.1 Restoration of the endbulb synapse

Cochlear implants are electronic neural prostheses that are able to restore functional hearing to most individuals who are profoundly deaf or severely hard of hearing. Cochlear implants achieve their effects through bypassing the nonfunctioning auditory hair cell receptors of the inner ear and directly stimulating the auditory nerve (Rauschecker & Shannon, 2002). Individuals who lose hearing after developing speech and congenitally deaf children who receive implants early in life are the best candidates for cochlear implants, although the level of benefit varies widely from one individual to the next. Young children under the age of 2 years who exhibit nonsyndromic sensorineural deafness are also excellent candidates (Waltzman et al., 1994, 1997). Because children who receive implants at progressively older ages tend to perform more poorly, it is hypothesized that uncorrected congenital deafness leads to irreversible abnormalities throughout the central auditory system.

The synaptic changes in auditory nerve endings associated with congenital deafness present an interesting test for thinking about sensory deprivation and brain plasticity. Restoration of auditory activity by unilateral electrical stimulation in deaf cats resulted in improvements in temporal processing at the level of the cortex (Klinke et al., 2001), the inferior colliculus (Vollmer et al., 2005) and the cochlear nucleus (Ryugo et al., 2005). We sought to determine whether synaptic abnormalities in the cochlear nucleus would represent the key to disrupting auditory processing throughout the central auditory system? Using miniaturized cochlear implants (Clarion II implants donated by Advanced Bionics Corporation) congenital deaf kittens were implanted at 3 and 6 months of age. The implants utilized a 6-electrode array. After a short period of recovery, each kitten was stimulated 7 hours a day, 5 days a week for 2-3 months. The device utilized a speech processor identical to that used with human patients (Kretzmer et al., 2004). During the period of stimulation animals learned to approach their food bowl in response to a specific "call" showing that the animals were processing signals of biological relevance. Synapse restoration was evident on the side of stimulation where the small size and dome-shaped curvature of the PSD returned (Ryugo et al., 2005, Figure 9) however, this was not observed in the 6-month late implanted group (O'Neil et al., 2010).

6.2 Trans-synaptic changes in the auditory pathway

Electrical stimulation of the auditory nerve via cochlear implantation restored many of the synaptic abnormalities associated with congenital deafness, including PSD size, distribution, and curvature, and synaptic vesicle density. The restored synapses, however, were not completely normal because intermembraneous cisternae that tend to flank release sites did not return (O'Neil et al., 2010). Moreover, electrically evoked ABRs differed from those in normal cats. Evoked peaks in the ABR waveform whose height and sharpness are indicative of synchronous ascending volleys, while more prominent in implanted cats compared to that of unstimulated congenitally deaf cats, were nonetheless delayed and flattened. These changes in ABR waveform suggest a loss of synchrony in the evoked responses, perhaps caused by an increase in transmission jitter or transmission failure. The ascending projections of SBCs are likely to sustain these abnormalities through the interaural time difference (ITD) circuitry.

6.3 Trans-synaptic effects on spherical bushy cells

Spike activity and neural transmission in spiral ganglion cells and their fibers appear essential for the normal development of cochlear nucleus neurons (Rubel & Fritzsch, 2002). It follows that procedure's that increase neuronal survival should boost cochlear implant benefits such as improving speech comprehension. Studies that used ototoxic deafening of normal hearing cats have reported small but positive effects of electrical stimulation on cochlear nucleus cell size (Stakhovskaya et al., 2008), whereas others using similar methods show no effects (Coco et al., 2007). Our data show that electrical stimulation of auditory nerve fibers via cochlear implants had no effect on the size of the SBC neurons in this model of hereditary deafness. Because spiral ganglion neurons die at a faster rate with ototoxic treatments compared to hereditary deafness (Anniko, 1985), it may be that the ototoxic treatment not only damages auditory hair cell receptors but also spiral ganglion neurons and central neurons. Hereditary deafness obviously represents a different model from ototoxic deafness so it remains to be determined to what extent the results from the separate animal models are comparable.

6.4 Changes in the Medial Superior Olive (MSO)

Excitatory inputs to MSO neurons are segregated such that ipsilateral input innervates lateral dendrites and contralateral inputs innervate medial dendrites (Russell et al., 1995; Kapfer et al., 2002). These neurons function as a "coincidence detector" for processing ITDs (Carr et al., 2004). In addition, inhibitory inputs tend to be confined to the MSO cell bodies of mammals specialized for low frequency hearing (e.g., gerbil, cat, chinchilla). This topographical arrangement differs in MSO cells of mammals specialized for high frequency hearing (e.g., rat, opossum, bat, juvenile gerbil) where there is an equal excitatory-inhibitory synapse distribution on both cell somata and dendrites. Inhibitory input to the MSO arise from the medial and lateral nucleus of the trapezoid body (MNTB, LNTB, Grothe & Sanes, 1993) and function to adjust the output signal of MSO neurons (Pecka et al., 2008). The spatial distribution of these excitatory and inhibitory inputs is sensitive to developmental abnormalities within the acoustic environment. Deafness causes a bilateral disruption in the spatially segregated inputs to the MSO principal neurons as seen in mammals with low frequency hearing. In congenitally deaf animals, inhibitory input at the cell somata is significantly less than what is observed in hearing controls (Kapfer et al., 2002; Tirko & Ryugo, 2012).

This change in axosomatic inhibition was inferred by a loss of staining for gephyrin, an anchoring protein for the glycine receptor (Kapfer et al., 2002) and the migration of terminals containing flattened and pleomorphic synaptic vesicles (indicative of inhibitory synapses) away from the cell body. Excitatory inputs to the dendrites were severely shrunken. Two-to-three months of electrical stimulation via cochlear implantation of the congenitally deaf cat resulted in a partial restoration of the size of excitatory inputs to dendrites and a restoration of inhibitory input onto the cell somata (Tirko & Ryugo, 2012).

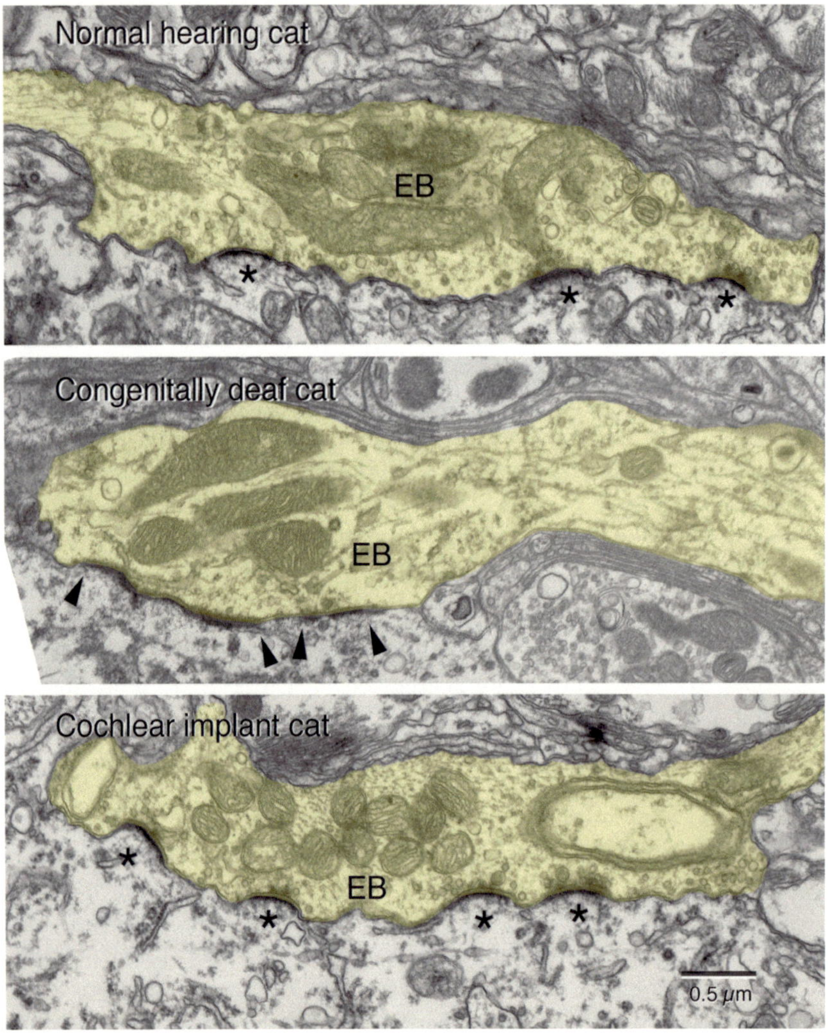

Fig. 9. Electron micrographs of endbulbs highlighted in yellow illustrating the restorative effect of activity on synapses. The endbulb of a congenitally deaf cat that received stimulation from a cochlear implant exhibits synapses with normal morphology. *Asterisks and arrowheads mark PSDs. (Adapted from Ryugo, D.K.; Kretzmer, E.A. & Niparko, J.K. (2005). Restoration of auditory nerve synapses in cats by cochlear implants. *Science*, Vol. 310, No. 5753, pp. 1490–1492).

6.5 Changes in the Lateral Superior Olive (LSO)

The LSO is involved in interaural level differences (ILDs, Tollin, 2003). This circuit measures the difference in sound level or intensity between the two ears, since the ear further from the sound source receives a relatively softer sound due to the "shadow" effect of the head. This binaural nucleus also plays a central role in sound localization, specifically in the processing of high frequency sounds. ILDs are encoded by integrating both excitatory and inhibitory input. The LSO receives excitatory input from ipsilateral SBCs and inhibitory input from the MNTB that in turn receives input from the contralateral globular bushy cells (Kandler et al., 2009).

The MNTB provides glycinergic input to the LSO. Glycine is a major inhibitory transmitter providing synaptic inhibition in the LSO and other nuclei within the superior olivary complex (Caspary et al., 1994; Grothe & Sanes, 1993). Inputs to the LSO are tonotopically organized similar to cochlear nuclei and are aligned so that a single neuron is excited and inhibited by the same sound frequency (Kandler et al., 2009).

Within the LSO, there is a remarkable degree of synaptic reorganization involving experience dependent plasticity that is important for normal auditory development (Kapfer et al., 2002; Kim & Kandler, 2003). In gerbils, development of the MNTB-LSO pathway begins with synaptic pruning of MNTB axon terminals in the LSO and a decrease in the spread of LSO dendrites occurring after hearing onset. This pruning depends in large part on auditory experience (Kandler et al., 2009). The specific elimination and strengthening of GABA/glycinergic synapses is essential for the formation of a precise tonotopic map (Gillespie et al., 2005).

Deafness-associated plasticity at the synapse level has long been observed in the auditory midbrain (Caspary et al., 1999; Sato et al., 2000; Holt et al., 2005). These synaptic changes influences the balance of excitation and inhibition and are reflected in neuronal response profiles (Francis & Manis, 2000; Syka et al., 2000; Syka & Rybalko, 2000) that vary with respect to cell type. A decrease in excitatory transmission to the LSO produces alterations in synaptic and membrane properties affecting the maturation of synaptic strength. This effect may be a result of a change in total synaptic contacts, presynaptic release or postsynaptic cell response (Buras et al., 2006).

6.6 Changes in the Inferior Colliculus (IC)

The IC is a tonotopically organized nucleus of the midbrain receiving ascending auditory inputs from many sources including both cochlear nuclei, superior olivary complex, as well as descending inputs from the auditory cortex and superior colliculus. It is a large nucleus, bilaterally located and representing the main station through which most ascending projections must pass before reaching the auditory forebrain. A rudimentary tonotopic organization within the IC has been shown to exist in long-term deafened animals (Snyder et al., 1990; Shepherd et al., 1999). This organization is maintained in the absence of auditory input (i.e., deafness) implying that connections are in place prior to hearing onset (Young & Rubel, 1986; Friauf & Kandler, 1990). Acute deafness did not increase temporal dispersion in spike timing to electric pulse trains in the auditory nerve nor impair ITD sensitivity (Shephard & Javel, 1997; Sly et al., 2007). Congenital deafness, however, did reduce ITD sensitivity in the responses of IC units. Single unit data in the IC showed that half as many neurons in the congenitally deaf cat showed ITD sensitivity to low pulse trains when compared to the acutely deafened animals. In neurons that showed ITD tuning, the tuning was found to be broader and more variable (Hancock et al., 2010). These findings reveal that ITD sensitivity is seriously affected by auditory deprivation and is consistent with what has been shown in humans with bilateral cochlear implants: these individuals perform better at distinguishing ILDs than ITDs. Collectively, the data imply that ITD discrimination is a highly demanding process and that even with near perfect synapse restoration, the task is sufficiently difficult that perhaps only complete restoration of synapses will enable the full return of function.

6.7 Changes in auditory cortex

Congenital deafness leads to functional and morphological changes in the auditory system from the cochlear nucleus, the first nuclei receiving auditory synaptic input to the auditory cortex (Kral et al., 2000, 2001). As clinical experience has shown, successful restoration of acoustic input to the auditory system depends on implantation age and sensitive periods in humans (Tyler et al., 1997; Busby & Clark, 1999) as well as cats (Klinke et al., 2001; O'Neil et al., 2010). In congenitally deaf cats, the auditory cortex does not receive any sound evoked input. However, it does display some rudimentary cortical representation of cochleotopy (Hartmann et al., 1997) and ITDs (Tillein et al., 2010). Investigations on the functional deficits of the auditory cortices in adult deaf cats were conducted where synaptic currents in cortical layers were compared between electrically stimulated congenitally deaf and electrically stimulated normal hearing animals (Kral et al., 2000). Marked functional deficits were found in the auditory cortex of the congenitally deaf cat believed to result from degeneration of the corticocortical and thalamocortical projections. Auditory experience through implantation was found to be necessary for recruitment and maturation of the auditory cortex, and such experience expanded the functional area of auditory cortex over that of animals who did not receive meaningful stimulation (Klinke et al., 2001).

7. Plasticity and binaural pathways

The ILD is the auditory cue used for localizing high-frequency sounds, whereas, ITD is the dominant auditory cue for localizing low-frequency sounds. These cues make up the binaural pathways important for sound-source localization. The endbulb synapse has been implicated in the ITD pathway that processes the precise timing features of sound that is crucial for binaural hearing. SBCs send projections from the AVCN to the superior olivary complex (Cant & Casseday, 1986). These projections terminate onto ipsilateral neurons of the LSO and bilaterally upon bipolar neurons of the MSO. In the MSO, inputs from the right cochlear nucleus terminate on the dendrites facing the right, whereas inputs from the left cochlear nucleus terminate on the dendrites facing left. The MSO is a key nucleus that processes synaptic input from both ears (Figure 10).

ITDs are crucial for localizing sounds on the horizontal plane. The ITD pathway utilizes the difference in arrival of a sound at the two ears to place a sound source. The general concept for this binaural sensitivity is the coincidence detection model where neurons would only respond when binaural excitatory inputs converged simultaneously (Jeffress, 1948). In this model, an array of MSO neurons receive systematically arranged inputs, each with a delay line such that it would only respond if a sound source were in a particular position off the midline. Some neurons would respond when the sound was directly in front of the animal, whereas others would respond when the sound moved away from the midline.

A delay line would compensate for a progressive shift in time of arrival at the two ears. The system is sensitive to differences in the range of tens of microseconds, so it is clear that precision in synaptic transmission is required (Grothe, 2000).

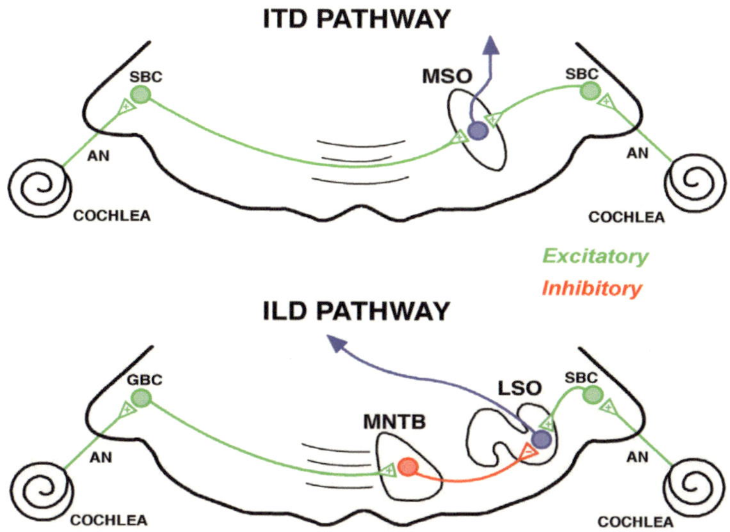

Fig. 10. Duplicity Theory Pathway (Adapted from Tollin, D.J. (2003). The lateral superior olive: a functional role in sound source localization. *Neuroscientist*, Vol. 9, No. 2, pp. 127-143 and O'Neil, J.N.; Connelly, C.J.; Limb, C.J. & Ryugo, D.K. (2011). Synaptic morphology and the influence of auditory experience. *Hear Res*, Vol. 279, No. 1-2, pp. 118-30).

The endbulb, therefore, is not only important for processing important timing cues for sound localization but also for time-varying cues in speech such as voice onset, stressed syllables, gaps, and amplitude modulation (Blackburn & Sachs, 1990). The point of this discussion is to emphasize that endbulbs and the timing of neural activity are linked and highly important to the proper processing and perception of sound.

8. Auditory function

Auditory experience has been shown to influence the maturation of the central auditory system throughout development. Auditory nerve activity in the form of spike discharges is necessary for the initial formation of precise synaptic structure, tonotopic organization, and proper distribution of terminals in the ascending auditory pathway. Abnormalities in organization result in a corruption of signal processing within the brain that ultimately impairs auditory perception. Structural changes occur in the brainstem and have been described in the congenitally deaf white cat model. The re-establishment of activity through electrical stimulation results in a remarkable recovery of the involved synapses and circuit organization. (O'Neil et al., 2011; Tirko & Ryugo, 2012).

Implants have allowed individuals with profound deafness, in particular children, to acquire speech understanding, language and social skills. Some benefits of binaural hearing can be accomplished with bilateral cochlear implants. Individuals affected with bilateral hearing loss implanted with sequentially cochlear implants benefit by having better speech understanding, especially in noise, and better sound localization. It allows the first ear that is implanted to preserve some of the benefits of binaural hearing somewhat avoiding the effects of auditory deprivation on the unimplanted ear. Auditory function can be somewhat restored by use of a cochlear implant depending on age at implant and upon how much auditory activity was available prior to implant.

9. Conclusion

Considerable progress has been made as a result of intensive cochlear implant research and development over the last forty years by adapting electronic technology for use in a physiological system. In doing so, the "world of hearing" have been opened to thousands of individuals in many countries. Even though the benefits of cochlear implants are many there is still progress to be made in addressing the extensive difficulties implant users have in localization of sound sources and the ability to enjoy music.

10. Acknowledgments

The authors gratefully acknowledge the support from NIH grants DC000232, DC005211, DC0023 and grants from the Office of Science and Medical Research, NSW, NMHRC grant #1009482, and the Garnett Passe and Rodney Williams Memorial Foundation.

11. References

Anniko, M. (1985). Principles in cochlear toxicity. *Arch Toxicol, Suppl*, Vol. 8, pp. 221-239

Babalian, A.L.; Ryugo, D.K. & Rouiller, E.M. (2003). Discharge properties of identified cochlear neurons and auditory nerve fibers in response to repetitive electrical stimulation of the auditory nerve. *Exp Brain Res*, Vol. 153, No. 4, pp. 452-460

Baker, C.A.; Montey, K.L.; Pongstaporn, T. & Ryugo, D.K. (2010). Postnatal development of the endbulb of Held in congenitally deaf cats. *Front Neuroanat*, Vol. 4, pp. 1-14

Blackburn, C.C. & Sachs, M.B. (1990). The representations of the steady-state vowel sound /e/ in the discharge patterns of cat anteroventral cochlear nucleus neurons. *J Neurophysiol*, Vol. 63, No. 5, pp. 1191-1212

Buras, E.D.; Holt, A.G.; Griffith, R.D.; Asako, M. & Altschuler, R.A. (2006). Changes in glycine immunoreactivity in the rat superior olivary complex following deafness. *J Comp Neurol*, Vol. 494, No. 1, pp. 179-189

Burwen, S.J. & Satir, B.H. (1977). Plasma membrane folds on the mast cell surface and their relationship to secretory activity. *J Cell Biol*, Vol. 74, No. 3, pp. 690-697

Busby, P.A. & Clark, G.M. (1999). Gap detection by early-deafened cochlear-implant subjects. *J Acoust Soc Am*, Vol. 105, No. 3, pp. 1841-1852

Cant, N.B. & Casseday, J.H. (1986) projections from the anteroventral cochlear nucleus to the lateral and medial superior olivary nuclei. *J Comp Neurol*, 247 No. 4, pp. 457-476

Carr, C.E. & Koppl, C. (2004). Coding interaural time differences at low best frequencies in the barn owl. *J Physiol*, Vol. 98, No. 1-3 pp. 99-112

Caspary, D.M.; Backoff, P.M.; Finlayson, P.G. & Palombi, P.S. (1994). Inhibitory inputs modulate discharge rate within frequency receptive fields of anteroventral cochlear nucleus neurons. *J Neurophysiol*, Vol. 72, No. 5, pp. 2124-2133

Caspary, D.M.; Holder, T.M.; Hughes, L.F.; Milbrandt, J.C.; McKerman R.M. & Naritoku, D.K. (1999). Age-related changes in GABA (A) receptor subunit composition and function in rat auditory system. *Neuroscience*, Vol. 93, No. 1, pp. 307-312

Chang, E.F., & Merzenich, M.M. (2003). Environmental noise retards auditory cortical development. *Science*, Vol. 300, No. 5618, pp. 498-502

Coco, A.; Epp, S.B.; Fallon, J.B.; Xu, J.; Millard, R.E. & Shepherd, R.K. (2007). Does cochlear implantation and electrical stimulation affect residual hair cells and spiral ganglion neurons? *Hear Res*, Vol. 225, No. 1-2, pp. 60-70

Djourno, A.; Eyries, C. & Vallancien, B. (1957). Premiers essays d'excitation électrique du nerf auditif chez l'homme, par microappareils incus a demeure. *Bull Natl Acad Med*, 141, pp. 481-483

Doyle, J.H.; Doyle, J.B. Jr. & Turnbull F.M. Jr. (1964). Electrical stimulation of eight cranial nerve. *Arch Otololaryngol*, Vol. 80, pp. 388-391

Eisen, M.D. (2009) The history of cochlear implants. In: *Cochlear implants: principles and practices* (2nd ed), J.K. Niparko, (Ed.), pp. 89-94, Lippincott Williams & Wilkins, Philadelphia, PA

Fay, R.R. (1988). *Hearing in vertebrates: a psychophysics databook*, Hill-Fay Associates, Winnetka, IL

Francis, H.W. & Manis, P.B. (2000). Effects of deafferentation on the electrophysiology of ventral cochlear nucleus neurons. *Hear Res*, Vol. 149, No. 1-2, pp. 91-105

Franklin, S.R.; Bruno-Bechtold, J.K. & Henkel, C.K. (2006). Unilateral cochlear ablation before hearing onset disrupts the maintenance of dorsal nucleus of the lateral lemniscus projection patterns in the rat inferior colliculus. *Neuroscience*, Vol. 143, No.1, pp. 105-115

Friauf, E. & Kandler, K. (1990). Auditory projections to the inferior colliculus of the rat are present by birth. *Neurosci Lett*, Vol. 120, No. 1, pp. 58-61

Gantz, B.J.; Tyler, R.S.; Woodworth, G.G.; Tye-Murray, N. & Fryauf-Bertschy, H., (1994). Results of multichannel cochlear implants in congenital and acquired prelingual deafness in children: five-year follow-up. *Am J Otol*, Vol. 15, *Suppl* 2, pp. 1-7

Gersuni, G.V. & Volokhov, A.A. (1936). On the electrical excitability of the auditory organ: On the effect of alternating currents on the normal auditory apparatus. *J Exp Psychol*, Vol. 19, pp. 370-382

Gillespie, D.C.; Kim, G. & Kandler, K. (2005). Inhibitory synapses in the developing auditory system are glutamatergic. *Nat Neurosci*, Vol. 8, No. 3, pp. 332-338

Grothe, B. (2000). The evolution of temporal processing in the medial superior olive, an auditory brainstem structure. *Prog Neurobiol*, Vol. 61, pp. 581-610

Grothe, B. & Sanes, D.H. (1993). Bilateral inhibition by glycinergic afferents in the medial superior olive. *J Neurophysiol*, Vol. 69, No.4, pp. 1192-1196

Gulley, R.L.; Landis, D.M. & Reese, T.S. (1978). Internal organization of membranes at endbulbs of Held in the anteroventral cochlear nucleus. *J Comp Neurol*, Vol. 180, No. 4, pp. 707-741

Hancock, K.; Noel, V.; Ryugo, D.K. & Delgutte, B. (2010). Neural coding of ITD with bilateral cochlear implants: Effects of congenital deafness. *J Neurosci*, Vol. 30, No. 42, pp. 14068-14079

Hartmann, R.; Shepherd, R.K.; Heid, S. & Klinke, R. (1997). Response of the primary auditory cortex to electrical stimulation of the auditory nerve in the congenitally deaf white cat. *Hear Res*, Vol. 112, No. 1-2, pp. 115-133

Held, H. (1893). Die centrale Gehorleitung. *Arch. Anat. Physiol. Anat. Abt.* 17, pp. 201-248

Holt, A.G.; Asako, M.; Lomax, C.A.; MacDonald, J.W.; Tong, L.; Lomax, M.I. & Altschuler, R.A. (2005). Deafness-related plasticity in the inferior colliculus: gene expression profiling following removal of peripheral activity. *J Neurochem*, Vol. 93, No.5, pp. 1069-1086

House, W.F. (1976). Cochlear implants. *Ann Otol Rhinol Laryngol*, Vol. 85, s27(3pt2), pp. 1-93

Jeffress, L.A. (1948). A place theory of sound localization. *J Comp Physiol Psychol*, Vol. 41, No. 1, pp. 35-39

Jerison, J.H. (1973). *Evolution of the Brain and Intelligence*, New York, Academic Press

Kandler, K. (2004). Activity-dependent organization of inhibitory circuits: lessons from the auditory system. *Curr Opin Neurobiol*, Vol. 14, No. 1, pp. 96-104

Kandler, K.; Clause, A. & Noh, J. (2009). Tonotopic reorganization of developing auditory brainstem circuits. *Nat Neurosci*, Vol. 12, No. 6, pp. 711-717

Kapfer, C.; Seidl, A.H.; Schweizer, H. & Grothe, B. (2002). Experience-dependent refinement of inhibitory inputs to auditory coincidence-detector neurons. *Nat Neurosci*, Vol. 5, No. 3, pp. 247-253

Kiang, N.Y.S.; Watanabe, T.; Thomas, E.C. & Clark, L.F. (1965). *Discharge Patterns of Single Fibers in the Cat's Auditory Nerve*, M.I.T. Press, Cambridge, MA

Kim, G. & Kandler, K. (2003). Elimination and strengthening of glycinergic/GABAergic connections during tonotopic map formation. *Nat Neurosci*, Vol. 6, No. 3, pp. 282-290

Klinke, R.; Hartmann, R.; Heid, S.; Tillein, J. & Kral, A. (2001). Plastic changes in the auditory cortex of congenitally deaf cats following cochlear implantation. *Audiol Neurootol*, Vol. 6, No. 4, pp. 203-206

Koerber, K.C., Pfeiffer, R.R., Warr, W.B. & Kiang, N.Y. (1966). Spontaneous spike discharges from single units in the cochlear nucleus after destruction of the cochlea. *Exp Neurol*, Vol. 16, No. 2, pp. 119-130

Kral, A.; Hartmann, R.; Tillein, J.; Heid, S. & Klinke, R. (2000). Congenital auditory deprivation reduces synaptic activity within the auditory cortex in a layer-specific manner. *Cereb Cortex*, Vol. 10, No. 7, pp. 714-726

Kral, A.; Hartmann, R.; Tillein, J.; Heid, S. & Klinke, R. (2001). Delayed maturation and sensitive periods in the auditory cortex. *Audiol Neurootol*, Vol. 6, No. 6, pp. 346- 362

Kral, A.; Hartmann, R.; Tillein, J.; Heid, S. & Klinke, R. (2002). Hearing after congenital deafness: central auditory plasticity and sensory deprivation. *Cereb Cortex*, Vol. 12, No. 8, pp. 797-807

Kral, A.; Tillein, J.; Heid, S.; Klinke, R. & Hartmann, R. (2006). Cochlear implants: cortical plasticity in congenital deprivation. *Prog Brain Res*, Vol. 157, pp. 283-313

Kretzmer, E.A.; Meltzer, N.E.; Haenggeli, C.A. & Ryugo, D.K. (2004). An animal model for cochlear implants. *Arch Otolaryngol Head Neck Surg*, Vol. 130, No. 5, pp. 499-508

Konishi, M. (1985). Birdsong: From behavior to neuron. *Ann Rev Neurosci*, Vol. 8, pp. 125- 170

Leake, P.A. & Hradek, G.T. (1988). Cochlear pathology of long term neomycin induced deafness in cats. *Hear Res*, Vol. 33, No. 1, pp. 11-33

Leake, P.A.; Hradek, G.T.; Chair, L. & Snyder, R.L. (2006). Neonatal deafness results in degrade topographic specificity of auditory nerve projections to the cochlear nucleus in cats. *J Comp Neurol*, Vol. 497, No.1, pp. 13-31

Lee, D.J.; Cahill, H.B. & Ryugo, D.K. (2003). Effects of congenital deafness in the cochlear nuclei of Shaker-2 mice: an ultrastructural analysis of synapse morphology in the endbulbs of Held. *J Neurocytol*, Vol. 32, No. 3, pp. 229-243

Lenn, N.J. & Reese, T.S. (1966). The fine structure of nerve endings in the nucleus of the trapezoid body and the ventral cochlear nucleus. *Am J Anat*, Vol. 118, No. 2, pp. 375-389

Limb, C.J. & Ryugo, D.K. (2000). Development of primary axosomatic endings in the anteroventral cochlear nucleus of mice. *J Assoc Res Otolaryngol*, Vol. 1, No. 2, pp. 103-119
Lorente de Nó, R. (1981). *The Primary Acoustic Nuclei*. Raven Press, New York
Lorenz, K. (1935). Der Kumpan in der Umwelt des Vogels. Der Artgenosse als auslosendes Moment sozialer Verhaltensweisen. *J fur Ornithologie*, 83, pp. 137-413
Manis, P.B. & Marx, S.O. (1991). Outward currents in isolated central cochlear nucleus neurons. *J Neurosci*, Vol. 11, No. 9, pp. 2865-2880
Michelson, R.P. (1971). The results of electrical stimulation of the cochlea in human sensory deafness. *Ann Otol Rhinol Laryngol*, Vol. 80, No. 6, pp. 914-919
Molnar, C.E. & Pfeiffer R.R. (1968). Interpretation of spontaneous discharge patterns of neurons in the cochlear nucleus. *Proc IEEE*, Vol. 56, No. 6, pp. 993-1004
Nicol, M.J. & Walmsley, B. (2002). Ultrastructural basis of synaptic transmission between endbulbs of held and bushy cells in the rat cochlear nucleus. *J Physiol*, Vol. 539(Pt 3), pp. 713-723
Niparko, J.K.; Lingua C. & Carpenter R.M. (2009). Assessment of Candidacy for Cochlear Implant Implantation, In: *Cochlear Implants: principles and practices*, (2nd ed), John K. Niparko (Ed.), pp. 137-146, Lippincott Williams & Wilkins, Philadephia, PA
Nordeen, K.W.; Killackey, H.P. & Kitzes, L.M. (1983). Ascending projections to the inferior colliculus following unilateral cochlear ablation in the adult gerbil, *Meriones unguiculatus*. *J Comp Neurol*, Vol. 214, No. 2, pp. 131-143
Oleskevich, S. & Walmsley, B. (2002). Synaptiic transmission in the auditory brainstem of normal and congenitally deaf mice. *J Physiol*, 540(Pt 2), pp. 447-455
Oleskevich, S.; Youssoufian, M. & Walmsley, B. (2004). Presynaptic plasticity at two giant auditory synapses in normal and deaf mice. *J Physiol*, Vol. 560(Pt 3), pp. 709-719
O'Neil, J.N.; Limb, C.J.; Baker, C.A. & Ryugo, D.K. (2010). Bilateral effects of unilateral cochlear implantation in congenitally deaf cats. *J Comp Neurol*, Vol. 518, No. 12, pp. 2382-2404
O'Neil, J.N.; Connelly, C.J.; Limb, C.J. & Ryugo, D.K. (2011). Synaptic morphology and the influence of auditory experience. *Hear Res*, Vol. 279, No. 1-2,pp. 118-130
Parks, T.N.; Rubel, E.W.; Popper, A.N. & Fay, R.R. (Eds), (2004). *Plasticity of the Auditory System*, Springer, New York
Pecka, M.; Brand, A.; Behrend, O. & Grothe, B. (2008). Interaural time difference processing in the mammalian medial superior olive: the role of glycinergic inhibition. *J Neurosci*, Vol. 28, No. 27, pp. 6914-6925
Qin, L.; Marrs, G.S.; McKim, R. & Dailey, M. (2001). Hippocampal mossy fibers induce assembly and clustering of PSD95 containing postsynaptic densities independent of glutamate receptor activation. *J Comp Neurol*, Vol. 440, No. 3, pp. 284-298
Rauschecker, J.P. & Shannon, R.V. (2002). Sending sound to the brain. *Science* Vol. 295, No. 5557, pp. 1025-1029
Rees, S.; Guldner, F.H. & Aitkin, L. (1985). Activity dependent plasticity of postsynaptic density structure in the ventral cochlear nucleus of the rat. *Brain Res*, Vol. 325, No. (1-2) pp. 370-374
Robbins, A.M. (2006). Language development in children with cochlear implants. In: *Cochlear Implants*, Waltzman, S.B., Roland Jr., J.R. (Eds.), pp. 153-166, Thieme Medical Publishers, New York

Rubel, E.W. & Fritzsch, B. (2002). Auditory system: primary auditory neurons and their targets. *Annu Rev Neurosci*, 25, pp. 51–101

Rubel, E. W. & Parks, T. N. (1988). Organization and development of the avian brain-stem auditory system. In: *Auditory Function: The Neurobiological Basis of Hearing*, Edelman, G. M., Gall, W. E., & Cowan, W. M. (Eds.), pp. 3–9, Wiley, NewYork

Russell, F.A. & Moore, D.R. (1995). Afferent reorganization within the superior olivary complex of the gerbil: development and induction by neonatal, unilateral cochlear removal. *J Comp Neurol*, Vol. 352, No. 4, pp. 607-625

Ryugo, D.K.; Baker, C.A.; Montey, K.L.; Chang, L.Y.; Coco, A.; Fallon, J.B. & Shepherd, R.K. (2010). Synaptic plasticity after chemical deafening and electrical stimulation of the auditory nerve in cats. *J Comp Neurol*, Vol. 518, No. 7, pp. 1046-1063

Ryugo, D.K. & Fekete, D. M. (1982). Morphology of primary axosomatic endings in the anteroventral cochlear nucleus of the cat: a study of the endbulbs of Held. *J Comp Neurol*, Vol. 210, No. 3, pp. 239-257

Ryugo, D.K.; Kretzmer, E.A. & Niparko, J.K. (2005). Restoration of auditory nerve synapses in cats by cochlear implants. *Science*, Vol. 310, No. 5753, pp. 1490-1492

Ryugo, D.K. & Parks, T.N. (2003). Primary innervation of the avian and mammalian cochlear nucleus. *Brain Res Bull*, Vol. 60, No. 5-6, pp. 435–456

Ryugo, D.K. & Spirou G.A. (2009). Auditory System: Giant Synaptic Terminals, Endbulbs and Calyces. In: *New Encyclopedia of Neuroscience*, Vol.1, Squire L.R. (Ed.), pp. 759-770, Academic Press, Oxford

Ryugo, D.K.; Pongstaporn, T.; Huchton, D.M. & Niparko, J.K. (1997). Ultrastructural analysis of primary endings in deaf white cats: morphologic alterations in endbulbs of Held. *J Comp Neurol*, Vol. 385, No. 2, pp. 230-244

Ryugo, D.K.; Rosenbaum, B.T.; Kim, P.J.; Niparko, J.K. & Saada, A.A. (1998). Single unit recordings in the auditory nerve of congenitally deaf white cats: morphological correlates in the cochlea and cochlear nucleus. *J Comp Neurol*, Vol. 397, No. 4, pp. 532-548

Ryugo, D.K. & Sento, S. (1991). Synaptic connections of the auditory nerve in cats: relationship between endbulbs of held and spherical bushy cells. *J Comp Neurol*, Vol. 305, No. 1, pp. 35-48

Ryugo, D.K.; Wu, M.M. & Pongstaporn, T. (1996). Activity-related features of synapse morphology: a study of endbulbs of Held. *J Comp Neurol*, Vol. 365, No. 1, pp. 141- 158

Saada, A.A.; Niparko, J.K. & Ryugo, D.K. (1996). Morphological changes in the cochlear nucleus of congenitally deaf white cats. *Brain Res*, Vol. 736, No. 1-2, pp. 315-328

Sato, K.; Shiraishi, S.; Nakagawa, H.; Kuriyama, H. & Altschuler, R.A. (2000). Diversity and plasticity in amino acid receptor subunits in the rat auditory brain stem. *Hear Res*, Vol. 147, No. 1-2, pp. 137-144

Scheibe, A. (1882). A case of deaf-mutism, with auditory atrophy and anomalies of development in the membraneous labyrinth of both ears. *Arch Otolaryngol*, Vol. 21, pp. 12-22

Schwartz, I.R. & Higa, J.F. (1982). Correlated studies of the ear and brainstem in the deaf white cat: changes in the spiral ganglion and the medial superior olivary nucleus. *Acta Otolaryngol*, Vol. 93, No. 1-2, pp. 9-18

Sento, S. & Ryugo, D.K. (1989). Endbulbs of Held and spherical bushy cells in cats: Morphological correlates with physiological properties. *J Comp Neuro*, Vol. 280, No. 4, pp. 553-562

Shepherd, R.K. & Javel, E. (1997). Electrical stimulation of the auditory nerve. I. Correlation of physiological responses with cochlear status. *Hear Res*, Vol. 108, No. 1-2, pp. 112-144

Shepherd, R.K. & Javel, E. (1999). Electrical stimulation of the auditory nerve: II. Effect of stimulus waveshape on single fibre response properties. *Hear Res*, 130, No. 1-2, pp. 171-188

Shepherd, R.K.; Meltzer, N.E.; Fallon, J.B. & Ryugo, D.K. (2006). Consequences of deafness and electrical stimulation on the peripheral and central auditory system. In: *Cochlear Implants*. Waltzman, S.B., Roland, J.T., (Eds.), pp. 25-39, Thieme Medical Publishers, New York

Simons, L.A.; Dunlop, C.W.; Webster, W.R. & Aitkin, L.M. (1966). Acoustic habituation in cats as a function of stimulus rate and the role of temporal conditioning of the middle ear musles. *Electroencephalogr Clin Neurophysiol*, Vol. 20, No. 5, pp. 485-493

Sly, D.J.; Heffer, L.F.; White, M.W.; Shepherd, R.K.; Birch, M.G.; Minter, R.L.; Nelson, N.E.; Wise, A.K. & O'Leary, S.J. (2007). Deafness alters auditory nerve fibre responses to cochlear implant stimulation. *Eur J Neurosci*, Vol. 26, No. 2, pp. 510-522

Snyder, R.L.; Rebscher, S.J.; Cao, K.L.; Leake, P.A. & Kelly, K. (1990). Chronic intracochlear electrical stimulation in the neonatally deafened cat. I: Expansion of central representation. *Hear Res*, Vol. 50, No. 1-2, pp. 7-33

Snyder, R.L.; Vollmer, M.; Moore, C.M.; Rebscher, S.J.; Leake, P.A. & Beitel, R.E. (2000). Responses of inferior colliculus neurons to amplitude-modulated intracochlear electrical pulses in deaf cats. *J Neurophysiol*, Vol. 84, No. 1, pp. 166-183

Stakhovskaya, O.; Hradek, G.T.; Snyder, R.L. & Leake, P.A. (2008). Effects of age at onset of deafness and electrical stimulation on the developing cochlear nucleus in cats. *Hear Res*, Vol. 243, No. 1-2, pp. 69-77

Stevens, S.S. & Jones, R.C. (1939). The mechanism of hearing by electrical stimulation. *J Acoust Soc Am*, Vol. 10, pp. 261-269

Suga, F. & Hattler, K.W. (1970). Physiological and histopathological correlates of hereditary deafness in animals. *Laryngoscope*, Vol. 80, No. 1, pp. 81-104

Syka, J.; Popelar, J.; Kvasnak, E. & Astl, J. (2000). Response properties of neurons in the central nucleus and external and dorsal cortices of the inferior colliculus in guinea pig. *Exp Brain Res*, Vol. 133, No. 2, pp. 254-266

Syka, J. & Rybalko, N. (2000). Threshold shifts and enhancement of cortical evoked responses after noise exposure in rats. *Hear Res*, Vol. 139, No. 1-2, pp. 59-68

Tillein, J.; Hubka, P.; Syed, E.; Hartmann, R.; Engel, A.K. & Kral, A. (2010). Cortical representation of interaural time difference in congenital deafness. *Cereb Cortex*, Vol. 20, No. 2, pp. 492-506

Tirko, N.N. & Ryugo, D.K. (2012). Synaptic plasticity in the medial superior olive of hearing, deaf, and cochlear-implanted cats. *J Comp Neurol*, (Epub ahead of print)

Tollin, D.J. (2003). The lateral superior olive: a functional role in sound source localization. *Neuroscientist*, Vol. 9, No. 2, pp. 127-143

Tyler, R.S.; Fryauf-Bertschy, H.; Gantz, B.J.; Kelsay, D.M. & Woodworth, G.G. (1997). Speech perception in prelingually implanted children after four years. *Adv Otorhinolaryngol*, Vol. 52, pp. 187-192

Tyler, R.S. & Summerfield, A.Q. (1996). Cochlear implantation: relationships with research on auditory deprivation and acclimatization. *Ear Hear*, Vol. 17, No. 3, pp. 38S-50S

Vale, C. & Sanes, D.H. (2002). The effect of bilateral deafness on excitatory and inhibitory synaptic strength in the inferior colliculus. *Eur J Neurosci*, Vol. 16, No. 12, pp. 2394–2404

Vollmer, M.; Leake, P.A.; Beitel, R.E.; Rebscher, S.J. & Snyder, R.L. (2005). Degradation of temporal resolution in the auditory midbrain after prolonged deafness is reversed by electrical stimulation of the cochlea. *J Neurophysiol*, Vol. 93, No. 6, pp. 3339-3355

Waltzmann, S.B.; Cohen, N.L. & Shapiro, W.H. (1991). Effects of chronic electrical stimulation on patients using cochlear prosthesis. *Otolaryngol Head Neck Surg*, Vol. 105, No. 6, pp. 797-801

Waltzman, S.B.; Cohen, N.L.; Gomolin, R.H.; Green, J.E.; Shapiro, W.H.; Hoffman, R.A. & Roland, J.T., Jr. (1997). Open-set speech perception in congenitally deaf children using cochlear implants. *Am J Otol*, Vol. 18, No. 3, pp. 342-349

Waltzman, S.B.; Cohen, N.L.; Gomolin, R.H.; Shapiro, W.H.; Ozdamar, S.R. & Hoffman, R.A. (1994). Long-term results of early cochlear implantation in congenitally and prelingually deafened children. *Am J Otol*, Vol. 15 Suppl 2, pp. 9-13

Waltzman, S.B. & Roland, J.T. Jr. (2005). Cochlear implantation in children younger than 12 months. *Pediatrics*, Vol. 116, No. 4, pp. 487-493

Wang, Y. & Manis, P.B. (2006). Temporal coding by cochlear nucleus bushy cells in DBA/2J mice with early onset hearing loss. *J Assoc Res Otolaryngol*, Vol. 7, No. 4, pp. 412-424

Weller, W.L. & Johnson, J.L. (1975). Barrels in cerebral cortex by receptor disruption in newborn, but not in five-day-old mice (*Cricetidoe* and *Muridae*). *Brain Res*, Vol. 83, pp. 504-508

Wever, E.G. & Bray, C.W. (1930). Auditory nerve impulses. *Science*, Vol. 71, No. 1834, pp. 215

Yasui, T.; Fujisawa, S.; Tsukamoto, M.; Matsuki, N. & Ikegaya, Y. (2005). Dynamic synapses as archives of synaptic history: state-dependent redistribution of synaptic efficacy in the rat hippocampal CA1. *J Physiol*, Vol. 566(Pt 1), pp. 143–160

Young, S.R. & Rubel, E.W. (1986). Embryogenesis of arborization pattern and topography of individual axons in N. laminaris of the chicken brain stem. *J Comp Neuro*, Vol. 254, No. 4, pp. 425-459

Zhou, X.; Nagarajan, N.; Mossop, B.J. & Merzenich, M.M. (2008). Influences of un-modulated acoustic inputs on functional maturation and critical-period plasticity of the primary auditory cortex. *Neuroscience*, Vol. 154, No. 1, pp. 390-396

http://www.nidcd.nih.gov/health/statistics/Pages/quick.aspx

http://www.nidcd.nih.gov/health/hearing/pages/coch.aspx

10

Cochlear Implants and the Right to Language: Ethical Considerations, the Ideal Situation, and Practical Measures Toward Reaching the Ideal

Tom Humphries[1], Poorna Kushalnagar[2], Gaurav Mathur[3], Donna Jo Napoli[4], Carol Padden[1], Christian Rathmann[5] and Scott Smith[6]

[1]University of California at San Diego
[2]Rochester Institute of Technology
[3]Gallaudet University
[4]Swarthmore College
[5]Universität Hamburg
[6]University of Rochester
[1,2,3,4,6]USA
[5]Germany

1. Introduction

Cochlear implants (CIs) in small children who do not yet have a firm footing in first language acquisition are an on-going experiment with human subjects, in the sense that the risks involved have not been properly identified, much less assessed, due to the failure to focus on the biology of language and its role in first language acquisition. Too often, the developmental cognitive milestones of the deaf child and the right to language are not considered, and we risk contributing to cases of linguistic deprivation with all the ensuing consequences. We propose an immediate remedy: to teach deaf children a sign language, along with training in speech and speech-reading. For many families, such as those that live far from a Deaf community, as in a rural situation, this presents practical problems, which we address.

2. Background on the problem

CIs as a rehabilitative technology to remediate hearing loss were approved before present-day information on the biology of first language acquisition was available. This mismatch of timing has led to the present problem.

2.1 History of cochlear implants

Research on transforming auditory information into electrical impulses that might deliver language to the brain began in the 1930s at the Military Academy in Leningrad, Russia. "Stimulating electrodes were inserted into the middle ear of patients with and without middle ear structures present" (Djourno et al., 1957, as cited in Eisen, 2000: 91). The disappointing results led to the rejection of the middle ear as the proper site of electrical stimulation.

In the 1950s at the Head and Neck Surgery section of the l'Institut Prophylactique in Paris, France, CIs were first developed, in which electrical stimulation was delivered to the auditory nerve. The first implant surgery was performed in 1957. Success was limited. The patient could only discriminate lower from higher frequency noises and could "appreciate environmental noises and several words, but could not understand speech" (Eisen, 2000: 91). Around 1960, American physicians attempted inserting gold wire electrodes through the skin, but local infections made this method unfeasible. In 1964, an electrode was implanted into the modiolus (the central axis of the cochlea) of a deaf patient at Stanford University Hospital. The potential for such an implant to deliver language was reported as "discouraging" (Simmons, 1966, as cited in Eisen, 2000: 92). Meanwhile, others elsewhere in California were implanting single electrode devices. Over the next decade, the attitude of the medical world was cautionary, but the concerns were about whether CIs would yield useful hearing. Importantly, the concerns were not about whether a CI could harm a patient.

In 1975, the National Institutes of Health sponsored an evaluation of thirteen patients who had been implanted with single-channel devices. They concluded that these devices "could not support speech understanding" but did support speech skills such as voicing and speech-reading, and these devices did enhance quality of life (Bilger, 1977, as cited in Eisen, 2000: 92). Immediately, testing began on a cat model in California, and other researchers in both California and Melbourne, Australia, capitalized on advancements in computer technology enabling them to miniaturize the various parts of the device. In 1972, the first U.S. Food and Drug Administration-approved devices were implanted, and by the mid-1980s 1000 individuals had been implanted. Of those first 1000 implant surgeries, several hundred were on children; the age criterion for use of the device was subsequently lowered from 18 years to 2 years old in 1980. In 1984, multiple channel devices (with multiple points of excitation to the cochlear nerve) were developed, and by the next year, the Food and Drug Administration approved their use in adults. In 1990, they extended their use to children as young as 2 years old, although children had been receiving these multiple channel devices in clinical trials since 1985 (Barnes, 1994). Since multiple channels "significantly boosted speech recognition performance", the push was to implant more children at a younger age (Wilson et. al., 1991, as cited in Eisen, 2000: 92). Optimism rose, and as one of the major pioneers in the development of CIs reported, "Limited open-set word and sentence recognition is possible for at least some children, perhaps as many as 30%" (House, 1991: 718).

Over the next decade, the advent of universal newborn hearing loss screenings coupled with studies showing that earlier implantation correlates to earlier development of auditory recognition and speech comprehension (Waltzman & Roland, 2005; Yoshinaga-Itano et al., 1998; Yoshinaga-Itano et al., 2000) resulted in more and more children being implanted at 12 months of age and even younger (Christensen & Leigh, 2002). By 2009 approximately 80% of deaf children in developed countries were implanted, many before the age of 1 year old (Brentari, 2010). In earlier days, if a child had better residual hearing in one ear, the ear with lower residual hearing would be implanted, so that the child could continue to use whatever residual hearing was available from the unimplanted ear (Brackmann et al., 2001). These days, however, CIs have become so overwhelmingly the standard of care that many children are binaurally implanted, which results in loss of whatever residual hearing benefits the unimplanted ear might offer (Snow & Wackym, 2008).

2.2 History of knowledge about first language acquisition

Multiple theories of language acquisition were in play in the decades before the 1990s. In 1967, Eric Lenneberg proposed that there was a language mechanism in the brain which allowed humans to acquire language naturally, without instruction, by being exposed to it. He further demonstrated that this mechanism changed over time, so that after a certain age the human brain no longer had this capacity (Lenneberg, 1967). The brain is hard-wired to acquire language, but the plasticity that allows this is lost early, around the age of five years old. This "critical-age" or "critical-period" hypothesis has since been exposed to a great deal of debate and testing. Discoveries of children who had grown up "wild", without being surrounded by human language (Shattuck, 1980), and discoveries of children who had been criminally abused to the point of being deprived of language (Curtiss, 1977), gave support to Lenneberg's hypothesis. Likewise, studies of deaf people who did not receive accessible language until after the critical period, either because they were denied hearing aids (Curtiss, 1994; Grimshaw et al., 1998) or because they were denied sign language (Mayberry & Eichen 1991; Newport, 1990), gave support to Lenneberg's hypothesis. Still, there were controversies over the biological nature of language.

However, with the advent of neuroimaging, there is even stronger evidence for a biological foundation for language (Pakaluk & Neville, 2010; and the references cited there). Initially, much of the work using neuroimaging was focused on language pathologies (Stemmer & Whitaker, 2008), but over time linguists, particularly those interested in the development of deaf children, have used it in studies of first language acquisition and of second language learning (Meisel, 2011; and the references cited there).

2.3 Summation of the problem

We now possess evidence for the following point, which we didn't know at the time that the Food and Drug Administration, a governmental agency in the United States, and similar governmental agencies in developed countries gave approval for the implantation of CIs in children: if a person does not acquire language before the age of five, that person is greatly at risk of not becoming fluent in any human language. Such a person is linguistically deprived.

In the abstract, this knowledge does not necessarily pose a dilemma with respect to CIs. In reality, however, some children who are implanted wind up linguistically deprived. CIs can actually lead to a harm that the Food and Drug Administration in the United States as well as governmental agencies in other countries were not aware existed at the time the devices were approved. Not only does new evidence challenge the basis of the FDA's approval, a recent commission established by the FDA concluded that existing procedures for implanted devices did not protect patients and recommended that these procedures be dropped (Institute of Medicine, 2011). Recent recalls of implant devices due to technical failures, such as the Sonova Holding AB's recall of its HiRes 90K device in 2010 and the Cochlear Ltd.'s recall of its Nucleus C1500 implants in 2011, raise the likelihood of repeat surgeries for implant recipients and cast further doubt on the wisdom of doing surgeries on infants and small children without a strong probability (not merely a possibility) of linguistic success (Lower, 2011). We will now establish our claim that CIs pose risk of harm to deaf infants and children.

3. Cochlear implants and linguistic deprivation

CIs lead to linguistic deprivation in some instances. This is due to two facts. First, CIs as a stand-alone technology do not provide accessible language. Second, health professionals typically either advise against or do not encourage giving a sign language to an implanted child, thus cutting them off from an accessible language during the years crucial to first language acquisition. There is not enough education in fields related to medicine about sign language and its role in language development. This leads to widespread misconceptions and misinformation, and thus, poor advice to parents and practitioners.

3.1 Variable success of cochlear implants

While many studies have tried to assess the success of CIs, it is difficult to know exactly what these studies mean in terms of what a family with a deaf newborn or newly deafened child can expect as they make decisions about language options. The first problem is that these studies report highly variable success (Bouchard et al., 2008; Fink et al., 2007; Peterson et al., 2010; Szagun, 2008), even in studies by enthusiastic promoters of CIs (such as Gulya et al., 2010). One would hope to be able to compare studies, to glean whatever reliable information they might offer to these families. However, many cannot be compared with each other because they use different methodologies and test for different auditory functions, some of which are only minimally related to language (Bouchard et al., 2008). Further, the children tested are a heterogeneous group with respect to the age of onset of hearing loss, the age of diagnosis of hearing loss, the age of implantation, the particular device implanted, the particular surgical technique used, the amount and type of rehabilitation after surgery, residual hearing in the unimplanted ear, socio-economic status of the family, and other factors, all of which will affect outcomes (Santarelli et al., 2008). This situation leaves families in a quandary as to what to do, and health professionals are unable to advise families effectively. Indeed, parents who are face for the first time with raising a child who is deaf are likely to report a higher level of stress and depressive symptomatology (Kushalnagar et al., 2007), although the stress level is ameliorated by perceived support from early intervention professionals or other parents who have deaf children (Hintermair, 2000; Lederberg & Goldbach, 2002; Meadow-Orlans, 1994).

In the next section, we make a strong recommendation about what families should do and about what health professionals should advise them. Here, we focus attention on one disturbing and sobering fact. While there is variability in the success rate and in standards for what constitutes success, there is agreement that some children receive no discernible auditory benefit from CIs. These children cannot distinguish speech sounds from environmental sounds, and they cannot distinguish between environmental sounds. The next group of children displaying more response to implants still do not gain linguistic benefit, but can distinguish among environmental sounds (such as distinguishing between a knock on a door and a fire alarm). The next group up gains only a minimal advantage in speech, such as being able to distinguish the number of syllables in a speech stream but not being able to distinguish words. We argue strenuously that this does not constitute linguistic benefit even if it involves speech units. The next group up can converse with family members and close friends, using speech-reading and context in addition to the auditory information that CIs provide. And the "stars," a term used often in the literature (e.g. David Pisoni), can converse with strangers, but they must use speech-reading and context in addition to auditory information. The numbers of children in each of these five groups is a point of controversy in the literature. A CI team (surgeon, psychologist, and rehabilitation therapist) from Alfred I. duPont Hospital for Children in Wilmington, Delaware, estimated that these groups were roughly equal in size (in a discussion at Swarthmore College in 2006). Multiple studies demonstrate that children implanted earlier, all other factors being equal, do better than children implanted later (O'Reilly et al., 2008, among many), hence the more recent practice of implanting children at twelve months or even earlier. But even children implanted early have a highly variable range of success. Additionally, initial gains in speech production and perception, as indicated through performance in hearing settings, are not maintained as children progress in school (Marschark et al., 2007). Websites of hospitals that perform CI surgery often report that they have "high success" rates, and websites that promote CI surgery often report that the "majority" of users are satisfied, but percentages are not given, and clear guidelines for what counts as success are elusive. Further, most of the evidence cited by these websites involve individuals who were implanted after the critical period. These websites do not give reliable statistics on children who rely on CIs for first language acquisition. The aspirations and expectations of deaf adults are quite different from those of a family who is considering implanting a small child and relying on the implant for first language acquisition.

As scientists who read CI literature and who are specialists in deaf matters, we suggest that a conservative estimate of the number of children who do not get enough linguistic input from CI usage to ensure acquisition of a first language is 20%, even assuming that the overall record has improved in recent years. We suspect the real percentage of lack of benefit is actually higher. In a study of more than 20,000 children implanted since 2000, 47% of them do not use their CIs (Watson & Gregory, 2005). Reported reasons for nonuse included lack of language satisfaction in addition to other reasons such as severe pain from the sounds and equipment, facial twitching, postsurgery scarring, and feelings of stigma. The human drive to communicate with others is so strong that if these children had actually found satisfaction in their linguistic abilities with the implants, we fully expect that most would not have stopped using them. There is a dearth of information about the experiences and language satisfactions of people with CIs (Valente, 2011), and those few people who do step forward to detail their experience (such as Snoddon, 2005) may find themselves the target of insult and ridicule for saying anything negative about CIs (Valente, 2011). The public's cultural belief in technology and its restorative powers make it difficult for many to risk telling their stories.

While an educated estimate of the true benefit of CIs is nothing more than that, we note two important facts. First, the burden should be on the promoters of CIs to provide reliable and understandable figures regarding success. In the absence of such information, we have stepped forward. Second, even if one argues that the failure rate is much lower, such as 5%, taking the risk that 5% of small children who are implanted will not get accessible language during the critical period and thus risk being linguistically deprived is unconscionable.

Many are unaware of this ethically problematic variability, or they dismiss it. Some people are optimistic about what CIs can do for the deaf child now; Stuart Blume gives a particularly telling account of his struggle to make language choices for his deaf son and the many positive things he was told about CIs being a "cure" for deafness, so much so that failure to implant a deaf child was considered a denial of best medical care by some (Blume, 2009). Others are optimistic that additional studies will clarify the rate of success of CIs (always in a context of consideration of multiple factors) so that families can make better informed decisions (indeed, an upcoming issue of the *International Journal of Otolaryngology* will be devoted to the "pearls and perils" of CIs). Still others suggest that the technology of CIs is improving so drastically that soon they will be so effective that the issue will become moot; on many websites we can read about CIs "curing" deafness, leading to a strong counter-response from members of the Deaf community fearing that such aspirations will lead to sign language becoming extinct and Deaf culture disappearing as CIs improve (a typical, if distorted, discussion is in Young, 2002).

Many present researchers, like us, take a more sober view of what technological improvements can accomplish. In describing advances up till now, Shannon et al. (2010: 369) write, "... technological advances may be nearing the point of diminishing returns, given the high costs involved and limited additional benefits they may provide. The next phase of improvement in CI performance may come not from further development of the implant hardware, but from understanding how implant speech processors may be more effectively programmed and customized for individual patients, so that the capabilities that are already available may be fully utilized."

This statement bears close reading, for it focuses our attention on an important fact: CIs are not computers. Computers sit on our desks and we instruct them what to do, and as technology improves, we can tell them more and more things to do. CIs are a different kind of technology. The implant device may add improvements but, unlike the processing power of a computer that we all consider beneficial, an improved implant device is unlikely to make substantial difference because the issue is getting the brain to interpret the input appropriately. Simply put, CIs do not hear. What they do is deliver electrical impulses directly to the cochlear nerve, bypassing the ordinary hearing channels of the ear. But the brain, which is hard-wired to receive auditory information that comes to us via the ear channels, is not hard-wired to interpret the electrical impulses that CIs deliver. That is why implanted people need "rehabilitation" (actually, training) following CI surgery. That rehabilitation goes on for years and years. In fact, long term users of CIs find that they must return to rehabilitation for a brush-up every so often. Kisor (1990: 166), who is what we call a "star" CI user, when describing what happens after his rehabilitative therapy, writes, "For more than a year, sometimes two, strangers will [come to] understand what I say the first time I say it at our first meeting, the benchmark by which I judge my speech." This benchmark should shatter ideas that functioning well in a hearing environment with a CI is easy. Many CI users cannot achieve the level of performance Kisor describes. Importantly, many hearing aid users (and non hearing aid users, for that matter) can surpass it, using an older technology.

The brain is complex, and hearing is complex. There is no reason to expect a quick and huge rise in success of CIs from an advance in technology. In any case, we must deal with the technology we presently have.

3.2 Strictly aural input

Many health care professionals advise against offering an implanted child a sign language (Krausneker, 2008; Lane, 2005; Lane & Grodin, 1997; Zimmerman, 2009) and instead urge therapies using aural input only, such as verbal-auditory therapy (AVT, as in Estabrooks, 2006 and earlier, evaluated in Rhoades, 2006). Sign language is turned to as a last resort when all else fails (Johnston, 2006). This view possibly derives from aural-oral only proponents' belief that with cochlear implants the aural-oral approach is much more effective then ever before and that sign language is not a place to expend valuable time and energy for the child, parents, or therapists. This may also be due to the fear that sign language use will interfere with oral language skills and/or that sign language is not perceived as a bona fide language so it cannot give the child the rich cognitive input necessary for language development.

The problem with this is that it still relies on a hope that the aural-oral environment and the CI technology will provide the language development that is crucial to the child's whole future. It does not consider the risk that the CI will not enhance an already risky approach.

The fears about sign language are unfounded. Deaf children who sign gain advanced language skills which they can then apply toward understanding spoken and written language (Dockrell & Messer, 1999), which may be why, among deaf children, a factor that correlates most reliably with good literacy skills is good signing abilities (Chamberlain & Mayberry, 2008; Fischer, 1998; Hoffmeister, 2000; McGuinness, 2005; Strong & Prinz, 2000; Wilbur, 2008; among many). Further, deaf children who sign identify themselves as being more confident and happy than deaf children who do not sign (Plaza Pust & Morales López, 2008; among many). In a recent quality of life study of 231 youths with mild to profound hearing loss, youths who used speech only as their preferred mode of communication were significantly more likely to report greater stigma associated to their hearing loss than youths who used a combination of speech and sign language (Kushalnagar et al., 2011). A similar conclusion was reported in a qualitative study of Australian children and adolescents with CIs (Punch & Hyde, 2011). Repeatedly, we find in the literature that when deaf people raised orally learn to sign as adults, they report unprecedented feelings of strong self esteem and an end to the psychological distress of having to constantly struggle at communication (Gao, 2007; Holte & Dinis, 2001; Restuccia, 2010). This suggests that the inclusion of sign language ability in deaf children's lives is beneficial and important for healthy development and overall well-being.

With respect to the second fear, sign languages have been found definitively to be natural human languages with all the complexity (including phonology, morphology, syntax, semantics, pragmatics and discourse considerations) and expressive potential as spoken languages (see a multitude of articles in many books (such as Brentari, 2010; Mathur & Napoli, 2010) and linguistics journals, including *Sign Language & Linguistics* and *Sign Language Studies*, particularly many on language acquisition (such as Chamberlain et al., 2000; Meier & Newport, 1990; Morgan & Woll, 2002; Petitto & Marentette, 1991), language processing (such as Emmorey, 2001), neurolinguistics (such as Neville, 1995; Poizner et al., 1987), second language learning (such as Newport, 1990), and sign literature (such as Sutton-Spence & Napoli, 2009)). The small child who, upon being diagnosed with a hearing loss, is exposed to a sign language with frequency and regularity, where good models of the language interact with the child, will acquire that language with full competency in all the language areas that hearing children have competency in - simply in a different modality (Schick et al., 2006).

In sum, there is no justification for advising children with CIs not to learn a sign language.

3.3 Harm done by cochlear implants

Any surgery involves risks, and CI surgery is no exception, where complications include infection, necrosis, injury during surgery to the facial nerve, post-surgical complications such as vertigo, meningitis, cerebrospinal fluid leakage, perilymph fluid leak, and tinnitus (Cohen & Roland, 2006; FDA, 2011; Steenerson et al., 2001; Walker, 2008). Further, residual hearing in the implanted ear is lost with many apparati, a significant harm since hearing loss is rarely total (Mogford, 1993), although new hybrid CIs stimulate only the basal end of the cochlea where the high frequency hearing has deteriorated, preserving the residual low-frequency hearing (Turner et al., 2007). Additionally, when the apparatus fails, a new surgery with repeated risks is called for (Borkowski et al., 2002). These risks are discussed elsewhere and we will not go into them further here since they are outside our focus.

Our focus is on language and cognitive development, an area where CI failure occurs in a significant percentage of children. Regardless of the exact percentage, every study we know of identifies failures and since this kind of failure is so destructive of the overall wellbeing of the child, this is ethically unacceptable. The advice of many health professionals to keep deaf children away from sign language compounds the problem. Since children are being implanted earlier and earlier, and more are receiving binaural implants (Snow & Wackym, 2008; Tyler et al., 2010), those who are not learning sign language often receive far too little linguistic input during the critical years of first language acquisition. We cannot put deaf children at risk of linguistic deprivation or even language delay. Furthermore, linguistic deprivation causes other disorders, since various cognitive functions depend upon first language acquisition, including the organization of memory (Ronnberg, 2010) and the manipulation of symbols (MacSweeney, 1998). Related are psychological harms; even the child who manages minimally well with a CI can experience psychosocial problems, e.g. identity issues, in the absence of sign language knowledge (Ramsey, 2000, among many).

CIs are an experiment with human subjects that is not protecting those subjects from a foreseeable and irreversible harm. This harm has the potential to isolate them in a drastic way from other people. Ethicists have presented the moral imperative to protect a child's right to an "open future" and to protect a child's "potential autonomy" when arguing Deaf parents should not have the right to genetically screen to ensure the birth of a deaf child; just so, these same arguments apply exactly here: deliberately putting a child in a position where she may have only limited options counts as a moral harm (Davis, 1997; Feinberg, 2007). Implantation should not continue until there is agreement about pairing implants with sign language in young children, and about the appropriate age for implantation beyond which it poses no risk of harm to language acquisition or cognitive development.

4. The remedy: Sign language

CIs have allowed many to function better (and sometimes very well) in a hearing environment, and being able to function in a hearing environment expands a deaf person's professional and personal opportunities. While we recognize this as an important part of the deaf person's life, the priority should be to ensure that the deaf child meets typical language and cognitive development milestones, as we have discussed. This is a medical concern. Without first language acquisition, children are at risk for language delay and associated cognitive difficulties, both having negative impact on psycho-social health.

Because of the initial failure to recognize the existence of the biological linguistic mechanism and the import of the critical period to language acquisition, the CI experiment began and gained momentum, so that it has been allowed to proceed without heed of some of the ethical principles for medical research involving human subjects. The technology developed faster than our understanding of first language acquisition. The result is that the linguistic rights and the cognitive health of deaf children have not been protected. Many implanted children fail to achieve fluency in receptive and expressive spoken language, and by the time lack of competence is recognized in the child, the child is past the critical period. Thus justice in human subjects research has not been ensured.

We offer an immediate remedy. Language is a human right. In order to protect that biological, cognitive, and psycho-social right, every deaf child should be raised with language that is completely accessible. Sign language is accessible to any deaf child (tactilely to the child who is both deaf and blind). This remedy does not exclude oral/aural training, however. Children with hearing aids and/or CI who do well at voicing and processing information received aurally will then be bilingual - a positive outcome. Children with hearing aids and/or CI who do not do well at voicing and processing information received aurally will nevertheless be assured of language acquisition, which is a prerequisite to many other cognitive activities like reading and which will assure them the right to participate in human activities that go forward largely via language, including self-expression, making friends, and fruitful employment. Given the present failure of CI to ensure fluency in a spoken language, providing access to sign language is a conservative approach that protects the right to language and is thus the morally just approach.

Raising a deaf child with a sign language when the parents are hearing calls for much proactive behavior on the part of the family, and we urge health professionals to advise in appropriate ways (which are discussed in Kushalnagar et al., 2010b, but which we outline in the next two sections). It is the responsibility of health professionals to do this because health professionals are the ones who families most often turn to first, given that they are the ones who usually deliver the diagnosis of hearing loss. And it is the responsibility of health professionals to do this particularly well and with utter thoroughness, since families receiving the information that their newborn or young child is deaf are in a vulnerable state, often of grief (Kurtzer-White & Luterman, 2003). Their lack of information about and familiarity with deafness can mean they initially suffer, and in this way, they have much in common with people experiencing illness. Hall & Schneider (2008) point out that sick people are more vulnerable for a variety of reasons beyond the fact that they are in pain, including the facts that they feel disabled and defeated by the illness; they are exhausted due to dealing with the illness; their control over their bodies (or, in the case of parents, over their child's body) is eroded; they are baffled by the condition and wonder about its origin, its trajectory, the uncertainty of everything; they are terrified of what they do not understand; they are isolated from others because they are suddenly different. Add it all up and the power of health professionals dealing with these families is huge; hence, their responsibility to give accurate and appropriate information and advice is likewise huge. True, the law gives families the right to make decisions about whether, when, and how to manage the physical and social needs of their child in most instances, and this applies to the language needs of deaf children (Ouelette, 2011), but the families rely heavily on consultation with their health professionals.

4.1 The ideal situation

In the ideal situation deaf children will be raised with sign language, regardless of their speech-producing and speech-processing skills, so that they will be bilingual in the bimodal sense (i.e. in both a sign language and a written language). All will have fluency and high literacy in both a sign language and a written language, and those who gain good speech skills will be bilingual and highly literate in both a sign language and a spoken/written language. Bilingualism is an added enormous benefit, since it has many cognitive advantages for everyone, including deaf people (Kushalnagar et al., 2010a). In developed countries (and in many underdeveloped countries), we have embraced the idea that our children should know more than one language. More and more elementary schools offer a second language, most middle schools do, and both high schools and colleges have foreign language requirements. Further, it has become popular in many countries to teach hearing babies some sign language, to further their expressive abilities. Given all this, it is difficult to understand how anyone could advise against offering deaf children sign language.

Health professionals can help to achieve this ideal situation by properly advising the families of deaf children about the biological nature of first language acquisition and by urging them to consult with experts in deaf matters (NAD, 2000). There are several recommendations they should make. First, the family of the deaf child needs to learn sign language; a deaf child whose hearing parents and siblings, particularly hearing mothers, sign with them demonstrate language expressiveness and theory of mind on a par with hearing children of the same age. (Schick et al. 2007; Spencer, 1993). But family is not enough. The deaf child needs to be brought into contact with a community of deaf signers so as to be exposed to good models of signing on a regular and frequent basis. The family should be in contact with signing community support groups in order to stay informed and be active in deaf issues and events: deaf advocacy groups, local deaf and hard of hearing community centers, and local and/or state deaf services bureaus. The family must advocate for their child's needs at school, including asking for an interpreter when necessary and whatever special aids or considerations are appropriate with respect to the instruction being given. And most of all, the family needs to affiliate and be active with parents of deaf children support groups, playgroups, and otherwise form friendships and provide visitation for themselves and their deaf child with other deaf parents and children. All of these activities have been reported to contribute to positive quality of life for deaf children.

Parents need to involve themselves in ways that help them develop clearer understanding of their deaf child. One of the greatest dangers to the emotional development of a young deaf child occurs when the parents (or one of them) do not understand the child's situation properly or project fear, concern, or other kinds of emotional distress into their relationship with the child or even into the larger environment of their child (Leigh, 2009; Marschark, 1997, 2009). Parents should be alerted to and helped to avoid the negativity of the "hearing impaired" discourse so rife among medical professionals and special educators. They should be encouraged to develop strong relationships with deaf people themselves as soon as possible and to get involved with the rich social and cultural lives of this community.

The advent of a deaf child into a family is a gateway to a new language and a rich culture. Families need to become informed, and there are good works out there to help, like Bauman (2008); Bauman & Murray (2009); Lane et al. (1996); Marschark (2009); Marschark et al. (2010a, 2010b); and Padden & Humphries (2005), all of which give substantial references.

4.2 The less than ideal situation

While what we have described in the last section is the ideal situation that a family should strive for, practical factors may inhibit achieving such a situation. In particular, the family of a deaf child may not have easy access to a signing community or perhaps even to an isolated signer. Rural families, in particular, may feel betrayed by advice to learn sign language. A family in this situation has little choice but to become more active in their child's proper development. There are a number of strategies that the family can adopt to maximize the potential for the child to acquire a first language, and there are websites to help (Enabling Education Network, n.d.).

First, the family must try to learn a sign language in the best way possible. It may require some driving time, but sign language classes are increasingly more popular and widespread. There are literally thousands of schools, colleges, or community centers offering courses today in many developed countries. And if the local community is small, the family can enlist the whole community in the effort to learn a sign language and to communicate with the deaf child in that sign language. Spiritual leaders (ministers, rabbis, etc.) can play a guiding role here, helping the community to understand both what it has to offer the deaf child and what the deaf child has to offer the community (Blankmeyer-Burke et al., 2011). A community might want to advertise for and hire a sign language teacher to come stay in their community for a prolonged period of time, teaching everyone who is willing to learn. There are also multiple online sites and DVDs to help someone learn a sign language (see the website of DawnSignPress in the United States or ForestBooks in the United Kingdom, for example).

Second, the family should find out about camps for deaf children, where their child can play with other deaf children and interact with adults who use a sign language as their most comfortable language (or among their most comfortable languages) and identify themselves as Deaf (that is, part of Deaf culture) or as very knowledgeable of Deaf culture (in the USA: Laurent Clerc National Deaf Education Center, n.d.). Many such camps exist: in the United States they are scattered across the states; in Germany the German Deaf Youth Association annually organizes camps for Deaf children and Deaf Youth. Some have scholarships available. Some are for the entire family (in the USA: Raising Deaf Kids, n.d.; in Canada: Deaf Children's Society of BC, n.d.; in Germany: Bundeselternverband gehörloser Kinder e.V., n.d.).

Third, the family must be resourceful. The family could start a sign language class with parents and children who are not deaf. Many hearing families are now encouraged about their hearing children learning to sign and communicating with them. If a parent can manage to learn enough sign language to get ahead of the others in the class, that parent can lead the class, along with the deaf child. Having others sign to the deaf child is important. If the family has relatives in a city with a thriving Deaf community arranging to spend time there, as hard as it may be on the family, may be the sacrifice that makes the world of difference to the child's development. The family might want to get online (using current video technology: Skype, iChat, gChat, ooVoo, etc.) with someone who knows many people in the Deaf community (perhaps a professor at a Deaf Studies program at some university or someone who works in a Deaf and Hearing Community Center in some urban area) and see if a Deaf family might like to come visit them for an extended period. The deaf child in one's home makes the home eligible to obtain a videophone setup from a video relay service or from welfare agencies. With this setup, the family can call directly via video to deaf people who they meet and form a stronger relationship. Sign language tutoring via VP (videophone) might even be arranged. Just social chatting via video with deaf people, other parents, advisors, etc. can help greatly. When the deaf child is old enough, he/she can use the videophone as well. This is a normal aspect of life among deaf people now and needs to be the same for the deaf child in any home as well as for the parents of that child.

If the family has opportunities to live in an urban area which has a Deaf community, now might be the time to realize those opportunities. While this may feel drastic, it was not too long ago that families with deaf children often moved to where there were schools for the deaf, so that their children could receive an education (Sacks, 1989).

4.3 The close-to-untenable situation

Another serious impediment to the ideal situation is posed by socioeconomic factors which are often unalterable. A family may not have the educational background to take on such proactive behavior or may not have the financial resources to do so; the family may not have the education or technological literacy needed to access and use the information available on sign language, and online access and webcam may not be available. Further, a family's home language may complicate the situation in ways that make the suggestions above infeasible (such as a Hmong family in Minnesota). Likewise, limited educational achievement may limit a family's ability to overcome cultural biases and learn another language, particularly one in a different modality. These are huge challenges, but if health professionals take a strong guiding role, they may not be insurmountable. People in these situations are already marginalized. If we allow the infeasibility of providing access to a sign language to stop us from making efforts in these situations, those children who do not find accessible language via an implant will be marginalized much further. The efforts might have to be extraordinary, but the damage risked by not making these efforts is also extraordinary.

4.4 The role of health professionals in achieving the ideal situation

A recent study by the United States Government Accountability Office (2011) concludes that parents of deaf children are ill-advised when it comes to matters of language and educational options. Families need to understand the crucial importance of first language acquisition for their children so that they can, in fact, be as resourceful as possible. And health professionals must help them understand. Both health professionals and families need to be very careful not to give in to low expectations as far as language and cognitive development are concerned. Deaf people, both as individuals, and as a social group, have been severely damaged by a history of expecting language delay and cognitive delay (Gregory, 1995; Gregory et al., 1995). This ideology of low expectation is unacceptable. There is no reason for it. With a signing environment and rich social world for the child, delayed development will not happen. Without sign language, there is a significant risk that it will. Equally important, however, is the fact that rosy scenarios of hopefulness from health professionals who ignore clear indications of language and cognitive development delay are not acceptable either. Parents need to know, via appropriate and whole-child assessment, if their child is developing well. Assessment focused exclusively on speech and auditory development, for example, is inadequate to measure overall language and cognitive development and cannot be equated with it.

5. The future

Presently many deaf implanted children do not feel at ease communicating in a hearing environment, and many do not succeed at it to the point where they can converse comfortably with strangers or even in a group of same-age peers. Further, a significant number simply do not thrive linguistically in a strictly aural/oral environment. We cannot look exclusively at the successful implanted children, who typically have a family that is economically and educationally able to provide them support in their rehabilitation and who have reliable ongoing rehabilitation. Many children are not in that situation, and even some who are in that situation do not experience success with respect to solid first language acquisition. We also cannot count on improvements in CI technology to ameliorate the social situation, language delay or the cognitive risk. What we need right now is studies of the most successful CI users. We need to understand what makes them stars that go beyond basic speech recognition and production. We must find out whether matters that we can easily control are most pertinent, such as surgical technique (Meshik et al., 2010). In the same vein, we must determine whether some methods of "rehabilitation" yield much better results than others. Then we must figure out whether some other factors are the keys. It is imperative to find out whether there are, in fact, predictable correlates to success and, if feasible, strive to ensure those correlates for all implanted children.

We need also to devise new protocols for young children with implants and evaluate them. For example, a protocol that calls for the parents and child to begin using a sign language from birth or as soon as possible after hearing-loss is detected, and well before the surgery, and continuing to use that sign language after the surgery, is supported by the research we have now. Such a protocol or other similar protocols is critically important for all implanted children, and it is the most conservative approach to protect the right to language for those children who receive little to no language input from the implant. We need a protocol that includes robust and frequent authentic assessments of the child's development (authentic in that it assesses language (not simply speech), communication, and literacy development) and monitors this development through a running record over time.

6. Conclusion

In order to ensure the typical cognitive development milestones, and hence the psycho-social health, of deaf children, we must make sure they acquire a first language. Since a sign language is the only type of language guaranteed to be accessible to deaf children, we must make sure they acquire a sign language. With a sign language, a deaf child who is implanted has the best chance at being cognitively healthy and of becoming bimodally-bilingual. It is well-recognized that bilingualism is positive for all people, children included. Around the world, educational systems require study of a second language before a child can graduate at the secondary level. Bilingualism can only be beneficial to the deaf child, as well. The acquisition of sign language provides a medical safety net for all deaf children. We simply cannot wait to see who does not thrive with an implant before offering sign language; for the child who does not thrive, the best result of such waiting is language delay, itself quite problematic, and the worst result is linguistic deprivation, a calamity.

It is the responsibility and obligation of health professionals to guide families of deaf newborns and newly deafened children toward choosing to raise their child with a sign language. If that is done, the harm that we presently see in some implanted deaf children who are raised without sign language experience will become a regret of the past.

7. References

Barnes, J. (1994). *Pediatric Cochlear Implants: An Overview of the Alternatives in Education and Rehabilitation,* Alexander Graham Bell Association for the Deaf, ISBN 978-0882002040, Washington, DC

Bauman, H-D. (Ed.). (2008). *Open Your Eyes: Deaf Studies Talking,* University of Minnesota Press, ISBN 978-0816646180, Minneapolis, MN

Bauman, H-D. & Murray, J. (2009). Reframing: From Hearing Loss to Deaf-gain. *Deaf Studies Digital Journal,* Vol.1, No.1. Retrieved from: http://dsdj.gallaudet.edu/

Bilger, R. (1977). Evaluation of Subjects Presently Fitted with Implanted Auditory Prostheses. *Annals of Otology, Rhinology, and Larygology,* Vol. 86, pp. 1-176

Blankmeyer-Burke, T.; Kushalnagar, P.; Mathur, G.; Napoli, D-J.; Rathmann, C. & VanGilder, K. (2011). The Language Needs of Deaf and Hard-of-hearing Infants and Children: Information for Spiritual Leaders and Communities. *Journal of Religion, Disability and Health,* Vol.15, pp. 272-295, ISSN 1522-8967

Blume, S. (2009). *The Artificial Ear: Cochlear Implants and The Culture of Deafness,* Rutgers University Press, ISBN 978-0813546605, Camden, NJ

Bouchard, M-E.; Ouellet, C. & Cohen, H. (2008). Speech Development in Prelingually Deaf Children with Cochlear Implants. *Language and Linguistics Compass,* Vol.2, pp. 1-18

Borkowski, G.; Hildmann, H. & Stark (2002). Surgical Aspects of Cochlear Implantation in Young and Very Young Children, In: *Cochlear Implants: An Update,* T. Kubo; Y. Takahashi; & T. Iwaki, pp. 223-226, Kugler Publications, ISBN 978-9062991914, The Hague, The Netherlands

Brackmann, D.; Shelton, C. & Arriaga, M. (2001). *Otologic Surgery,* (2nd edition), Saunders, ISBN 978-0721689760, Philadelphia, PA

Brentari, D. (Ed.). (2010). *Sign Languages,* Cambridge University Press, ISBN 978-0521883702, Cambridge, UK

Bundeselternverband gehörloser Kinder e.V. (n.d.). 18.07.11, Available from http://www.gehoerlosekinder.de/

Chamberlain, C. & Mayberry, R. (2008). American Sign Language Syntactic and Narrative Comprehension in Skilled and Less Skilled Readers: Bilingual and Bimodal Evidence for the Linguistic Basis of Reading. *Applied Psycholinguistics,* Vol.29, No.3, pp. 367-388, ISSN: 0142-7164

Chamberlain, C.; Morford, J. & Mayberry, R. (Eds.). (2000). *Language Acquisition by Eye,* Lawrence Erlbaum Associates, ISBN 978-0805829372, Mahwah, NJ

Christensen, J. & Leigh, I. (2002). *Cochlear Implants in Children: Ethics and Choices,* Gallaudet University Press, ISBN 978-1563681165, Washington, DC

Cohen , N. & Roland, J. (2006). Complications of Cochlear Implant Surgery, In: *Cochlear Implants,* (2nd edition), S. Waltzman & T. Roland, (Eds.), pp. 205-213, Thieme Medical Publishers, ISBN 978-1588904133, New York, NY

Curtiss, S. (1977). *Genie: A Psycholinguistic Study of a Modern-day "Wild Child",* Academic Press, ISBN 978-0121963507, New York, NY

Curtiss, S. (1994). Language as a Cognitive System: Its Independence and Selective Vulnerability, In: *Noam Chomsky: Critical Assessments: 4*, C. Otero, (Ed.), pp. 211-255, Routledge, ISBN 978-0415010054, London, UK

Davis, D. (1997). Cochlear Implants and the Claims of Culture? A Response to Lane and Grodin. *Kennedy Institute of Ethics Journal*, Vol.7, No.3, pp. 253-258, ISSN 1054-6863

Deaf Children's Society of BC. (n.d.). Learning Vacation Experience, 18.07.11, Available from http://www.deafchildren.bc.ca/about-us/history

Djourno, A.; Eyries, C. & Vallancien, B. (1957). De L'excitation Electrique du Nerf Cochleaire Chez L'homme, Par Induction a Distance, a L'aide D'un Micro-bobinage Inclus à Memeure. *La Presse Médicale*, Vol.65, No.63, pp. 31 (cited in Eisen, 2000)

Dockrell, J., & Messer, D. (1999). *Children's Language and Communication Difficulties: Understanding, Identification, and Intervention*, Cassell, ISBN 978-0304336579, New York, NY

Emmorey, K. (2001). *Language, Cognition and the Brain: Insights from Sign Language Research*, Lawrence Erlbaum Associates, ISBN 978-0805833980, Mahwah, NJ

Eisen, M. (2000). The History of Cochlear Implants, In: *Cochlear Implants: Principles and Practices*, J. Niparko, (Ed.), pp. 89-93, Lippincott Williams & Wilkins, ISBN 978-0781717823, Philadelphia, PA

Enabling Education Network. (n.d.). Services for Deaf People in a Rural Setting: Issues and Recommendations for Sign Language, 18.07.11, Available from http://www.eenet.org.uk/resources/docs/signlang.php

Estabrooks, W. (2006). Auditory-verbal Therapy and Practice, Alexander Graham Bell Association for the Deaf, ISBN 978-0882002231, Washington, DC

Federal Drug Administration. (2011). Benefits and Risks of Cochlear Implants, 18.07.11, Available from http://www.fda.gov/MedicalDevices/ProductsandMedicalProcedures/ImplantsandProsthetics/CochlearImplants/ucm062843.htm

Feinberg, J. (2007). The Child's Right to an Open Future, In: *Philosophy of Education: An Anthology*, R. Curren, (Ed.), pp. 112-123, Wiley-Blackwell, ISBN 978-1405130226, Malden, MA

Fink, N.; Wang, N-Y.; Visaya, J.; Niparko, J.; Quittner, A. & Eisenberg, L. (2007). Childhood Development after Cochlear Implantation Study: Design and Baseline Characteristics. *Cochlear Implants International*, Vol.8, No.2, pp. 92-116, ISSN 1467-0100

Fischer, S. (1998). Critical Periods for Language Acquisition: Consequences for Deaf Education, In: *Issues Unresolved: New Perspectives on Language and Deaf Education*, A. Weisel, (Ed.), pp. 9-26, Gallaudet University Press, ISBN 978-1563680670, Washington, DC

Gao, T. (2007). A Neglected Culture: How Cochlear Implants Affect Deaf Children's Self-Esteem, In: DIAGLOGUES@RU, 18.07.11, Available from http://dialogues.rutgers.edu/vol_06/essays/documents/gao.pdf

Gregory, S. (1995). *Deaf Children and Their Families*, Cambridge University Press, ISBN 978-0521438476, Cambridge, UK

Gregory, S.; Bishop, J. & Sheldon, L. (1995). *Deaf Young People and Their Families*, Cambridge University Press, ISBN 978-0521429986, Cambridge, UK

Grimshaw, G.; Adelstein, A.; Bryden, M. & MacKinnon, G. (1998). First-language Acquisition in Adolescence: Evidence for a Critical Period for Verbal Language Development. *Brain and Language*, Vol.63, No.2, pp. 237-255, ISSN 0093-934X

Gulya, A.; Minor, L. & Poe, D. (2010). *Glasscock-Shambaugh's Surgery of the Ear*, (6th edition), People's Medical Publishing House USA, ISBN 978-1607950264, Shelton, CT

Hall, M. & Schneider, C. (2008). Patients as Consumers: Courts, Contracts, and the New Medical Marketplace. *Michigan Law Review*, Vol.106, pp. 643-689

Hintermair, M. (2000). Hearing Impairment, Social Networks, and Coping: The Need for Families with Hearing-Impaired Children to Relate to Other Parents and to Hearing-Impaired Adults. *American Annals of the Deaf,* Vol.*145*, pp. 41–53, ISSN 0002-726X

Hoffmeister, R. (2000). A Piece of the Puzzle: The Relationship between ASL and English Literacy in Deaf Children, In: *Language Acquisition by Eye,* C. Chamberlain; J. Morford, & R. Mayberry, (Eds.), pp. 143-163, Lawrence Erlbaum Associates, ISBN 978-0805829372, Mahwah, NJ

Holte, M. & Dinis, M. (2001). Self-esteem Enhancement in Deaf and Hearing Women: Success Stories. *American Annals of the Deaf,* Vol.146, No.4, pp. 348-354, ISSN 0002-726X

House, W. (1991). Cochlear Implants and Children. The Western Journal of Medicine, Vol.154, No.6, pp. 717-718

Institute of Medicine. (2011). *Medical Devices and the Public's Health: The FDA 510(k) Clearance Process at 35 years,* National Academies Press, ISBN 978-0309212427, Washington, DC

Johnston, T. (2006). Response to Comments. *Sign Language Studies,* Vol.6, No.2, pp. 225-243, ISSN 0302-1475

Kisor, H. (1990). *What's That Pig Outdoors?: A Memoir of Deafness,* Hill and Wang, ISBN 978-0809096893, New York, NY

Krausneker, V. (2008). The Protection and Promotion of Sign Languages and the Rights of Their Users in Council of Europe Member States: Needs Analysis, In: *Council of Europe – Partial Agreement in the Social and Public Health Field,* 15.07, 11, Available from http://www.coe.int/t/DG3/Disability/Source/Report_Sign_languages_final.pdf

Kurtzer-White, E. & Luterman, D. (2003). Families and Children with Hearing Loss: Grief and Coping. *Mental Retardation and Developmental Disabilities Research Reviews,* Vol.9, No.4, pp. 232-235, ISSN 1940-5529

Kushalnagar, P.; Krull, K.; Hannay, H.; Mehta, P.; Caudle, S. & Oghalai, J. (2007). Intelligence, Parental Depression and Behavior Adaptability in Deaf Children Being Considered for Cochlear Implantation. *Journal of Deaf Studies and Deaf Education,* Vol.12, No.3, pp. 335-349, ISSN 1081-4159

Kushalnagar, P.; Hannay, H. & Hernandez, A. (2010a). Bilingualism and Attention: A Study of Balanced and Unbalanced Bilingual Deaf Users of American Sign Language and English. *Journal of Deaf Studies and Deaf Education,* Vol.15, No.3, pp. 263–273, ISSN 1081-4159

Kushalnagar, P.; Mathur, G.; Moreland, C.; Napoli, D-J.; Osterling, W.; Padden, C. & Rathmann, C. (2010b). Infants and Children with Hearing Loss Need Early Language Access. *Journal of Clinical Ethics,* Vol.21, No.2, pp. 143-154, ISSN 1046-7890

Kushalnagar, P.; Topolski, T.; Schick, B.; Edwards, T.; Skalicky, A. & Patrick, D. (2011). Mode of Communication, Perceived Level of Understanding, and Perceived Quality of Life in Youth Who are Deaf or Hard of Hearing. *Journal of Deaf Studies and Deaf Education,* Vol.16, No.4, pp. 512-523, ISSN 1081-4159

Lane, H. (2005). Ethnicity, ethics, and the Deaf-World. *Journal of Deaf Studies and Deaf Education*, Vol.10, No.3, pp. 291–310, ISSN 1081-4159

Lane, H. & Grodin, M. (1997). Ethical Issues in Cochlear Implant Surgery: An Exploration into Disease, Disability, and the Best Interests of the Child. *Kennedy Institute of Ethics Journal*, Vol.7, No.3, pp. 231-251, ISSN 1054-6863

Lane, H.; Hoffmeister, R. & Bahan, B. (1996). *A Journey into the Deaf-World*, Dawn Sign Press, ISBN 978-0915035632, San Diego, CA

Laurent Clerc National Deaf Education Center. (n.d.) Summer Camps for Deaf and Hard of Hearing Children and Teens, 18.07.11, Available from http://www.gallaudet.edu/x17375.xml

Lederberg, A. & Goldbach, T. (2002). Parental Stress and Social Support in Hearing Parents: Pragmatic and Dialogic Characteristics. *Journal of Deaf Studies and Deaf Education*, Vol.7, No.4, pp. 330-345, ISSN 1081-4159

Leigh, I. W. (2009). *A Lens on Deaf Identities*, Oxford University Press, ISBN 978-0195320664, Oxford, UK

Lenneberg, E. (1967). *Biological Foundations of Language*, John Wiley & Sons, ISBN 978-0471526261, New York, NY

Lower, Gavin. (2011). Cochlear Recalls Implants: Top manufacturer's action affects latest range of devices after rise in failures. *The Wall Street Journal*, Corporate News Section B 5, Tuesday, September 13, 2011.

MacSweeney, M. (1998). Cognition and Deafness, In: *Issues in Deaf Education*, S. Gregory, P. Knight, W. MacCracken, S. Powers & L. Watson, (Eds.), pp. 20-27, David Fulton Publishers, ISBN 978-1853465123, London, UK

Marschark, M. (1997). *Psychological Development of Deaf Children*, Oxford University Press, ISBN 978-0195115758, Oxford, UK

Marschark, M. (2009). *Raising and Educating a Deaf Child: A Comprehensive Guide to the Choices, Controversies, and Decisions Faced by Parents and Educators*, Oxford University Press, ISBN 978-0195376159, Oxford, UK

Marschark, M.; Rhoten, C. & Fabich, M. (2007). Effects of Cochlear Implants on Children's Reading and Academic Achievement. *Journal of Deaf Studies and Deaf Education*, Vol.12, No.3, pp. 269-282, ISSN 1081-4159

Marschark, M. & Spencer, P. (Eds.) (2010a). *The Oxford Handbook of Deaf Studies, Language, and Education, Vol.1*, (2nd edition), Oxford University Press, ISBN 978-0199750986, Oxford, UK

Marschark, M. & Spencer, P. (Eds.) (2010b). *The Oxford Handbook of Deaf Studies, Language, and Education, Vol.2*, Oxford University Press, ISBN 978-0195390032, Oxford, UK

Mathur, G. & Napoli, D-J. (Eds.). (2010). *Deaf Around the World: The Impact of Language*, Oxford University Press, ISBN 978-0199732531, Oxford, UK

Mayberry, R. & Eichen, E. (1991). The Long-lasting Advantage of Learning Sign Language in Childhood: Another Look at the Critical Period for Language Acquisition. *Journal of Memory and Language*, Vol.30, No.4, pp. 486-512, 0749-596X

McGuinness, D. (2005). *Language Development and Learning to Read: The Scientific Study of How Language Development Affects Reading Skill*, MIT Press, ISBN 978-0262633406, Cambridge, MA

Meadow-Orlans, K. (1994). Stress, Social Support, and Deafness: Perceptions of Infants' Mothers and Fathers. *Journal of Early Intervention*, Vol.18, No.1, pp. 91–102, ISSN 1053-8151

Meier, R. & Newport, E. (1990). Out of the Hands of Babes: On a Possible Sign Advantage. *Language*, Vol.66, No.1, pp. 1-23

Meisel, J. (2011). *First and Second Language Acquisition: Parallels and Differences*, Cambridge University Press, ISBN 978-0521557641, Cambridge, UK

Meshik, X.; Holden, T.; Chole, R. & Hullar, T. (2010). Optimal Cochlear Implant Insertion Vectors. *Otology and Neurotology*, Vol.31, No.1, pp. 58-63, ISSN 1531-7129

Mogford, K. (1993). Oral Language Acquisition in the Prelingually Deaf, In: *Language Development in Exceptional Circumstances*, D. Bishop & K. Mogford, (Eds.), pp. 110-131, Lawrence Erlbaum Associates, ISBN 978-0863773082, Hillsdale, NJ

Morgan, G. & Woll, B. (Eds.). (2002). *Directions in Sign Language Acquisition*, John Benjamins, ISBN 978-1588112354, Amsterdam, The Netherlands

National Association of the Deaf. (2000). NAD Position Statement on Cochlear Implants, 18.07.11, Available from http://www.nad.org/issues/technology/assistive listening/cochlear-implants

Neville, H. (1995). Developmental Specificity in Neurocognitive Development in Humans, In: *The Cognitive Neurosciences*, M. Gazzaniga, (Ed.), pp. 219-231, MIT Press, ISBN 978-0262071574, Cambridge, MA

Newport, E. (1990). Maturational Constraints on Language Learning. *Cognitive Science*, Vol. 14, No.1, pp. 11-28

O'Reilly, R.; Mangiardi, A. & Bunnell, T. (2008). Cochlear Implants, In: *Access: Multiple Avenues for Deaf People*, D. DeLuca, I. Leigh, K. Lindgren, & D-J. Napoli, (Eds.), pp. 38-74, Gallaudet University Press, ISBN 978-1563683930, Washington, DC

Ouellette, A. (2011). Hearing the Deaf: Cochlear Implants, the Deaf Community, and Bioethical Analysis. *Valparaiso University Law Review*, Vol.45, No.3, pp. 1247-1270

Padden, C. & Humphries, T. (2005). Inside Deaf Culture, Harvard University Press, ISBN 978-0674015067, Cambridge, MA

Pakaluk, E. & Neville, H. (2010). Biological Bases of Language Development. In: *Encyclopedia of Early Childhood Development*, R. Tremblay, R. Peters, M. Boivin & R. Barr, (Eds.), pp. 1-7, Center of Excellence for Early Child Development, Retrieved from http://www.child-encyclopedia.com/documents/Pakulak-NevilleANGxp.pdf

Peterson, N.; Pisoni, D. & Miyamoto, R. (2010). Cochlear Implants and Spoken Language Processing Abilities: Review and Assessment of the Literature. *Restorative Neurology and Neuroscience*, Vol.28, No.2, pp. 237-250, ISSN 0922-6028

Petitto, L. & Marentette, P. (1991). Babbling in the Manual Mode: Evidence for the Ontogeny of Language. *Science*, Vol.251, No.5000, pp. 1493-1496, ISSN 0036-8075

Plaza Pust, C. & Morales López, E. (2008). *Sign Bilingualism: Language Development, Interaction, and Maintenance in Sign Language Contact Situations*, John Benjamins, ISBN 978-9027241498, Amsterdam, The Netherlands

Poizner, H.; Klima, E. & Bellugi, U. (1987). *What the Hands Reveal about the Brain*, MIT Press, ISBN 978-0262161053, Cambridge, MA

Punch, R. & Hyde, M. (2011). Social Participation of Children and Adolescents With Cochlear Implants: A Qualitative Analysis of Parent, Teacher, and Child Interviews. *Journal of Deaf Studies and Deaf Education*, Vol.16, No.4, pp. 474-493, ISSN 1081-4159

Raising Deaf Kids. (n.d.). Summer camps, 18.07.11, Available from http://www.raisingdeafkids.org/growingup/camp.php

Ramsey, C. (2000). Ethics and Culture in the Deaf Community Response to Cochlear Implants. *Seminars in Hearing*, Vol.21, No.1, pp. 75-86, ISSN 0734-0451

Restuccia, A. (2010). Michael Schwartz: Multiple Communication Methods Assist Deaf Law Professor In and Outside of the Classroom, In *The Daily Orange: The Independent Student Newspaper of Syracuse, New York*, 07.03.11, Available from http://www.dailyorange.com/2.8691/michaelschwartz-multiple-communication-methods-assist-deaf-law-professor-in-and-outside-ofthe-classroom-1.1237578

Rhoades, E. (2006). Research Outcomes of Auditory-Verbal Intervention: Is the Approach Justified? *Deafness and Education International*, Vol.8, No.3, pp. 125-143, ISSN 1464-3154

Ronnberg, J. (2010). Working Memory, Neuroscience, and Language: Evidence from Deaf and Hard-of-hearing Individuals, In: *The Oxford Handbook of Deaf Studies, Language, and Education, Vol.1*, (2nd edition), M. Marschark & P. Spencer, (Eds.), pp. 478-490, Oxford University Press, ISBN 978-0199750986 , Oxford, UK

Sacks, O. (1989). *Seeing Voices: A Journey into the World of the Deaf*, University of California Press, ISBN 978-0520060838, Berkeley, CA

Santarelli, R.; De Filippi, R.; Genovese, E. & Arslan, E. (2008). Cochlear Implantation Outcome in Prelingually Deafened Young Adults. *Audiology and Neurotology*, Vol.13, No.4, pp. 257-265, ISSN 1420-3030

Schick, B.; Marschark, M. & Spencer, P. (Eds.). (2006). *Advances in the Sign Language Development of Deaf Children*, Oxford University Press, ISBN 978-0195180947, New York, NY

Schick, B.; de Villiers, P.; de Villiers, J. & Hoffmeister, R. (2007). Language and Theory of Mind: A Study of Deaf Children. *Child Development*, Vol.78, No.2, pp. 376-396, ISSN 0009-3920

Shannon, R.; Fu, Q-J.; Galvin, J. &. Friesen, L. (2010). Speech Perception with Cochlear Implants, In: *Cochlear Implants: Auditory Prostheses and Electrical Hearing*, F-G. Zeng, A. Popper & R. Fay, (Eds.), pp. 334-376, Springer, ISBN 978-0387225852, New York, NY

Shattuck, R. (1980). *The Forbidden Experiment: The Story of the Wild Boy of Aveyron*, Farrar, Straus and Giroux, ISBN 978-0436458750, New York, NY

Simmons, F. (1966). Electrical Stimulation of the Auditory Nerve in Man. *Archives of Otolaryngology*, Vol.84, No.1, pp. 2–54 (cited in Eisen, 2000)

Snoddon, K. (2005). Return, In: *Between Myself and Them: Stories of Disability and Difference, C.* Krause, (Ed.), pp. 179-188, Second Story Press, ISBN 978-1896764993, Toronto, Canada

Snow, J. & Wackym, P. (2008). *Ballenger's Otorhinolaryngology*, (17th edition), People's Medical Publishing House, ISBN 978-1550093377, Shelton, CT

Spencer, P. (1993). The Expressive Communication of Hearing Mothers and Deaf Infants. *American Annals of the Deaf*, Vol.138, No.3, pp. 275-283, ISSN 0002-726X

Steenerson, R.; Cronin, G. & Gary, L. (2001). Vertigo after Cochlear Implantation. *Otology and Neurotology*, Vol.22, No.6, pp. 842-843, ISSN 1531-7129

Stemmer, B. & Whitaker, H. (Eds.) (2008). *Handbook of the Neuroscience of Language*, Academic Press, ISBN 978-0080453521, London, UK

Strong, M. & Prinz, P. (2000). Is American Sign Language Skill Related to English Literacy? In: *Language acquisition by eye*, C. Chamberlain, J. Morford & R. Mayberry, (Eds.), pp. 131-142, Lawrence Erlbaum Associates, ISBN 978-0805829372, Mahwah, NJ

Sutton-Spence, R. & Napoli, D-J. (2009). *Humour in Sign Languages: The Linguistic Underpinnings,* Centre for Deaf Studies, Trinity College, ISSN: 2009-1680, Dublin, Ireland

Szagun, G. (2008). The Younger the Better? Variability in Language Development of Young German-speaking Children with Cochlear Implants, In: *Proceedings of the Child Language Seminar 2007 – 30th Anniversary,* T. Marinis, A. Papangeli & V. Stojanovik, (Eds.), pp. 183-194, University of Reading Press, Reading, UK

Turner, C.; Reiss, L. & Gantz, B. (2007). Combined Acoustic and Electric Hearing: Preserving Residual Acoustic Hearing. *Hearing Research,* 42, pp. 164-171

Tyler, R.; Witt, S.; Dunn, C.; Perreau, A.; Parkinson, A. & Wilson, B. (2010). An Attempt to Improve Bilateral Cochlear Implants by Increasing the Distance Between Electrodes and Providing Complementary Information to the Two Ears. *Journal of the American Academy of Audiology,* Vol.21, No.1, pp. 52–65

United States Government Accountability Office. (2011). Deaf and Hard-of-hearing Children: Federal Support for Developing Language and Literacy, 18.07.11, Available from http://www.gao.gov/products/GAO-11-357

Valente, J. (2011). Cyborgization: Deaf Education for Young Children in the Cochlear Implantation Era. *Qualitative Inquiry,* Vol.17, No.7, pp. 639–652, ISSN 1077-8004

Walker, G. (2008). A Conversation with Grace Walker: Personal Experiences with a Cochlear Implant, In: *Access: Multiple Avenues for Deaf People,* D. DeLuca, I. Leigh, K. Lindgren, & D-J. Napoli, (Eds.), pp. 140-145, Gallaudet University Press, ISBN 978-1563683930, Washington, DC

Waltzman, S. & Roland, T. (2005). Cochlear Implantation in Children Younger Than 12 Months. *Pediatrics,* Vol.116, No.4, pp. e487-e493, ISSN 0031-4005

Watson, L. & Gregory, S. (2005). Non-use of Implants in Children: Child and Parent Perspectives. *Deafness and Education International,* Vol.7, No.1, pp. 43-58, ISSN 1464-3154

Wilbur, R. (2008). How to Prevent Educational Failure, In: *Signs and Voices: Deaf Culture, Identity, Language and Arts,* K. Lindgren, D. DeLuca & D-J. Napoli, (Eds.), pp. 117-138, Gallaudet University Press, ISBN 978-1563683633, Washington, DC

Wilson, B.; Finley, C.; Lawson, D.; Wolford, R.; Eddington, D. & Rabinowitz, W. (1991). Better Speech Recognition with Cochlear Implants. *Nature,* Vol.352, No.6332, pp. 236-238 (cited in Eisen, 2000)

Yoshinaga-Itano, C.; Sedey, A.; Coulter, D. & Mehl, A. (1998). Language of Early- and Later-Identified Children with Hearing Loss. *Pediatrics,* Vol.102, No.5, pp. 1161 –1171, ISSN 0031-4005

Yoshinaga-Itano, C.; Coulter, D. & Thomson, V. (2000). The Colorado Hearing Screening Program: Effects on Speech and Language for Children with Hearing Loss. *Journal of Perinatology,* Vol.20, No.8s, pp. s132 –s142, ISSN 0743-8346

Young, C. (2002). Sound Judgement: Does Curing Deafness Really Mean Cultural Genocide? In: *The CBS Interactive Business Network,* 18.07.11, Available from http://findarticles.com/p/articles/mi_m1568/is_11_33/ai_84246679/

Zimmerman, A. (2009). Do You Hear the People Sing? Balancing Parental Authority and a Child's Right to Thrive: The Cochlear Implant Debate. *Journal of Health and Biomedical Law,* Vol.5, No.2, p. 309

11

Cochlear Implantation in Auditory Neuropathy Spectrum Disorder

C. M. McMahon[1,2], K. M. Bate[1,2,3], A. Al-meqbel[1,2,4] and R. B. Patuzzi[5]
[1]HEARing CRC,
[2]Centre for Language Sciences, Macquarie University,
[3]Cochlear Ltd,
[4]College of Allied Health Sciences, Kuwait University,
[5]School of Biomedical, Biomolecular and Chemical Sciences,
University of Western Australia,
[1,2,3,5]Australia
[4]Kuwait

1. Introduction

With the implementation of newborn hearing screening programs, permanent congenital hearing loss is typically diagnosed in babies within six weeks of age (JCIH, 2007). Many hearing screening programs use a two-stage transient-evoked otoacoustic emissions (TEOAEs) screen because of the ease-of-use and time- and cost-effectiveness (Hayes, 2003). Because infants are unable to provide reliable behavioural responses to sound stimuli, hearing thresholds are estimated using the auditory brainstem response (ABR), a measure of synchronous neural activity that correlates well with behavioural thresholds in infants with normal hearing and conductive and sensorineural hearing loss (Hyde et al., 1990). As a result, early intervention is targeted, resulting in spoken language development that is similar to normally hearing peers and significantly better than later identified peers, irrespective of the magnitude of loss (Yoshinaga-Itano et al., 1998).

On the other hand, Auditory Neuropathy Spectrum Disorder (ANSD) describes a unique type of permanent hearing loss that is not identified with newborn hearing screening programs that utilise otoacoustic emissions (OAEs) as a first-line screen, unless the impairment is detected through alternative risk-based screening programs (which occurs for individuals with additional and/or associated neonatal problems such as anoxia and hyperbilirubinemia; Rance et al., 2002). ANSD is characterised by significantly disordered auditory afferent neural conduction with preservation of cochlear outer hair cell function (Starr et al., 1996), based on clinical findings of normal OAEs and/or cochlear microphonic (CM) potentials with the absence or marked abnormality of the ABR. Despite poor afferent responses, individuals with ANSD have pure tone thresholds that may vary from normal to profound hearing loss in a variety of audiometric configurations (Starr et al., 2000). Therefore OAE screening would inaccurately "pass" these individuals and, while ABR screening would detect them, diagnostic ABR testing would not provide an accurate estimate of hearing thresholds.

The estimation of hearing thresholds in infancy is only one of the challenges that are faced in selecting the most appropriate intervention pathways and hearing devices for these individuals. Unlike standard sensorineural hearing losses which show impaired spectral processing, largely resulting from the loss of outer hair cells (OHCs), individuals with ANSD show distinct deficits in auditory temporal processing. Presumably, this results from the disordered or temporally jittered neural activity. This is the ability of the auditory system to detect and analyze temporal cues within an acoustic signal that occur within milliseconds (Green, 1971). Auditory temporal processing plays an important role in the development of speech perception, language and reading skills in all children and it has been speculated that this underpins most auditory processing capabilities (Benasich & Tallal, 2002; Musiek, 2003). Both fast (20-40Hz) and slow (<2-16Hz) temporal processing is needed to: (i) detect and resolve relevant phonetic sounds and the speech envelope within segregated speech; and (ii) extract speech sounds from noisy environments, where it is the perception of the sound onset that is most critical to detect speech-in-noise (Drullman et al. 1994a,b; Kaplan-Neeman et al., 2006; Shannon et al., 1995). Rapid temporal processing abilities are important for the development of phonological awareness (Nittrouer, 1999), which is significantly correlated with language and reading ability in children (Stark & Tallal, 1979; Benasich & Tallal, 2002; Catts et al., 2002), although not exclusively related (Bretherton & Holmes, 2003). In particular, this is highlighted in many cases of dyslexia and specific language impairment (SLI) which show impaired temporal processing abilities compared with children with normal language and reading development (Farmer & Klein, 1995). However the temporal processing deficits in individuals with dyslexia and SLI appear less severe in comparison with most individuals with ANSD (see Figure 1).

2. Temporal processing & speech perception

Psychoacoustic measures in adults and children with ANSD show impairments of pitch discrimination (particularly at lower frequencies), temporal integration, gap detection, temporal modulation detection, backward and forward masking, perception of speech-in-noise and sound localization using inter-aural time differences (Rance et al., 2004; Starr et al., 1996; Zeng et al., 1999; Zeng et al., 2005). It is assumed that these deficits are caused by the disrupted temporal perception. Several studies have demonstrated that the magnitude of the disruption of temporal processing in individuals with ANSD varies considerably and it is this which determines speech perception outcomes, rather than hearing thresholds *per se* (Rance et al., 2004; Zeng et al., 1999, 2005; Kumar & Jayaram, 2005). Using amplitude modulated-broadband noise with varying modulation depths at three frequencies (10, 50 and 150 Hz), Rance and colleagues (2004) compared differences in temporal processing abilities between three populations of children; normal hearing (n=10), ANSD (n=14) and sensorineural hearing loss (n=10) and compared this with speech perception outcomes using Consonant-Nucleus-Consonant (CNC) words. The latter two groups with hearing loss showed pure tone thresholds within a mild-moderate range. While no difference existed in temporal processing abilities for individuals with normal hearing and sensorineural hearing loss, significant differences existed between these populations and children with ANSD. When the ANSD population was stratified into good (≥30% phoneme recognition; n=7) and poor performers (<30% phoneme recognition; n=7), the disruption was only mild for those with good speech perception scores, and disruptions to low frequency modulations (10 Hz) only occurred in those with very poor speech discrimination. Similar outcomes have been demonstrated by Zeng et al. (2005) who examined temporal modulation detection as a

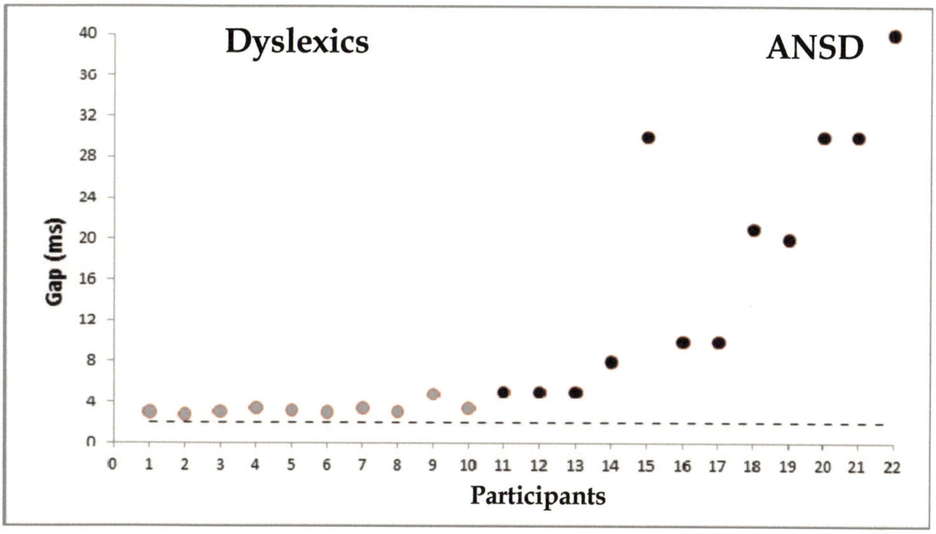

Fig. 1. Thresholds of gap detection for adults with ANSD (black circles; from Michalewski et al., 2005) and children with dyslexia (grey circles; from Van Ingelghem et al., 2001) compared to adults and children (120–144 months) without ANSD or dyslexia (dashed line).

function of modulation frequency (ranging from 2-2000 Hz) in 16 ANSD adult participants, with hearing thresholds varying from normal to severe. Additionally, Kumar and Jayaram (2005) evaluated temporal modulation detection abilities at six modulation frequencies, (4, 16, 32, 64, 128 and 200 Hz), in 14 adult ANSD participants and compared the results with 30 normally hearing participants, matched by age and gender. Results were stratified by speech perception abilities and demonstrated that ANSD participants who had speech perception scores of greater than 50% showed greater sensitivity to the temporal modulations when compared to those who had speech perception scores of less than 20%. While the results from Rance et al. (2004) indicate that those individuals with good speech perception scores show good temporal processing at low-frequency rates of modulation (10 Hz), Kumar and Jayaram's (2005) study showed poor temporal processing at all frequencies for adults with good (>50%) and poor (>20%) speech perception scores using open-set Kannada words. Nonetheless, if averaged, temporal resolution scores for all ANSD participants seemed to be similar at 10 Hz for all three studies discussed above, of an approximate -10 dB detection threshold. In contrast to temporal modulation detection, gap detection thresholds (psychoacoustic measure of temporal resolution) are consistently impaired in individuals with ANSD. While normal-hearing listeners require 2–3 ms at supra-threshold levels (40–50 dB SPL) to detect a brief gap in noise, ANSD individuals require 20–28 ms (Starr et al., 1996; Zeng et al., 1999; Zeng et al., 2005).

In any case, for individuals with ANSD, it seems that it is the temporal processing ability that is paramount to the development of speech and language and, therefore, the success of hearing aid fitting, rather than pure tone thresholds *per se*. While objective measures of temporal processing are beginning to emerge in the literature, these are clearly needed to guide timely decisions about device fitting, particularly in view of the critical period of language development.

3. Cochlear implantation and site-of-lesion

It is clear that early detection of hearing loss minimises the longer-term consequences of auditory deprivation on speech perception, language and socio-emotional development (Geers, 2006; Moog & Geers 2010; Moog, Geers Gustus & Brenner, 2011). For individuals with severe to profound sensorineural hearing loss, cochlear implantation is commonly part of an effective intervention program, providing greater access to speech than conventional hearing aids. Earlier implantation as well as early educational placement and / or intensive habilitation facilitates more rapid and extensive language development as well as improved speech perception and production (Hayes et al., 2009; Nicholas & Geers, 2007; Svirsky et al., 2004; Tomblin, et al., 2005). Animal models of sound deprivation highlight the extent of anatomical changes that can occur within the auditory pathways and cortex with congenital hearing loss (Fallon et al., 2008). However, the effects of early implantation appear to facilitate normal synaptic and cortical development through restored sound input (Kral et al., 2001, 2002; O'Neill et al., 2010; Ryugo et al., 2005). Kral and Eggermont (2007) suggest that the sensitive period for language learning in children with pre-lingual hearing loss fitted with a cochlear implant correlates with the age of significant reduction in synaptic density in normally hearing subjects (4-5 years of age). This is consistent with electrophysiological data from Sharma and colleagues (2002a&b; 2005, 2009) who show that later implanted children (over 7 years of age) show significant and sustained delays in the latency of the P1 peak of the cortical auditory evoked potential (CAEP). On the other hand, delays in the P1 peak of earlier implanted children (under 3.5 years of age) are resolved within 6-8 months after implant surgery. It is assumed, therefore, that the comparatively better functional outcomes from earlier implantation partly result from greater synaptic development and maturity occurring within the critical period (Hammes et al., 2002; Harrison et al., 2005). While early identification and intervention are also important for children with ANSD, identifying *who* will benefit from cochlear implants and deciding *when* to implant is more challenging than for individuals with sensorineural hearing loss.

The term "auditory neuropathy" was initially used to describe this disorder, consistent with the findings from a longitudinal study of 10 individuals, 8 of which later developed concomitant peripheral neuropathies (Starr et al., 1996). In this case, it was assumed that the lesion existed at the auditory nerve resulting from demyelination of peripheral neurons. However, subsequent studies have shown that proportionally large numbers of individuals diagnosed with ANSD do not develop additional neuropathies and good functional outcomes have been reported in many cases after cochlear implantation (Mason et al., 2003; Gibson & Sanli, 2007; Shannon et al., 2001), which suggest that the lesion is pre-neural. Therefore the term has been widely contested because of the potentially negative impact this might hold for clinical decision-making, such as cochlear implantation (that is, this may be considered a deterrent for implantation). While other terms including auditory dys-synchrony (Berlin et al., 2001) were suggested as alternatives, the physiological mechanisms underpinning this disorder are unclear and are likely to be many. Certainly genetic, electrophysiological and imaging data show that multiple sites of lesion can exist (Cacace & Pinheiro, 2011; Manchaiah et al., 2010; Santarelli, 2010; Varga et al., 2003) and this is supported by the variability in objective measurements, such as electrically-evoked ABR (EABR), after cochlear implantation (McMahon et al., 2008; Shallop et al., 2001). To encompass the breadth of different lesions (whether synaptic, neural or brainstem) that could lead to the clinical classification of this disorder and the wide range of functional outcomes, an alternative term "auditory neuropathy spectrum disorder", or ANSD, was proposed at the International Conference of Newborn Hearing Screening (Como, 2008), although this term also has little prognostic information about functional outcomes within this population. Broadening the term may also lead to greater inclusion of identifiable lesions of the auditory nerve, such as cochlear nerve deficiency (CND; Buchman et al., 2006), or hereditary conditions of known late-onset auditory neural demyelination, such as Freidreich's Ataxia (Rance et al., 2008) and Charcot-Marie Tooth disease, which will certainly have poorer outcomes with cochlear implantation (Madden et al., 2002; Song et al 2010) than the population of ANSD without known neural lesions.

Various studies have shown that the prevalence of this disorder ranges from 0.23-24% in the at-risk neonatal population (Rance et al., 1999; Berg et al., 2005) to 5.1-15% of children with sensorineural hearing loss (Madden et al., 2002b; McFadden et al., 2002). While many cases of ANSD occur with infectious diseases, perinatal and postnatal insults and genetic disruptions (Madden et al., 2002), some have no co-morbid medical problems or familial hearing loss. Common medical insults assumed to cause ANSD include hyperbilirubinaemia (which may account for up to 48.8% of cases; Berlin et al., 2010) and/or perinatal anoxia, prematurity and low birth-weight (Berlin et al., 2010; Beutner, et al., 2007; Salujaet al., 2010). Each of these can have widespread effects on the auditory system as well as other neurodevelopment consequences, including cerebral palsy and cognitive or neurodevelopmental delay (Johnson & Bhutani, 2011; Schlapbach et al., 2011). Additionally, some infants diagnosed with ANSD within this high-risk category show full or partial recovery of ABR waveforms within 12 months of diagnosis or following medical intervention (such as exchange transfusion), which indicates that some cases of ANSD may be due to neuromaturational delay or reversible transient brainstem encephalopathy (Amin et al., 1991; Krumholz et al., 1985; Granziani et al., 1967). While ANSD can be detected early through newborn hearing screening programs or through targeted screening of the "at-risk" populations in the NICU, no uniform management plan exists because of the variability in hearing thresholds, temporal processing abilities and sites-of-lesion that cannot be measured using behavioural tests at that age. Early intervention and fitting of hearing aids, particularly high-powered aids, or cochlear implants is considered, with caution, to avoid permanently damaging normally functioning outer hair cells and neural structures, that may be immature rather than permanently disordered (Maddon et al., 2002a,b). As many individuals with ANSD show hearing thresholds within a normal to moderate range (Starr et al., 2000; Berlin et al., 2010), it is clear that neural information is being transmitted to the auditory cortex. However, the sound quality of the auditory input is variable amongst this population, with speech discrimination scores disproportionate to the pure tone audiogram (Rance et al., 2002), and often significantly poorer in noisy environments (Starr et al., 1996).

Hyperbilirubinaemia describes the high concentrations of unconjugated bilirubin that can occur in the newborn, which is a neurotoxin that can cause irreversible neurological damage, including auditory, motor and ocular movement impairments (Shapiro & Popelka, 2011). The Gunn rat pup provides a model of the effects of kernicterus in the neonate. Electrophysiological and anatomical studies have shown that severe cases of kernicterus in the Gunn rat lead to disruption of the auditory pathway from the cochlear nucleus to the higher auditory brainstem, including the inferior colliculus (Uziel et al., 1983). While both inner and outer hair cells appear to be spared by high levels of bilirubin, the spiral ganglion cells of auditory neurones can be disrupted (Shapiro, 2005), indicating a neuronal cause of ANSD. Improvements in auditory brainstem responses in infants with hyperbilirubinemia, particularly after exchange transfusions, have been noted by a number of authors (Deliac et al., 1990; Perlman et al., 1983; Rhee et al., 1999; Roberts et al., 1982). Rhee and colleagues (1999) evaluated TEOAEs and ABR responses in 11 neonates after exchange transfusions for hyperbilirubinemia. All infants showed normal OAE responses but 3 showed absent ABR responses to clicks at stimulus levels of 90dBnHL and, within 12 months of follow-up 1 showed significant improvements in hearing thresholds, estimated using ABR.

Prematurity is identified as another major cause of ANSD. However, it is likely that it is not the prematurity *per se* that underpins the damage to the auditory system but associated conditions of low-birth weight, hypoxia from respiratory failure, hyperbilirubinemia, presence of fetal pathology (infection or retarded intrauterine growth) or perinatal pathology, or ototoxicity from antibiotics given for hyaline membrane disease (Ferber-Viart et al., 1996). Extremely low birth-weight infants are at risk of developing ANSD (Xoinis et al., 2007). A retrospective study by Xoinis and colleagues (2007) showed that the prevalence of ANSD was 5.6/1000 in the NICU (n=24) compared with 16.7/1000 infants with sensorineural hearing loss (n=71). They identified that infants with ANSD were born more prematurely (mean gestational age 28.3±4.8 weeks compared with 32.9±5.2 weeks of SNHL infants) and showed significantly lower birth weights (mean 1.318±0.89 kg compared with 1.968±1.00 kg of those with SNHL). Psarommatis and colleagues (2006) retrospectively reviewed medical records of 1150 NICU neonates and identified 25 infants with ANSD. Of these, 20 were re-examined at approximately 5 months of age and 12 showed full recovery of the ABR with 1 infant showing partial recovery (with click ABR thresholds measured to 50dBnHL). A significant difference in mean birth-weight and gestational age (GA) was found between infants who recovered (BW= 1.89±0.90 kg and GA= 32.9±1.1 weeks) and those who showed no recovery (BW= 3.0±0.66 kg and GA= 36.4±1.25 weeks), suggesting that those born more prematurely and with lower birth weight may be more at risk of delayed neuromaturational development rather than ANSD. Amatuzzi and colleagues (2001) evaluated the temporal bones of 15 non-surviving NICU infants, 12 who failed the ABR screen bilaterally and 2 who passed bilaterally. Of those who failed, 3 infants (all born prematurely) showed bilateral selective inner hair cell loss whereas both infants who passed the ABR screen showed no cochlear histopathologic abnormalities. This may suggest that pathologies related to prematurity are more likely to target inner hair cells than neural elements, making these individuals good candidates for cochlear implantation.

Two large-scale studies of individuals with ANSD both conducted in 2010 by Teagle et al. (n=140) and Berlin et al. (n=260) have provided the most comprehensive information to date about the etiologies of ANSD and outcomes of individuals fitted with hearing aids and / or cochlear implants. Berlin and colleagues reported that only 11 of 94 individuals who used hearing aids showed good speech and language development. 60% of the 258 subjects reported had pure tone thresholds characterised as being between normal to moderate-severe (within a very aidable range) and the remaining 40% had thresholds described as either moderate-profound, severe, severe-profound or profound, presumably fitting within the more typical range of CI candidacy. On the other hand, 85% of those fitted with a CI showed successful outcomes (evaluated by parent and teacher report) and 8% were too young to conclude this. Teagle and colleagues reported that of the 52 individuals with ANSD who were implanted, 50% demonstrated open-set speech perception abilities, although 30% were not tested because of their young actual or developmental age and individuals identified with CND showed 0% open-set speech perception scores. Therefore it is clear that ANSD is heterogeneous in cochlear implantation outcomes, possibly partly related to the high incidence of co-morbidity and multiple disabilities as well as differences in the site-of-lesion.

4. Role of evoked potentials in decision-making

Given the variability in the magnitude of temporal processing disruption and in the sites-of-lesion in ANSD, which is important for CI outcomes, the focus of our research has been in the development and/or evaluation of objective measures to better quantify temporal processing ability (Al-meqbel & McMahon, 2011) and identify the site-of-lesion (McMahon et al., 2008) in ANSD. Cortical auditory evoked potentials (CAEPs) have been shown to be important in the measurement of temporal processing ability because they are less reliant on rapid neural timing than the auditory brainstem responses. Rance and colleagues (2002) were the first to show that the presence of CAEPs in ANSD with a mild to moderate hearing loss correlated well with good aided speech perception outcomes. In this study, 8 of 15 children showed good aided functional outcomes, identified as >30% correctly identified phoneme scores using Phonetically-Balanced Kindergarten Words, and each of these showed present CAEP waveforms to either a pure tone (440Hz for 200ms) and/or a synthesised speech token (/daed/) presented at a comfortable level using headphones or insert earphones. The remaining 7 children who showed poor aided speech perception results also showed absent CAEP waveforms to either the pure-tone or speech stimuli. This important finding highlighted the role of evoked potentials in guiding management decisions in this population. Michalewski and colleagues (2005) used CAEPs measured with an active and passive gap-in-noise paradigm to determine temporal processing acuity in 14 adults with ANSD. They obtained CAEP responses from 11 subjects, with active responses measured in all 11 subjects but passive responses in only 7 subjects. No response was measured for 3 individuals who showed profound hearing loss. In 7 subjects who showed present passive responses to gap detection, good correlations were found between psychoacoustic and objective CAEP measures of gap detection. In 3 of 4 subjects with only active responses, a good correlation was also found. This unexpected appearance of the CAEP in response to attention may shed some light into the role of attention in the synchronisation of responses in some individuals with ANSD.

Subsequently, our retrospective study (McMahon et al., 2008) showed that the frequency-specific electrocochleographic waveforms, measured from the round-window of 14 implanted children with ANSD with severe-profound hearing loss, correlated well with the EABR measured immediately after implantation. This supports the use of frequency-specific electrocochleography (ECochG) in enabling better delineation of site-of-lesion. Electrocochleography is a useful tool in the identification of cochlear lesions because it enables more accurate recording of the summed extracellular currents from cochlear hair cells (the cochlear microphonic, CM; Figure 2A in the guinea-pig and Figure 2E in the human, and summating potential, SP; Figure 2B in the guinea-pig and Figure 2G in the human), the excitatory post-synaptic currents (known as the dendritic potential, DP) arising from the primary afferent dendrites, the terminal endings of the primary afferent neurones that synapse with the inner hair cells (Figure 2C), and the compound action potential (CAP) from the primary afferent neurones which is described by three dominant peaks, labelled N_1, P_1 and N_2 (Figure 2D; see Sellick et al., 2003 for a review). Because there is a cascade of events that leads to the generation of an action potential (see Fuchs, 2005 for a review), the presence or absence of these potentials can indicate where a lesion is located. That is, depolarisation of inner hair cells leads to the opening of L-type calcium channels in the basolateral wall of these cells and, ultimately, the mobilisation and release of neurotransmitter from the base of these cells. This process involving the gene otoferlin that is implicated in some types of ANSD (Roux et al., 2006). Neurotransmitter diffuses across the synaptic cleft and binds to the α-amino-3-hydroxy-5-methyl-4-isoxazolepropionic acid receptor (AMPA) channels on the dendrite which allows an influx of positive ions, generating an excitatory post-synaptic potential (EPSP) inside

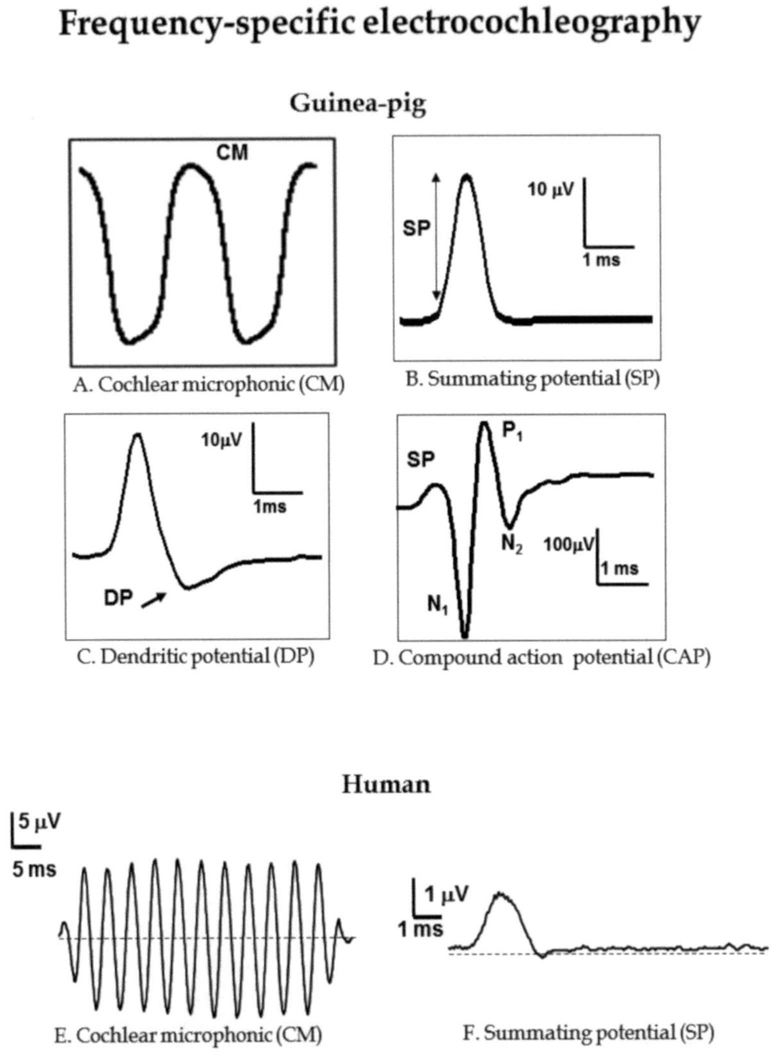

Fig. 2. Using a round-window electrode, local hair cell, dendritic and neural potentials can be measured using frequency-specific electrocochleography in the anaesthestised guinea pig (A-D) or human (E-F). A single polarity low-frequency tone-burst clearly shows the cochlear microphonic (CM) waveform (A&E). A high-frequency alternating polarity tone-burst is used to elicit the summating potential (SP; B&F), dendritic potential (DP; C) and compound action potential (CAP; D). The presence of the CAP obscures the DP, which is only observed in pathological cases such as ANSD in human. Note that the differences observed between the guinea-pig and human CM and SP are largely because of the different stimulus-frequencies and time-scales used to elicit and display the response.

the dendrite. If this voltage is large enough, it will trigger an action potential, which is often considered an all-or-none event. Selective disruption of these potentials using pharmacological block in an anaesthetised guinea-pig model demonstrates this point (Figure 2A-D). Intracochlear perfusion of the excitotoxic drug kainite which blocks the ligand-gated AMPA channels, abolishes both the CAP and the DP, whereas the SP amplitude is unchanged (Figure 2B). On the other hand, intracochlear perfusion of tetrodotoxin (TTX), a spider venom which blocks the voltage-gated Na^+ channels, abolishes the CAP, but the SP remains and the DP can be observed in the average waveform (Figure 2C which previously was masked by the much larger CAP observed in the normal hearing guinea-pig (Figure 2D).

There are two main limitations to this technique. Firstly, the currents measured from the recording electrode are local currents (i.e. those generated within the proximity of the recording electrode) and, in our study, were measured from the cochlear round window. Therefore, to a first approximation, we assumed that any disruption identified at the round window (which has a best frequency of about 8kHz in humans) was the same throughout the cochlea. Secondly, a disruption at a particular site along the auditory pathway might be one of multiple disruptions that could occur. As previously discussed, many of the underlying causes of ANSD cause widespread disruption that may impact cochlear and brainstem structures and are not highly localised to a single site. In any case, in the study conducted by McMahon et al. (2008), we identified two types of ECochG waveforms in 14 individuals with ANSD, each who showed normal Magnetic Resonance Imaging (MRI) recordings (with no identifiable neural abnormalities): (i) a delayed latency SP that showed little or no compound action potential, suggestive of a pre-synaptic or synaptic lesion, and (ii) a normal latency SP with a clear DP waveform that was more visible at lower sound levels (where it was assumed that the much larger SP distorted the DP waveform at higher sound levels), suggestive of a neural or post-synaptic lesion (see Figure 3). In 6 of 7 ears implanted with the pre-synaptic or synaptic ECochG waveform, normal morphology EABR waveforms were measured from electrical stimulation of the majority of the 22 electrodes of the cochlear implant. Additionally, in 6 of 6 ears implanted with post-synaptic ECochG waveforms, the EABR waveforms were grossly abnormal or absent for all 22 electrodes (see Figure 3).

The physiological mechanisms underlying spike failure in cases of ANSD and leading to a pre-synaptic or synaptic mechanism of disruption could be numerous. Assuming a normal distribution of EPSP amplitudes results from the quantal release of neurotransmitter (Fuchs, 2005), then a reduction in the amplitude (or number) of EPSPs would reduce the probability of spike initiation (see Figure 4A). This might occur due to disruption of transmitter-release (possibly mediated by otoferlin deficiency, Roux et al., 2006) or a scattered loss of IHCs (Amatuzzi et al., 2001). Alternatively, an increase in the trigger-level voltage could reduce the probability of EPSPs reaching this critical voltage (see Figure 4B), or, depolarisation of the dendrite itself (possibly from lateral efferent modulation; Brown, 1987) would also reduce the chance of EPSPs generating spikes (see Figure 4C).

Santarelli and colleagues (2008) also measured ECochG waveforms in 8 children and adults with ANSD, using a forward masking paradigm of rapidly presented click stimuli to differentiate between cochlear and neural sites-of-lesion. Given that neural potentials decay significantly with faster rates of stimulation due to neural refractoriness (Miller et al., 2001), the amount of adaption in the measured response enables differential diagnosis of the site-of-lesion. In this study, 3 patterns were identified: (i) presence of the SP without a CAP, consistent with a pre-synaptic lesion; (ii) presence of the SP and CAP, consistent with a post-synaptic lesion and (iii) significantly prolonged latency potentials (up to 12 ms), which the authors suggest may result from slowed neural conduction and/or reduced action potential generation. Since implantation in cases of cochlear nerve deficiency is known to have poorer outcomes (Buchman et al., 2006), then ECochG provides a useful tool in the differential diagnosis of ANSD.

Types of ECochG waveforms in ANSD

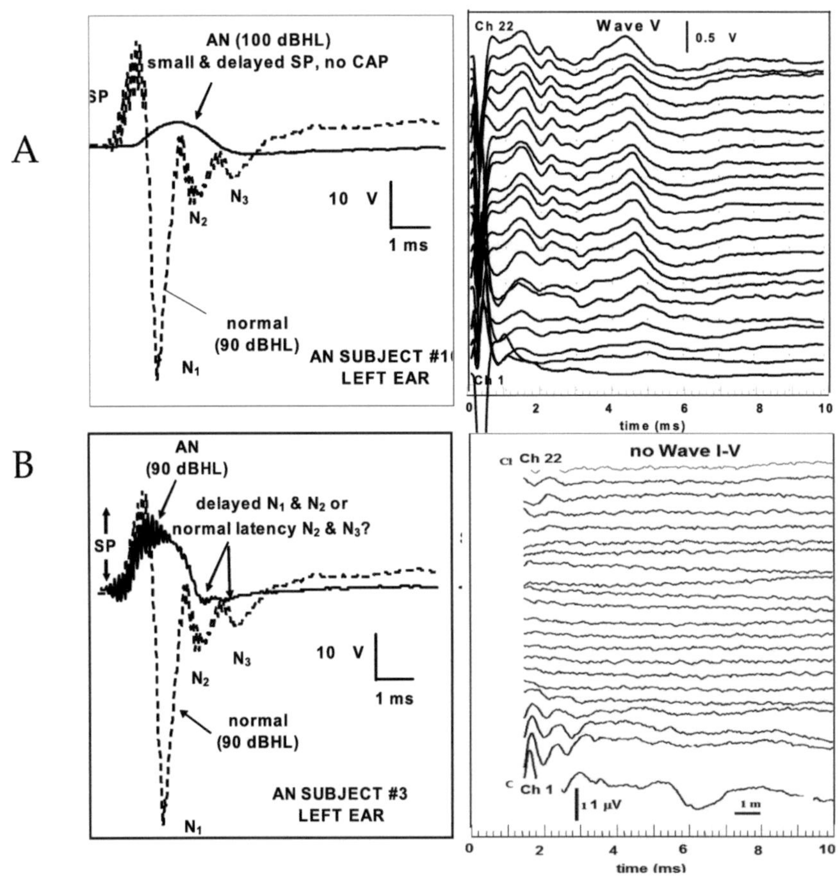

Fig. 3. Electrocochleographic recordings using an 8kHz alternating time-burst show two types of waveforms exist in the 14 ANSD individuals in this study: (A) a delayed SP with either a small or absent CAP present, consistent with normal implanted EABR waveforms suggesting a pre-synaptic lesion and (B) a normal latency SP with a DP present at lower sound levels, consistent with absent or grossly abnormal implanted EABR responses, consistent with a post-synaptic lesion.

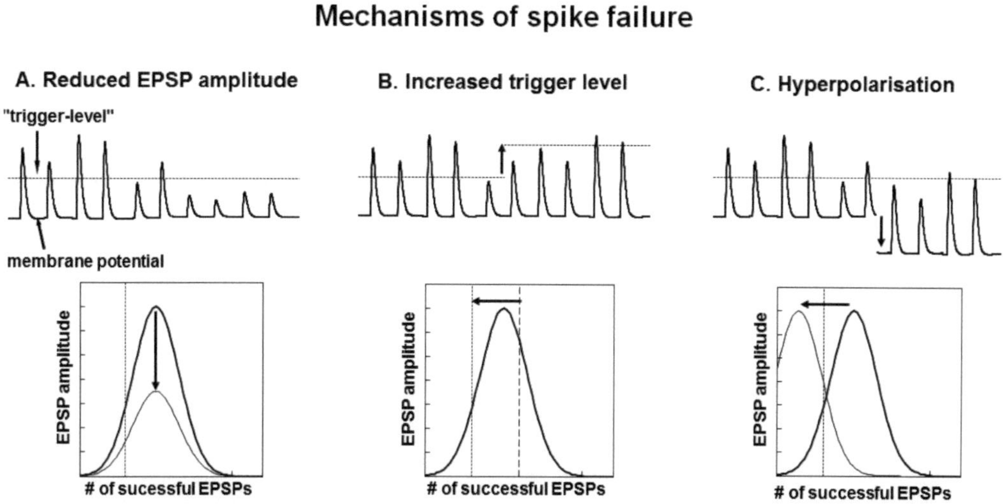

Fig. 4. Physiological mechanisms of spike failure from pre-synaptic or synaptic disruptions might include: (A) a reduction in the amplitude of the EPSPs; (B) an increase in the voltage need to reach trigger-level; or (C) hyperpolarisation of the membrane potential of the primary afferent dendrites (possibly from lateral efferent modulation).

Our next study aimed to identify whether EABR provided a good measure of functional performance in implanted individuals with ANSD and severe-profound hearing loss. In this study (Bate & McMahon, in preparation), we compared speech perception outcomes using the phoneme scores of age-appropriate word lists (either CNC words or Manchester Junior Words) presented at 65dBSPL in the free-field with a speaker located at 0 degrees azimuth with electrically-evoked CAEP (ECAEP) waveforms measured at least 1 year after implantation and EABR waveforms measured immediately after implantation. Ten individuals with ANSD diagnosed by present CM but absent ABR waveforms and with normal MRI participated in this study and each showed good speech perception (scoring >50% phonemes correct) and normal motor and cognitive development. Interestingly, only 40% of these individuals showed good EABR waveform morphology but 80% showed good ECAEP waveforms when elicited by direct electrical stimulation at a comfortably loud level from at least 2 of 3 spatially separated electrodes (representing an apical, mid- and basal position of the electrode array). This suggests that even in cases where cochlear implantation may not by-pass the lesion underpinning ANSD, it may provide the necessary amplification needed for the individual to access the speech signal. We did not perform further complex speech, language or reading testing to determine age equivalence, however, we suspect that differences between individuals with present EABR and absent EABR may exist if we evaluated the broader population base and if our testing was more extensive. Nonetheless, these results do suggest that cochlear implantation can benefit some individuals with a post-synaptic site-of-lesion. It is important to highlight that both studies we have conducted included only those individuals with normal MRI scans, indicating no structural abnormality of the auditory nerve (although it is acknowledged that even high resolution MRI cannot identify all structural abnormalities). Previous studies have shown that individuals with a known lesion on the auditory nerve (which would also be defined as a post-synaptic or neural lesion) including neural demyelination (Miyamoto et al., 1999) and auditory nerve agenesis or hypoplasia (Maxwell et al., 1999; Gray et al., 1998; Buchman et al

2006) have significantly poorer outcomes following cochlear implantation. While some authors strongly pursue the differentiation of terminology for a true neuropathy of the auditory nerve and an endocochlear disruption that produces the same clinical results (Loundon et al., 2005), the more inclusive term of ANSD seems to be generally used within the literature. We agree that such a differentiation is important to better understand the mechanisms that underpin this disorder and to develop targeted intervention strategies.

Figure 5 shows three case studies that highlight the variability in evoked potentials and functional outcomes that occur in cases of ANSD, either with normal or abnormal MRI. Case 1 illustrates the electrophysiological test battery as being a good predictor of a good outcome after cochlear implantation in the first ear implanted (4.5 years of age), but not in the second (10 years of age). The electrophysiological test result pre-implantation measured by ECochG and trans-tympanic EABR indicate a pre-synaptic site of lesion (as described by McMahon et al., 2008). Specifically, as shown in Figure 5A, the ECochG results of a delayed latency SP and no evidence of a DP in both ears are consistent with a pre-synaptic lesion (McMahon et al., 2008). The preoperative test results, coupled with the evidence of normal anatomy as shown on preoperative imaging allow prediction of a good outcome. Electrophysiology post-cochlear implant insertion was measured using an intraoperative EABR which showed good responses from all channels in the left and right (data not shown) ears. No other disabilities are noted with this individual and as predicted an open set speech perception ability as measured by was achieved at 6 months post cochlear implantation. These results are consistent with those seen in other studies such as Gibson and Sanli (2007) who showed 32/39 children with good EABR results and good functional outcomes. It is possible that the poorer functional outcomes measured in the subsequently implanted ear arose from the prolonged delay in implanting the second ear (Ramsden et al., 2005; Gordon et al., 2008) although conflicting evidence exists about the impact of duration of sequential implantation on functional outcomes (Zeitler et al., 2008). In any case, in contrast to Case 1, Case 2 provides an example of a subset of individuals identified as having ANSD with additional confounding factors, including cerebral palsy, developmental delay, Autism Spectrum Disorder. While the electrophysiological test results may be similar in both cases, it is presumed that the addition of significant other factors, including cognitive or developmental impairment, may be the cause of the poorer functional outcomes. Poor morphology or the absence of wave V on an EABR post cochlear implantation has been shown to be associated with poor speech perception outcomes (Rance, 1999; Gibson & Sanli, 2007; Song et al., 2010). Case 3, shows ECochG results with a present SP and SP and very poor morphology EABR, consistent with a post-synaptic site-of-lesion (McMahon et al., 2008). Despite this, functional assessment shows a good Manchester Words Junior phoneme score 4 years after implantation. Given the results of these studies, we present an evoked-potential protocol that might be utilised to better inform device and management decisions in individuals with ANSD (see Figure 6). It is not intended that this protocol be used alone. Intensive monitoring of auditory behaviours and receptive and expressive language development is important in providing complementary information to determine the most appropriate way to manage a child with ANSD. On the other hand, this protocol intends to support the decision-making process by providing information about the individual's temporal processing ability, needed to develop speech and language, and the location of the lesion, which might influence cochlear implantation outcomes. Roush (2008) highlights the types of speech perception and behavioural questionnaires that are useful in obtaining behaviourally relevant information in this population.

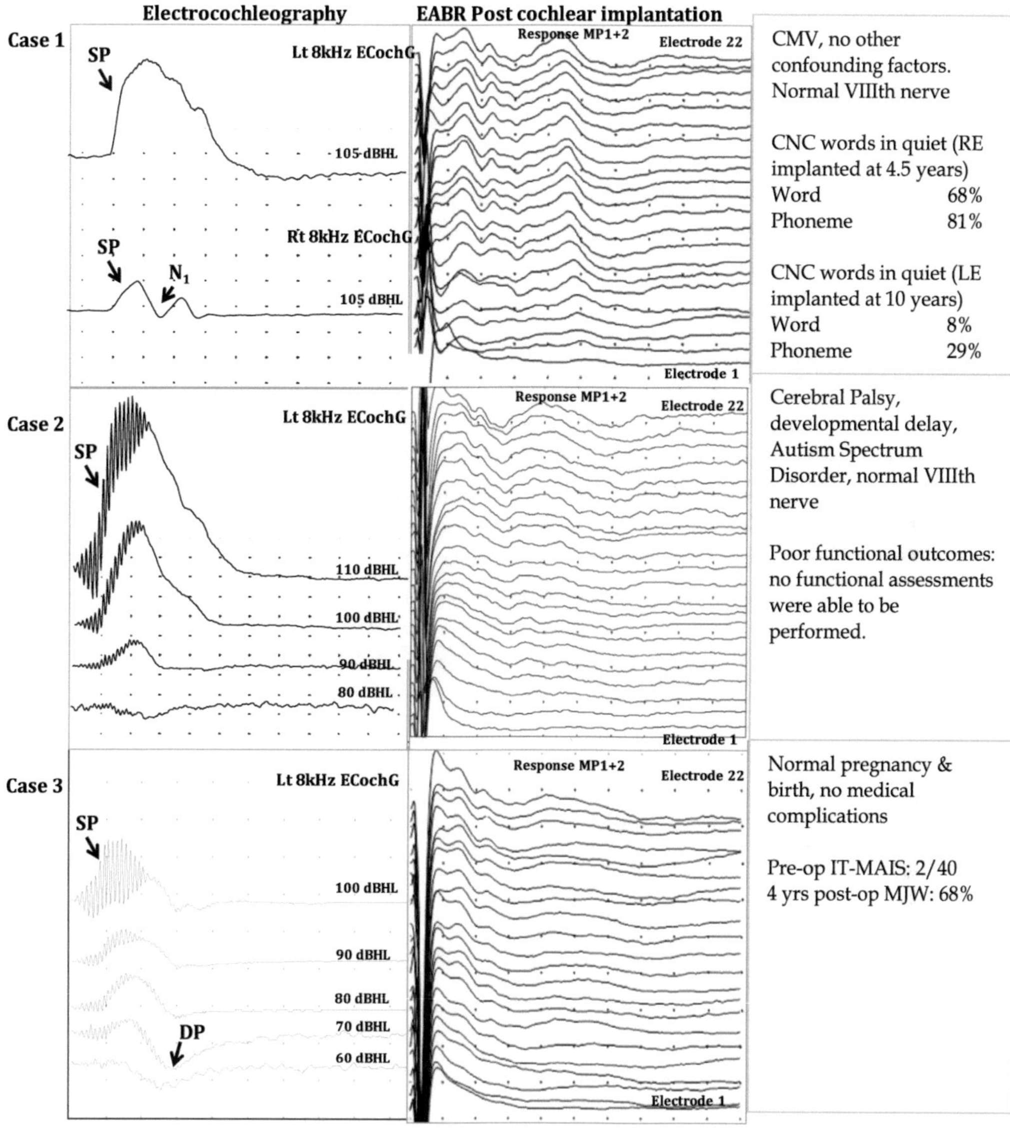

Fig. 5. Electrocochleography and EABR testing provides information useful in understanding the likely site of lesion in ANSD (McMahon et al., 2008; Gibson & Sanli, 2007). These specific cases have been used to demonstrate the variability of outcomes in this population. Case 1: a child with normal neonatal medical history who was bilaterally sequentially implanted, and electrocochleography and EABR results on both sides (EABR RE not shown) are consistent with a pre-synaptic lesion. The right ear was fitted at 4.5 years and the left at 10 years of age. Good functional outcomes were measured using CNC words in quiet with the right ear alone but poor functional outcomes were measured in the left. Case 2: a child with a significant medical history but with normal VIIIth nerve. ECochG waveforms show a normal latency SP but no evidence of a DP, suggestive of a pre-synaptic lesion. EABR waveforms are good for basal electrodes but poorer for apical electrodes. Poor functional outcomes were reported and no functional assessments were

able to be performed. Case 3: a child born with no medical history of complications. ECochG waveforms showed the presence of the SP and DP, suggestive of a post-synaptic lesion. EABR results showed poor morphology waveforms for all channels. Despite this, good functional outcomes were measured using Manchester Junior Words.

1. To determine if sufficient hearing or timing cues exist for hearing aids to be effective measure CAEP to pure tones, speech stimuli or gaps in noise.
If CAEPs are present, then sufficient timing cues and hearing thresholds exist
If CAEPs are absent - poor timing cues and hearing thresholds

2. To determine whether the lesion is located at before or at the level of the auditory nerve measure ECochG response to an 8kHz alternating tone-burst.
Currently we are unsure of the predictive value of this so the presence of a post-synaptic - like lesion should not alone prevent implantation from taking place.

3. To determine the likely speech outcomes of implantation for children without additional disabilities, use EABR to confirm the site-of-lesion and ECAEP to determine potential functional outcomes.
The presence of the ECAEP is a better indicator of speech perception outcomes than the EABR.

Fig. 6. A possible protocol for the use of evoked potentials in directing management of ANSD. It is important to note that evoked potentials should not be used in isolation of behavioural testing and observations.

In conclusion, while the variability of ANSD presents a challenge to audiological management, a structured approach using parental questionnaires to evaluate auditory behaviours as well as objective testing may assist in guiding effective decision-making in this population in infancy.

5. Acknowledgements

The authors acknowledge the financial support of the HEARing CRC, established and supported under the Australian Government's Co-operative Research Centres program and the generous support from the Sydney Cochlear Implant Centre and their clients, without them this research would not have been possible.

6. References

Almeqbel A. McMahon CM. Auditory cortical temporal processing abilities in young adults. Clin. Neurophys (under review).

Al-meqbel A. McMahon CM. Cortical auditory temporal processing abilities in elderly listeners and young adults with normal hearing. *International Evoked Response Audiometry Study Group Conference*, Moscow, Russia, 26-30 June 2011

Amatuzzi MG. Northrop C. Liberman, C. Selective inner hair cell loss in premature infants and cochlear pathological patterns from neonatal intensive care unit autopsies. *Arch. Otolaryngol – Head & Neck Surgery*. 127, 629-636.2001

Amin SB Ahlfors C, Orlando MS, Dalzell LE, Merle KS, Guilette R. Bilirubin and serial auditory brainstem responses in premature infants. *Pediatrics*, 107, 664-670. 2001.

Beutner D, Foerst A, Lang-Roth R, von Wedel H, Walger M. Risk factors for auditory neuropathy/auditory synaptopathy. *ORL J Otorhinolaryngol Relat Spec.* 69(4):239-44. 2007

Benasich A. Tallal P. Infant discrimination of rapid auditory cues predicts later language impairment. *Behav. Brain Res.* 136, 31-49. 2002

Berg AL, Spitzer JB, Towers HM, Bartosiewicz C, Diamond BE.Newborn hearing screening in the NICU: profile of failed auditory brainstem response/passed otoacoustic emission. *Pediatrics*. 116(4):933-8. 2005

Berlin C, Hood L, Rose K. On renaming auditory neuropathy as auditory dys-synchrony: Implications for a clearer understanding of the underlying mechanisms and management options. *Audiology Today*, 13, 15-17. 2001.

Berlin CI, Bordelon J. Hurley A. Autoimmune inner ear disease: Basic science and audiological issues. In: CI Berlin (Ed). *Neurotransmission and Hearing Loss: Basic Science, Diagnosis and Management* (p137-146). San Diego: Singular Publishing Group.1997

Berlin CI, Hood LJ, Morlet T, Wilensky D, Li L, Mattingly KR, Taylor-Jeanfreau J, Keats BJ, John PS, Montgomery E, Shallop JK, Russell BA, Frisch SA. Multi-site diagnosis and management of 260 patients with auditory neuropathy/dys-synchrony (auditory neuropathy spectrum disorder). *Int J Audiol*.49(1):30-43. 2010

Beutner D, Foerst A, Lang-Roth R, von Wedel H, Walger M. Risk factors for auditory neuropathy/auditory synaptopathy. *ORL J Otorhinolaryngol Relat Spec.* 2007;69(4):239-44. 2007

Bretherton L. Holmes VM. The relationship between auditory temporal processing, phonemic awareness, and reading disability. *J Exp Child Psych*, 84, 218-243.

Brown M.C. Morphology of labeled efferent fibers in the guinea pig cochlea. *J. Comp. Neurol.*, 260 (1987), pp. 605–618

Buchman A, Roush PA, Teagle H F. B, Brown CJ, Zdanski CJ, Grose JH. Auditory Neuropathy Characteristics in Children with Cochlear Nerve Deficiency. *Ear & Hear*, 27, 399-408. 2006.

Cacace AT, Pinheiro JM. The Mitochondrial Connection in Auditory Neuropathy. *Audiol Neurootol.* 16(6):398-413. 2011

Catts HW, Gillespie M, Leonard LB, Kail RV, Miller CA. The role of speed of processing, rapid naming and phonological awareness in reading achievement. *J Learning Disabilities*, 35, 510-525. 2002.

Coenraad S, Goedegebure A, van Goudoever JB, Hoeve LJ. Risk factors for auditory neuropathy spectrum disorder in NICU infants compared to normal-hearing NICU controls. *Laryngoscope*. 121(4):852-5 2011

Deliac P, Demarquez JL, Barberot JP, Sandler B. Paty J. Brainstem auditory evoked potentials in icteric fullterm newborns: Alternations after exchange transfusion. *Neuropediatrics*, 21, 115-118. 1990.

Drullman R, Festen JM, Plomp R. Effect of temporal envelope smearing on speech reception. *J. Acoust. Soc. Am*, 95, 1053-1064. 1994a

Drullman R, Festen JM, Plomp R. Effect of reducing slow temporal modulations on speech reception. *J. Acoust. Soc. Am*, 95, 2670-2680. 1994b

Fallon JB Irvine DRF Shepherd RK Cochlear implants and brain plasticity. *Hearing Research* 238 110-117, 2008.

Farmer ME, Klein RM. The evidence for a temporal processing deficit linked to dyslexia: A review. *Psychonomic Bulletin & Review*, 2, 460-493. 1995

Ferber-Viart C, Morlet T, Maison S. Duclaux R, Putet G, Dubrieuil C. Type of initial brainstem auditory evoked potentials (BAEP) impairment and risk factors in premature infants. *Brain & Development*, 18, 287-293. 1996

Fryauf-Bertschy, H., Tyler, R.S., Kelsay, D.M., Gantz, B.J., Woodworth, G.G., 1997. Cochlear implant use by prelingually deafened children: the influences of age at implant and length of device use. *J. Speech Lang. Hear. Res.* 40, 183–199.

Fuchs P (2005). Time and intensity coding at the hair cell's ribbon synapse. *J Physiol*, 566, 7-12.

Fulmer SL, Runge CL, Jensen JW, Friedland DR. Rate of neural recovery in implanted children with auditory neuropathy spectrum disorder. *Otolaryngol Head Neck Surg.* 144(2):274-9. 2010

Gáborján A, Lendvai B, Vizi ES. Neurochemical evidence of dopamine release by lateral olivocochlear efferents and its presynaptic modulation in guinea-pig cochlea. *Neurosci*, 90, 131-138. 1999

Geers AE. Factors influencing spoken language outcomes in children following early cochlear implantation. *Adv Otorhinolaryngol.* 64:50-65; 2006

Gibson WPR, Sanli H. Auditory Neuropathy: An update. *Ear & Hear*, 28, 102s-106s. 2007

Gordon KA, Valero J, vanHoesel R, Papsin BC. Abnormal timing delays in auditory brainstem responses evoked by bilateral cochlear implant use in children. Otol & Neurotol. 29, 193-198. 2008

Granziani LJ, Weitzman ED, Velasco MSA. Neurologic maturation and auditory evoked responses in low birth weight infants. *Pediatrics*, 41, 483-494. 1968.

Gray RF, Ray J, Baguley DM, Vanat Z, Begg J, Phelps PD. Cochlear implant failure due to an unexpected absence of the eighth never – a cautionary tale. *J Laryngol & Otology*, 112, 646-49. 1998.

Green DM. Temporal auditory acuity. *Psych Rev*, 78, 540-551. 1971

Greisiger R, Tvete O, Shallop J, Elle OJ, Hol PK, Jablonski GE. Cochlear implant-evoked electrical auditory brainstem responses during surgery in patients with auditory neuropathy spectrum disorder. *Cochlear Implants Int.*12 Suppl 1:S58-60. 2011

Hammes DM, Novak MA, Rotz LA, Willis M, Edmondson DM, Thomas JF. Early identification and cochlear implantation: critical factors for spoken language development. *Ann Otol Rhinol Laryngol Suppl.* 189:74-8 2002

Harrison RV, Gordon KA, Mount RJ. Is there a critical period for cochlear implantation in congenitally deaf children? Analyses of hearing and speech perception performance after implantation. *Dev Psychobiol* 46:252-61. 2005

Hayes D. Screening methods: current status. *Ment Retard Dev Disabil Res Rev.* 9(2):65-72. 2003

Hayes H, Geers AE, Treiman R, Moog JS. Receptive vocabulary development in deaf children with cochlear implants: achievement in an intensive auditory-oral educational setting. *Ear Hear.* 128-35, 2009

Hyde ML, Riko K, & Malizia K. Audiometric accuracy of the click ABR in infants at risk for hearing loss. *J Am Acad Audiol* 1:59-74, 1990

Johnson L, Bhutani VK. The clinical syndrome of bilirubin-induced neurologic dysfunction. *Semin Perinatol.* 35:101-13. 2011

Joint Committee on Infant Hearing. Position Statement: Principles and Guidelines for Early Hearing Detection and Intervention Programs. *Pediatrics* 120:898-921, 2007

Kapman-Neeman RK, Kishon-Rabin L, Muchnik C. Identification of syllables in noise: Electrophysiological and behavioral correlates. *J. Acoust. Soc. Am.* 120, 926-933, 2006.

Kral A, Eggermont JJ. What's to lose and what's to learn: development under auditory deprivation, cochlear implants and limits of cortical plasticity. *Brain Res Rev.* 56(1):259-69. 2007

Kral, A., Hartmann, R., Tillein, J., Heid, S., Klinke, R. Delayed maturation and sensitive periods in the auditory cortex. *Audiol. Neuro-otol.* 6, 346–362. 2001

Kral, A., Hartmann, R., Tillein, J., Heid, S., Klinke, R.. Hearing after congenital deafness: central auditory plasticity and sensory deprivation. *Cereb. Cortex* 12, 797–807. 2002

Krumholz A, Feliz JK, Goldsein PJ, McKenzie E. Maturation of the brains-stem auditory evoked potential in premature infants. *Electroencephalog. & Clin Neurophys*, 62, 124-134. 1985.

Kumar AU, Jayaram M. Auditory processing in individuals with auditory neuropathy. *Behavioural & Brain Functions*, 1: 21, 2005

Loundon N, Marcolla A, Roux I, Rouillon I, Denoyelle F, Feldmann D, Marlin S, Garabedian EN. Auditory neuropathy or endocochlear hearing loss? *Otology & Neurology*, 26, 748-54, 2005

Madden C, Hilbert L, Rutter M, Greinwald J, Choo D. Pediatric cochlear implantation in auditory neuropathy. *Otol Neurotol*.163-8. 2002a

Madden C, Rutter M, Hilbert L, Greinwald JH Jr, Choo DI. Clinical and audiological features in auditory neuropathy. *Arch Otolaryngol Head Neck Surg*.128(9):1026-30. 2002b

Manchaiah VK, Zhao F, Danesh AA, Duprey R. The genetic basis of auditory neuropathy spectrum disorder (ANSD). *Int J Pediatr Otorhinolaryngol.* 75(2):151-8. 2010

Mason DC, Michelle A, Stevens C. Cochlear implantation in patients with auditory neuropathy of varied etiologies. *Laryngoscope*, 113, 45-9. 2003

Maxon AB, White KR, Behrens TR, Vohr BR. Referral rates and cost efficiency in a universal newborn hearing screening program using transient evoked otoacoustic emissions. *J Am Acad Audiol.* 271-7. 1995

Maxwell A, Mason SM, O'Donoghue G. Cochlear nerve aplasia: It's importance in cochlear implantation. *Otology & Neurotology*, 20, 293-408. 1999

McMahon C, Patuzzi R, Gibson WP, Sanli H. Frequency-specif ic electrocochleography indicates that presynaptic and postsynaptic mechanisms of auditory neuropathy exist. *Ear Hear* 29:314-25. 2008

Michalewski HJ, Starr A, Nguyen TT, Kong YY, Zeng FG. Auditory temporal processes in normal-hearing individuals and in patients with auditory neuropathy. *Clin Neurophys*, 116, 669-680, 2005

Miller CA, Abbas PJ, Robinson BK. Response properties of the refractory auditory nerve fiber. *J. Assoc. Res. Otolaryngol*, 2, 216-232.2001

Miyamoto RT, Kirk KH, Renshaw J, Hussain D. Cochlear implantation in auditory neuropathy. *Laryngoscope*, 109, 181-185, 1999

Moog JS, Geers AE, Gustus CH, Brenner CA. Psychosocial adjustment in adolescents who have used cochlear implants since preschool. *Ear Hear.* Feb;32(1 Suppl):75S-83S. 2011

Moog JS, Geers AE. Early educational placement and later language outcomes for children with cochlear implants. *Otol Neurotol.* Oct;31(8):1315-9. 2010

Musiek F. Temporal processing: The basics. *Hearing Journal*, 56, 52. 2003

Nicholas JG, Geers AE. Will they catch up? The role of age at cochlear implantation in the spoken language development of children with severe to profound hearing loss. *J Speech Lang Hear Res.* 50(4):1048-62. 2007

Nittrouer S. Do temporal processing deficits cause phonological processing problems? *JSLHR*, 42, 925-942. 1999.

O'Neil JN, Connelly CJ, Limb CJ, Ryugo DK. Synaptic morphology and the influence of auditory experience. *Hearing Research*, 297, 118-130, 2011.

Perlman M, Fainmesser P, Sohmer H, Tamari H, Wax Y & Pevsmer. Auditory nerve-brainstem evoked responses in hyperbilirubinemic neonates. *Pediatrics*, 72, 658-664. 1983.

Prabhu P, Avilala V, Barman A. Speech perception abilities for spectrally modified signals in individuals with auditory dys-synchrony. *Int J Audiol.* 50(5):349-52. 2011

Psarommatis I, Riga M, Douros K, Koltsidopoulos P, Douniadakis D, Kapetanakis I, Apostolopoulos N. Transient infantile auditory neuropathy and its clinical implications. *Int J Ped Otorhinolayrngol*, 70, 1629-1637.2006

Ramsden R. Greenham P. O'Driscoll M. Mawman D, Proops D, Craddock L, Fielden C, Graham J, Meerton L, Verschuur C, Toner J, McAnallen S, Osbourne J, Doran M, Gray R, Pickerill. Evaluation of bilaterally implanted adult subjects with the Nucleus 24 cochlear implant. *Otol & Neurotol*, 26, 988-998. 2005.

Rance G, Barker E, Mok M, Dowell R, Rincon A, Garratt R. Speech perception in noise for children with auditory neuropathy/dys-synchrony type hearing loss. *Ear Hear.* 28(3):351-60. 2007a

Rance G, Barker EJ, Sarant JZ, Ching TY. Receptive language and speech production in children with auditory neuropathy/dyssynchrony type hearing loss. *Ear Hear.* Sep;28(5):694-702. 2007b

Rance G, Barker EJ. Speech and language outcomes in children with auditory neuropathy/dys-synchrony managed with either cochlear implants or hearing aids. *Int J Audiol.*48(6):313-20. 2009

Rance G, Beer D, Cone-Wesson B, Shepherd R, Dowell R, King A, Rickards F, Clark G. Clinical findings for a group of infants and young children with auditory neuropathy, *Ear Hear*, 20, 238- 1999

Rance G, Cone-Wesson B, Wunderlich J, Dowell R. Speech Perception and Cortical Event Related Potentials in Children with Auditory Neuropathy. *Ear Hear* 23:239-54, 2002

Rance G Fava R, Baldock H, Chong A, Barker E, Corben L, Delatycki MB. Speech perception ability in individuals with Friedreich ataxia. *Brain*, 131, 2002-2012. 2008b

Rance G, McKay C, Grayden D. Perceptual characterization of children with auditory neuropathy. *Ear Hear*, 25, 34-46. 2004.

Rhee CK, Park HM, Jang YY. Audiologic evaluation of neonates with severe hyperbilirubinemia using transiently evoked otoacoustic emissions and auditory brainstem responses. *Laryngoscope*, 109, 2005-2008. 1999

Roberts JL, Davis H, Phon GL, Reichert TJ, Stutevant EM, Marshall RE. Auditory brainstem responses in preterm neonates: maturation and follow-up. *Pediatrics*, 101. 257-263. 1982.

Rodríguez-Ballesteros M, del Castillo FJ, Martín Y, Moreno-Pelayo MA, Morera C, Prieto F, Marco J, Morant A, Gallo-Terán J, Morales-Angulo C, Navas C, Trinidad G, Tapia MC, Moreno F, del Castillo I. Auditory neuropathy in patients carrying mutations in the otoferlin gene (OTOF). *Hum Mutat.* 22, 451-6. 2003.

Rodríguez-Ballesteros M, Reynoso R, Olarte M, Villamar M, Morera C, Santarelli R, Arslan E, Medá C, Curet C, Völter C, Sainz-Quevedo M, Castorina P, Ambrosetti U, Berrettini S, Frei K, Tedín S, Smith J, Cruz Tapia M, Cavallé L, Gelvez N,

Primignani P, Gómez-Rosas E, Martín M, Moreno-Pelayo MA, Tamayo M, Moreno-Barral J, Moreno F, del Castillo I. A multicenter study on the prevalence and spectrum of mutations in the otoferlin gene (OTOF) in subjects with nonsyndromic hearing impairment and auditory neuropathy. *Hum Mutat.* 823-3, 2008

Rouillon I, Marcolla A, Roux I, Marlin S, Feldmann D, Couderc R, Jonard L, Petit C, Denoyelle F, Garabédian EN, Loundon N. Results of cochlear implantation in two children with mutations in the OTOF gene. *Int J Pediatr Otorhinolaryngol.*;70(4):689-96. 2005

Roush P. Auditory neuropathy spectrum disorder: Evaluation and management. *Hearing J,* 61, 36-41. 2008

Roux I, 8, Safieddine S, Nouvian R, Grati M, Simmler MC, Bahloul A, Perfettini I, Le Gall M, Rostaing P, Hamard G, Triller A, Avan P, Moser T, Petit C. Otoferlin, defective in a human deafness form, is essential for exocytosis at the auditory ribbon synapse. *Cell* 127, 277-289. 2006.

Ryugo DK, Kretzmer EA, Niparko JK. Restoration of auditory nerve synapses in cats by cochlear implants. *Science.* 2;310(5753):1490-2. 2005

Saluja S, Agarwal A, Kler N, Amin S. Auditory neuropathy spectrum disorder in late preterm and term infants with severe jaundice. *Int J Pediatr Otorhinolaryngol.* 74(11):1292-7. 2010

Santarelli R. Information from cochlear potentials and genetic mutations helps localize the lesion site in auditory neuropathy. *Genome Med.* 22; 91, 2010

Santarelli R, Arslan E. Electrocochleography in auditory neuropathy. *Hear Res;* 170: 32-47. 2002

Santarelli R, Starr A, Michalewski H, Arslan E. Neural and receptor cochlear potentials obtained by transtympanic electrocochleography in auditory neuropathy. *Clin. Neurophys,* 1028-41, 20008.

Schlapbach LJ, Aebischer M, Adams M, Natalucci G, Bonhoeffer J, Latzin P, Nelle M, Bucher HU, Latal B; the Swiss Neonatal Network and Follow-Up Group. Impact of Sepsis on Neurodevelopmental Outcome in a Swiss National Cohort of Extremely Premature Infants. *Pediatrics.* 128, e348-e357. Epub 2011.

Sellick P Patuzzi R Robertson D. Primary afferent and cochlear nucleus contributions to extracellular potentials during tone-bursts. *Hear Res.* 176; 42-58, 2003.

Shallop JK. Peterson A, Facer GW, Fabry LB, Driscoll CLW. Cochlear implants in five cases of auditory neuropathy: postoperative findings and progress. *Laryngoscope,* 111, 555-562. 2001.

Shannon RV, Zeng FG, Kamath V, Wygonski J, Ekelid M. Speech recognition with primarily temporal cues. Science, 270 303-305. 1995

Shapiro S. Definition of the clinical spectrum of kernicterus and bilirubin-induced neurologica dysfunction (BIND*). J. Perinatology,* 25, 54-49. 2005

Shapiro SM, Popelka GR. Auditory impairment in infants at risk for bilirubin-induced neurologic dysfunction. *Semin Perinatol.* 35(3):162-70. 2011

Sharma A, Cardon G, Henion K, Roland P. Cortical maturation and behavioral outcomes in children with auditory neuropathy spectrum disorder. *Int J Audiol.* 50(2):98-106. 2011

Sharma A, Dorman MF, Kral A. The influence of a sensitive period on central auditory development in children with unilateral and bilateral cochlear implants. *Hear Res.* 203 134–143. 2005.

Sharma A, Nash AA, Dorman M. Cortical development, plasticity and re-organization in children with cochlear implants. *J Commun Disord.* 42(4):272-9. 2009

Sharma, A., Dorman, M.F., Spahr, A.J. Rapid development of cortical auditory evoked potentials after early cochlear implantation. *Neuroreport* 13 (10), 1365–1368. 2002a

Sharma, A., Dorman, M., Spahr, T. A sensitive period for the development of the central auditory system in children with cochlear implants. *Ear Hear.* 23 (6), 532–539. 2002b

Song MH, Bae MR, Kim HN, Lee WS, Yang WS, Choi JY. Value of intracochlear electrically evoked auditory brainstem response after cochlear implantation in patients with narrow internal auditory canal. *Laryngoscope*, 120, 1625-31.

Stark RE, Tallal P. Analysis of stop consonant production errors in developmentally dysphasic children. *J. Acoust. Soc. Am*, 66, 1703-1712. 1979

Starr A. Picton TW. Sininger Y. Hood L Berlin C. Auditory Neuropathy. *Brain*, 119, 741-753. 1996

Starr A, Sininger YS, Pratt H. The varieties of auditory neuropathy. J Basic & Clin Physiol. & Pharmacol. 11, 215-230. 2000

Svirsky MA, Teoh SW, Neubirger H. Development of language and speech perception in congentially, profound deaf children as a function of age at cochlear implantation. *Audiol & Neurotol*, 9; 224-233. 2004

Teagle HFB, Roush PA, Woodard JS, Hatch D, Zdanski CJ, Buss E, Buchman CA. Cochlear implantation in children with auditory neuropathy. *Ear Hear*, 31, 325-335. 2010

Tomblin JB, Barker, BA, Spencer LJ, Zhang X, Gantz BJ. The effect of age at cochlear implant initial stimulation on expressive language growth in infants and toddlers. *J Speech, Lang & Hear Research* Vol.48 853-867 2005.

Uziel A, Marot M, Pujol R. The Gunn rat: An experimental model for central deafness. *Acta Oto-laryngologica* 95, 651-656. 1983.

Van Ingelghem MCA, van Wieringen A, Wouters J, Vandenbussche E, Onghena P, Ghesquière P.

Psychophysical evidence for a general temporal processing deficit in children with dyslexia. *Neuroreport*, 12, 3603-3607. 2001

Varga R, Avenarius MR, Kelley PM, Keats BJ, Berlin CI, Hood LJ, Morlet TG, Brashears SM, Starr A, Cohn ES, Smith RJ, Kimberling WJ. OTOF mutations revealed by genetic analysis of hearing loss families including a potential temperature sensitive auditory neuropathy allele. *J Med Genet.* 43(7):576-81. Epub 2005

Varga R, Kelley PM, Keats BJ, Starr A, Leal SM, Cohn E, Kimberling WJ. Non-syndromic recessive auditory neuropathy is the result of mutations in the otoferlin (OTOF) gene. *J Med Genet.* 40(1):45-50. 2003

Xoinis K, Weirather Y, Mavoori H, Shaha SH, Iwamoto LM. Extremely low birth weight infants are at risk for auditory neuropathy. *J Perinatology*, 27, 718-723. 2007.

Yoshinaga-Itano C, Sedley A, Coulter D, Mehl A. Language of early- and later- identified children with hearing loss . *Pediatrics* 5:1161-71. 1998

Zeitler DM, Kessler MA, Terushkin V, Roland JT, Svirsky MA, Lalwani AK, Watlzman SB. Speech perception benefits of sequential bilateral cochlear implantation in children and adults: a retroscpetive analysis. *Otol & Neurotol.* 29; 314-325. 2008.

Zeng FG, Oba S, Garde S, Sininger Y, Starr A. Temporal and speech processing deficits in auditory neuropathy. *Neuroreport*, 10, 3429-3435. 1999

Zheng FG, Kong YY. Michalewski HJ. Starr A. Perceptual consequences of disrupted auditory nerve activity. *J Neurophys*, 93, 3050-3063. 2005